PSYCHOLOGY FOR NURSES

and allied health professionals

RICHARD GROSS
NANCY KINNISON

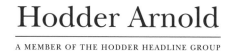
Hodder Arnold

A MEMBER OF THE HODDER HEADLINE GROUP

Photo credits

p.5 Zephyr/Science Photo Library; **p.6** © Bubbles/Angela Hampton; **p.9** Sally Greenhill; **p.11** © Bob Battersby/BDI Images Ltd.; **p.18** From *Opinions and Social Pressure* by Solomon Asch, Scientific American, Nov. 1955, Vol 193(5), pp.31–35, photos © William Vandivert, Dennis, MA, USA.; **p.25** AP/Empics; **p.28** © Bettmann/Corbis; **p.31** © Bettmann/Corbis; **p.36** © The Independent (newspaper supplied by John Frost Newspapers); **p.57** Anthea Sieveking/Wellcome Photo Library; **p.65** Henning Christoph/Still Pictures; **p.82** © Sam Tanner/Photofusion; **p.86** © Mark M. Lawrence/Corbis; **p.88** © Bettmann/Corbis; **p.92** Photofusion Picture Library/Alamy; **p.123** Robin Jones/Rex Features; **p.138** British Film Institute; **p.153** Anglo Amalgamated/The Kobal Collection; **p.154** British Film Institute; **p.164** Rex Features; **p.170** British Film Institute; **p.184** AP/Empics; **p.189** Reproduced with the permission of the British Heart Foundation; **p.202** © Bettmann/Corbis; **p.205** Rex Features; **p.208** Empics; **p.223** From *Opinions and Social Pressure* by Solomon Asch, Scientific American, Nov. 1955, Vol 193(5), pp.31–35, photos © William Vandivert, Dennis, MA, USA; **p.225** © Bettmann/Corbis; **p.240** Copyright 1965 by Stanley Milgram from the film *Obedience*, distributed by Pennsylvania State University, Audio Visual Services, reproduced by permission of Alexandra Milgram; **p.243** Getty Images; **p.257** © Rob Goldman/Corbis; **p.262** © Bubbles/Jennie Woodcock; **p.268** Concord Video & Films Council/Joyce Robertson www.robertsonfilms.info/www.concordemedia.co.uk; **p.278** © Farrell Grehan/Corbis; **p.291** © Julie Houck/Corbis; **p.300** Tim Rooke/Rex Features; **p.306** © Steve Azzara/Corbis; **p.307** © Bonaventura Apicella/Photofusion; **p.311** Ronald Grant Archive; **p.315** © Bubbles/Angela Hampton; **p.319** © Bubbles/David Robinson; **p.321** © David H. Wells/Corbis; **p.322** © Royalty Free/Corbis; **p.327** © Bubbles; **p.339** © Crispin Hughes/Photofusion; **p.347** Anthea Sieveking/Wellcome Photo Library; **p.352** © Parrot Pascal/Corbis Sygma; **p.359** British Film Institute; **p.360** Alfred Pasieka/Science Photo Library; **p.371** © Russell Underwood/Corbis; **p.380** Brian Bell/Science Photo Library; **p.384** CC Studio/Science Photo Library; **p.385** AP/Empics.

Every effort has been made to obtain necessary permission with reference to copyright material. The publishers apologise if inadvertently any sources remain unacknowledged and will be glad to make the necessary arrangements at the earliest opportunity.

To Jan, the ultimate carer. – R.G.

To Theresa and Michael, with love and gratitude
and
to 'those who care'. – N.K.

Orders: please contact Bookpoint Ltd, 130 Milton Park, Abingdon, Oxon OX14 4SB. Telephone: (44) 01235 827720. Fax: (44) 01235 400454. Lines are open from 9.00–5.00, Monday to Saturday, with a 24 hour message answering service. You can also order through our website www.hoddereducation.co.uk.

British Library Cataloguing in Publication Data
A catalogue record for this title is available from the British Library

ISBN 978 0 340 93011 3

First Published 2007
Impression number   10 9 8 7 6 5 4 3 2
Year   2012 2011 2010 2009 2008 2007

Copyright © 2007 by Richard Gross and Nancy Kinnison

Cover: Brian Hagiwara/Brand X Pictures RF/Jupiter Images

Hodder Headline's policy is to use papers that are natural, renewable and recyclable products and made from wood grown in sustainable forests. The logging and manufacturing processes are expected to conform to the environmental regulations of the country of origin.

Typeset by Phoenix Photosetting, Chatham, Kent
Printed in Great Britain for Hodder Arnold, an imprint of Hodder Education and a member of the Hodder Headline Group an Hachette Livre UK company, 338 Euston Road, London NW1 3BH by Martins the Printers, Berwick-upon-Tweed.

PSYCHOLOGY FOR NURSES

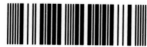

CONTENTS

CONTENTS

CONTENTS

ACKNOWLEDGEMENTS

Special thanks to Emma Woolf for believing in this project and giving me the encouragement to pursue it. Thanks also to Nina Hyland and the rest of the team at Hodder.

I'm also grateful to Julie Apps, Graham Macintosh (and some of his students), Lynne Brunyee and Janet Bolton, for reviewing sample chapters or providing feedback on the proposal.

Last but not least ... thank you, Nancy, for providing what I couldn't – the essential ability to 'translate' psychological theory and research into the language of Nursing practice.

R.G.

I join Richard in his acknowledgments above. My own extend further: thanks also to Heather Warrad, Helen Chalmers and Penny Mukherji for information and helpful comments, and to the tutors, care practitioners (from novice to expert) and patients for sharing so generously with me their thoughts, experiences and feelings. For reasons of confidentiality you must remain anonymous – but you know who you are. Particular thanks to Alison for her long-suffering support throughout!

I owe a very special debt of gratitude to Richard Gross for his general textbook (an unrivalled reference throughout my teaching career) and for his patient guidance and encouragement during our work on this book. It has been a privilege and a pleasure.

N.K.

INTRODUCTION

This book has had an unusually long gestation period, something approaching 30 years. Richard Gross began his teaching career in Psychology in 1973 (which included teaching on a Diploma of Nursing and Nursing degree in Oxford), married his nurse-to-be wife the following year, and while teaching in London worked with his fellow-author-to-be and experienced ex-nurse Nancy Kinnison. The combination of all these factors made it almost inevitable that a book such as the present one would be born at some point, and so it has proved. But the kind of book it would turn out to be, and how it would change during the protracted period of labour, were far more difficult to predict. And, indeed, just how difficult the labour would be was also unpredictable.

What we have delivered, we hope, is a text that engages the reader in a novel way. The psychological theory and research is interpreted and digested through the eyes of an imaginary student, Surena, whose 'From my diary' extracts (indicated by the open book and pen icon in the margin) provide the scenarios that relate to the chapter. The chapters are arranged in a conventional way, grouped into parts and sections as any psychology text would be. Surena doesn't make her 'appearance' until Chapter 3 when she begins to use the book to help her understand her experiences in her placements. As in your own practice, these don't follow the sequence of the chapters. To help you find your way around the book, we've provided a 'map' in the form of a grid (on page xiii) which shows how Surena's placements and the chapters are related.

Throughout each chapter, Surena makes notes indicated by the notepad icon in the margin. These may reflect on her feelings about and behaviour towards her patients* (Level 1) or apply the psychological material to the patients' and her own behaviour (Level 2). Sometimes she comments on or evaluates the psychological material itself, or reflects on ethical and social issues (displaying Level 3 skills). Note that in all chapters, the psychology text includes critical evaluation of theory and research, which demonstrates the higher level academic skills you are expected to develop during your course.

In addition to Surena's diary extracts and reflections, a recurring feature are the 'Ask Yourself...' breaks. These usually appear in the margin and are designed to encourage you to think about the text that follows, and to have questions (if not always answers) in your mind to help you understand and digest the studies and theories that you read about. So, instead of just reading in a rather passive way, you'll adopt a more critical approach, equipped with some idea of what to expect and what to look out for.

Sometimes the questions are quite specific and the answers are given directly in the text that immediately follows. At other times, the questions are more general and abstract, and the answers unfold throughout the next few paragraphs. Another kind of question will require you to reflect on your own experiences and views on a particular issue - in these cases, of course, there's no 'correct' answer.

*Goodman J (1984), in Jasper M. Beginning Reflective Practice. Nelson Thornes 2003

Occasionally, these 'Ask Yourself...' breaks appear as 'Research Question...', where you're asked to think about methodological issues arising from a particular piece of research described in the text.

These breaks are one of the features 'borrowed' from *Psychology: The Science of Mind and Behaviour* by Richard Gross. This is referred to at regular intervals, pointing you in the direction of more detailed discussion of a particular theory or study, or discussion of something that space doesn't allow in the present text at all.

Other features include 'Key Study' and 'Critical Discussion' boxes. Every chapter begins with an introduction and overview, which tells you what's covered in the chapter and sets the scene, and ends with a comprehensive summary, useful for revision.

The need for nurses and all health professionals to have a theoretical knowledge and understanding of psychology seems self-evident. Knowing how to apply it within a textbook is less obvious (and, of course, there's no one best or correct way to do it). We believe that our approach is unique and hope that you will find it both useful and enjoyable. The 'for' in the title explicitly relates to nurses and allied health professionals in their different roles; but implicitly, and as is demonstrated throughout the text, it also relates to you as an individual. Our 'child' is for you the person, as well as you the professional.

Richard Gross and Nancy Kinnison

WHAT IS PSYCHOLOGY?

1

INTRODUCTION AND OVERVIEW

When a psychologist meets someone for the first time at, say, a party and replies truthfully to the standard opening line, 'What do you do for a living?', the reaction of the newly made acquaintance is likely to fall into one of the following categories:

◎ 'Oh, I'd better be careful what I say from now on' (partly defensive, partly amused)
◎ 'I bet you meet some right weirdos in your work' (partly intrigued, partly sympathetic)
◎ 'What exactly is psychology?' (partly inquisitive, partly puzzled).

What these reactions betray – especially the first two – is an inaccurate and incomplete understanding of the subject. The first seems to imply that psychologists are mind readers and have access to other people's thoughts (they *don't*), while the second seems to imply that psychologists work mainly with people who are 'mentally ill' or 'mad' (again, they *don't*, although many do). The third reaction perhaps implies that the boundaries between psychology and other subject disciplines aren't clearly drawn (they *aren't*), but what this chapter aims to do is make them sufficiently clear to enable you, the reader, who may be 'visiting' psychology for the first time, to find your way around this book – and the subject – relatively easily.

The opening chapter in any textbook is intended to 'set the scene' for what follows, and this normally involves defining the subject or discipline. In most disciplines, this is usually a fairly simple task. With psychology, however, it's far from straightforward. Definitions of psychology have changed frequently during its relatively short history as a separate field of study. This reflects different, and sometimes conflicting, theoretical views regarding the nature of human beings and the most appropriate methods for investigating them. While most psychologists would consider themselves to be scientists, they disagree about exactly what science involves, and the appropriateness of using certain scientific methods to study human behaviour.

A BRIEF HISTORY

The word 'psychology' is derived from the Greek *psyche* (mind, soul or spirit) and *logos* (knowledge, discourse or study). Literally, then, psychology is the 'study of the mind'.

The emergence of psychology as a separate discipline is generally dated at 1879, when Wilhelm Wundt opened the first psychological laboratory at the University of Leipzig in Germany. Wundt and his co-workers were attempting to investigate 'the mind' through *introspection* (observing and analysing the structure of their own conscious

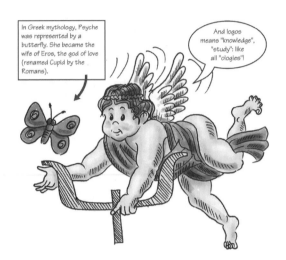

mental processes). Introspection's aim was to analyse conscious thought into its basic elements and perception into its constituent sensations, much as chemists analyse compounds into elements. This attempt to identify the structure of conscious thought is called *structuralism*.

Wundt and his co-workers recorded and measured the results of their introspections under *controlled conditions*, using the same physical surroundings, the same 'stimulus' (such as a clicking metronome), the same verbal instructions to each participant, and so on. This emphasis on measurement and control marked the separation of the 'new psychology' from its parent discipline of philosophy.

Philosophers had discussed 'the mind' for thousands of years. For the first time, *scientists* (Wundt was a physiologist by training) applied some of scientific investigation's basic methods to the study of mental processes. This was reflected in James's (1890) definition of psychology as 'the Science of Mental Life, both of its phenomena and of their conditions … The Phenomena are such things as we call feelings, desires, cognition, reasoning, decisions and the like.'

However, by the early twentieth century, the validity and usefulness of introspection were being seriously questioned, particularly by an American psychologist, John B. Watson. Watson believed that the results of introspection could never be proved or disproved, since if one person's introspection produced different results from another's, how could we ever decide which was correct? *Objectively*, of course, we cannot, since it's impossible to 'get behind' an introspective report to check its accuracy. Introspection is *subjective*, and only the individual can observe his/her own mental processes.

Consequently, Watson (1913) proposed that psychologists should confine themselves to studying *behaviour*, since only this is measurable and observable by more than one person. Watson's form of psychology was known as *behaviourism*. It largely replaced introspectionism and advocated that people should be regarded as complex animals and studied using the same scientific methods as those used in chemistry and physics. For Watson, the only way psychology could make any claim to being scientific was to emulate the natural sciences and adopt its own objective methods. He defined psychology as 'that division of Natural Science which takes human behaviour – the doings and sayings, both learned and unlearned – as its subject matter' (Watson, 1919). The study of inaccessible, private, mental processes was to have no place in a truly scientific psychology.

Especially in America, behaviourism (in one form or another) remained the dominant force in psychology for the next 40 years or so. The emphasis on the role of *learning* (in the form of *conditioning*) was to make that topic one of the central areas of psychological research as a whole (see Chapter 2, pages 23–27).

Box 1.1 Psychoanalytic theory and Gestalt psychology

- In 1900, Sigmund Freud, a neurologist living in Vienna, first published his *psychoanalytic theory* of personality in which the *unconscious* mind played a crucial role. In parallel with this theory, he developed a form of psychotherapy called *psychoanalysis*. Freud's theory (which forms the basis of the *psychodynamic* approach) represented a challenge and a major alternative to behaviourism (see Chapter 2, pages 27–31).

- A reaction against both structuralism and behaviourism came from the *Gestalt* school of psychology, which emerged in the 1920s in Austria and Germany. Gestalt psychologists were mainly interested in perception, and believed that perceptions couldn't be broken down in the way that Wundt proposed and behaviourists advocated for behaviour. Gestalt psychologists identified several 'laws' or *principles of perceptual organisation* (such as 'the whole is greater than the sum of its parts'), which have made a lasting contribution to our understanding of the perceptual process (see Gross, 2005, for a detailed discussion).

In the late 1950s, many British and American psychologists began looking to the work of computer scientists to try to understand more complex behaviours which, they felt, had been either neglected altogether or greatly oversimplified by learning theory (conditioning). These complex behaviours were what Wundt, James and other early scientific psychologists had called '*mind*' or mental processes. They were now called *cognition* or *cognitive processes*, and refer to all the ways in which we come to know the world around us, how we attain, retain and regain information, through the processes of perception, attention, memory, problem-solving, decision-making, language and thinking in general.

Cognitive psychologists see people as *information-processors*, and cognitive psychology has been heavily influenced by computer science, with human cognitive processes being compared with the operation of computer programs (the *computer analogy*). Cognitive psychology now forms part of *cognitive science*, which emerged in the late 1970s (see Figure 1.1).

Although mental or cognitive processes can be *inferred* only from what a person does (they cannot be observed literally or directly), mental processes are now accepted as being valid subject matter for psychology, provided they can be made 'public' (as in memory tests or problem-solving tasks). Consequently, what people say and do are perfectly acceptable sources of information *about* their cognitive processes, the processes themselves remain inaccessible to the observer, who can study them only *indirectly*.

The influence of both behaviourism and cognitive psychology is reflected in Clark and Miller's (1970) definition of psychology as 'the scientific study of behaviour. Its subject matter includes behavioural processes that are observable, such as gestures, speech and physiological changes, and processes that can only be inferred, such as thoughts and dreams'. Similarly, Zimbardo (1992) states that, 'Psychology is formally defined as the scientific study of the behaviour of individuals and their mental processes.'

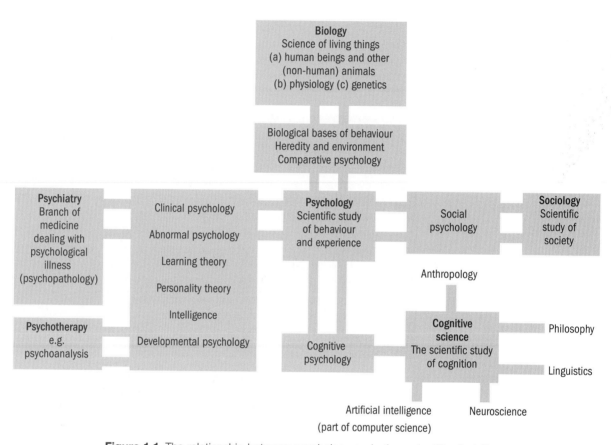

Figure 1.1 The relationship between psychology and other scientific disciplines

CLASSIFYING THE WORK THAT PSYCHOLOGISTS DO

Despite behaviourist and cognitive psychology's influence on psychology's general direction in the last 90 years or so, much more goes on within psychology than has been outlined so far. There are other theoretical approaches or orientations, other aspects of human (and non-human) activity that constitute the special focus of study, and different kinds of work that different psychologists do.

A useful, but not hard and fast, distinction can be made between the *academic* and *applied* branches of psychology. Academic psychologists carry out research and are attached to a university or research establishment, where they'll also teach undergraduates and supervise the research of postgraduates. Research is both *pure* (done for its own sake and intended, primarily, to increase our knowledge and understanding) and *applied* (aimed at solving a particular problem). Applied research is usually funded by a government institution like the Home Office, National Health Service (NHS) or the Department for Education and Skills (DfES), or by some commercial or industrial institution. The range of topics that may be investigated is as wide as psychology itself, but they can be classified as focusing either on the processes or *mechanisms* underlying various aspects of behaviour, or more directly on the *person* (Legge, 1975).

THE PROCESS APPROACH

This is divided into three main areas: physiological, cognitive, and comparative psychology.

Physiological (or bio)psychology

Physiological (or bio)psychologists are interested in the physical basis of behaviour, how the functions of the *nervous system* (in particular the brain) and the *endocrine (hormonal)* system are related to and influence behaviour and mental processes. For example, are there parts of the brain specifically concerned with particular behaviours and abilities (*localisation of brain function*)? What role do hormones play in the experience of emotion and how are these linked to brain processes? What is the relationship between brain activity and different *states of consciousness* (including sleep)?

A fundamentally important biological process with important implications for psychology is *genetic transmission*. The *heredity and environment* (or *nature–nurture*) issue draws on what geneticists have discovered about the characteristics that can be passed from parents to offspring, how this takes place, and how genetic factors interact with environmental ones (see Gross, 2005). Other topics within physiological psychology include motivation and stress (an important topic within *health psychology* – see Chapters 3–7).

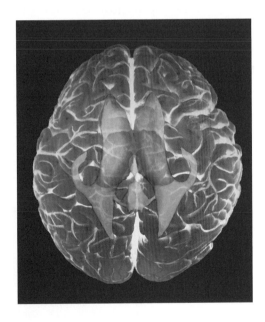

Cognitive psychology

As we saw earlier, cognitive (or mental) processes include *attention, memory, perception, language, thinking, problem-solving, decision-making, reasoning* and *concept-formation* ('higher-order' mental activities). Social psychology (classified here as belonging to the person approach) is heavily cognitive in flavour: for example many social psychologists study the mental processes we use when trying to explain people's behaviour (*social cognition*). Also, Piaget's theory (again, belonging to the person approach) is concerned with *cognitive development*.

Comparative psychology

Comparative psychology is the study of the behaviour of non-human animals, aimed at identifying similarities and differences between species. It also involves studying non-human animal behaviour to gain a better understanding of human behaviour. The basis of comparative psychology is *evolutionary theory*. Research areas include classical and operant conditioning, and evolutionary explanations of human behaviour (see Chapter 2, pages 25–29, and Gross and Rolls, 2006).

THE PERSON APPROACH

Social psychology (Chapters 8–13)

Some psychologists would claim that 'all psychology is social psychology', because all behaviour takes place within a social context and, even when we're alone, our behaviour continues to be influenced by others. However, other people usually have a more immediate and direct influence upon us when we're actually in their presence (as in *conformity* and *obedience* – see Chapters 12 and 13).

Social psychology is also concerned with *interpersonal perception* (forming impressions of others), *interpersonal attraction*, and *interpersonal relationships*, *prejudice* and *discrimination*, and *pro-* and *anti-social behaviour* (especially *aggression*).

Developmental psychology (Chapters 14–20)

Developmental psychologists study the biological, cognitive, social and emotional *changes* that occur in people over time. One significant change within developmental psychology during the past 30 years or so is the recognition that development isn't confined to childhood and adolescence, but is a lifelong process (the *lifespan approach*). It's now generally accepted that development continues beyond childhood and adolescence into adulthood and late adulthood.

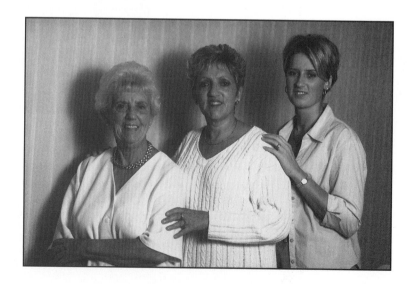

Individual differences

This is concerned with the ways in which people can differ from one another, including *personality* (see Chapter 6), *intelligence* and *psychological abnormality*. Major mental disorders include schizophrenia, depression, anxiety disorders and eating disorders. *Abnormal psychology* is closely linked with *clinical psychology*, one of the major *applied* areas of psychology (see below). Psychologists who study abnormality and clinical psychologists are also concerned with the effectiveness of different forms of treatment and therapy. Each major theoretical approach has contributed to both the explanation and treatment of mental disorders (see Chapter 2).

Comparing the process and person approaches

In practice, it's very difficult to separate the two approaches, even if it can be done theoretically. However, there are important relative differences between them.

Box 1.2 Some important differences between the process and person approaches

- **The process approach** is typically confined to the laboratory (where experiments are the method of choice). It makes far greater experimental use of non-human animals and assumes that psychological processes (particularly learning) are essentially the same in all species and that any differences between species are only *quantitative* (differences of degree).

- **The person approach** makes much greater use of field studies (such as observing behaviour in its natural environment) and of non-experimental methods (e.g. correlational studies: see Gross and Rolls, 2006). Typically, human participants are studied and it's assumed that there are *qualitative* differences (differences in kind) between humans and non-humans.

AREAS OF APPLIED PSYCHOLOGY

Discussion of the person/process approaches has been largely concerned with the *academic* branch of psychology. Since the various areas of applied psychology are all concerned with people, they can be thought of as the *applied* aspects of the person approach.

According to Hartley and Branthwaite (1997), most applied psychologists work in four main areas: *clinical, educational* and *occupational psychology*, and *government service* (such as *forensic psychologists*). In addition, Coolican *et al.* (1996) identify *forensic* (or *criminological*), *sport, health* and *environmental psychologists*. Hartley and Branthwaite argue that the work psychologists do in these different areas has much in common: it's the *subject matter* of their jobs that differs, rather than the skills they employ. Consequently, they consider an applied psychologist to be a person who can deploy specialised skills appropriately in different situations.

Box 1.3 Seven major skills (or roles) used by applied psychologists

- **The psychologist as counsellor:** helping people to talk openly, express their feelings, explore problems more deeply, and see these problems from different perspectives. Problems may include school phobia, marriage crises and traumatic experiences (such as

---

being the victim of a hijacking), and the counsellor can adopt a more or less directive approach (see Chapter 2, pages 32–33).

- **The psychologist as colleague:** working as a member of a team and bringing a particular perspective to a task, namely drawing attention to the human issues, such as the point of view of the individual end-user (be it a product or a service of some kind).

- **The psychologist as expert:** drawing upon psychologists' specialised knowledge, ideas, theories and practical knowledge to advise on issues ranging from incentive schemes in industry to appearing as an 'expert witness' in a court case.

- **The psychologist as toolmaker:** using and developing appropriate measures and techniques to help in the analysis and assessment of problems. These include questionnaire and interview schedules, computer-based ability and aptitude tests, and other *psychometric tests* (mental measurement) (see Chapter 6).

- **The psychologist as detached investigator:** many applied psychologists carry out evaluation studies to assess the evidence for and against a particular point of view. This reflects the view of psychology as an objective science, which should use controlled experimentation whenever possible. The validity of this view is a recurrent theme throughout psychology (see below).

- **The psychologist as theoretician:** theories try to explain observed phenomena, suggesting possible underlying mechanisms or processes. They can suggest where to look for causes and how to design specific studies that will produce evidence for or against a particular point of view. Results from applied psychology can influence theoretical psychology, and vice versa.

- **The psychologist as agent for change:** applied psychologists are involved in helping people, institutions and organisations, based on the belief that their work will change people and society for the better. However, some changes are much more controversial than others, such as the use of psychometric tests to determine educational and occupational opportunities, and the use of behaviour therapy and modification techniques to change abnormal behaviour (see Chapters 2 and 5).

(Based on Hartley and Branthwaite, 2000)

ASK YOURSELF ...

- Which, if any, of the skills identified by Hartley and Branthwaite do you consider to be relevant to nursing (or allied health professions)?

- How do they apply (it might be useful to think in terms of whether they apply *formally* or *informally*, *implicitly* or *explicitly*)?

- Are there any major skills that are used in nursing (or allied health professions) that *aren't* included by Hartley and Branthwaite?

Clinical psychology

Clinical psychologists are the largest single group of psychologists, both in the UK (Coolican *et al.*, 1996) and the USA (Atkinson *et al.*, 1990). A related group is 'counselling psychologists', who tend to work with younger clients in colleges and universities rather than in hospitals.

Box 1.4 The major functions of the clinical psychologist

The functions of a clinical psychologist include:

- assessing people with learning difficulties, administering psychological tests to brain-damaged patients, devising rehabilitation programmes for long-term psychiatric patients and assessing elderly people for their fitness to live independently

- planning and carrying out programmes of therapy, usually *behaviour therapy/modification* (both derived from learning theory principles) or *psychotherapy* (group or individual) in preference to, or in addition to, behavioural techniques (see Chapter 2)
- carrying out research into abnormal psychology, including the effectiveness of different treatment methods ('outcome' studies); patients are usually adults, many of whom will be elderly, in psychiatric hospitals, psychiatric wards in general hospitals and psychiatric clinics
- involvement in community care, as psychiatric care in general moves out of the large psychiatric hospitals
- teaching other groups of professionals, such as nurses, psychiatrists and social workers.

Clinical psychologists work largely in health and social care settings, including hospitals, health centres, community mental health teams, child and adolescent mental health services, and social services. They usually work as part of a team with, for example, social workers, medical practitioners and other health professionals. Most work in the National Health Service, but some work in private practice.

Psychotherapy is usually carried out by psychiatrists (medically qualified doctors specialising in psychological medicine) or psychotherapists (who've undergone special training, including their own psychotherapy). In all its various forms, psychotherapy is derived from Freud's psychoanalysis (see Chapter 2), and is distinguished both from behavioural treatments and physical (somatic) treatments (those based on the medical model – see Chapter 3, pages 41–42, and Gross, 2005).

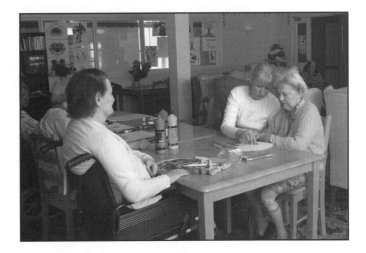

Forensic psychology

This is a branch of psychology that attempts to apply psychological principles to the criminal justice system. Areas of research interest include jury selection, the presentation of evidence, eyewitness testimony, improving the recall of child witnesses, false memory syndrome and recovered memory, offender profiling, stalking, crime prevention, devising treatment programmes (such as anger management) and assessing the risk of releasing prisoners.

Educational psychology

Educational psychologists are mostly employed by Local Education Authorities (LEAs), working in schools, colleges, child and family centre teams (previously called 'child guidance'), the Schools Psychological Service, hospitals, day nurseries, nursery schools, special schools (day and residential), and residential children's homes. Their functions include:

◎ administering psychometric tests (particularly intelligence/IQ tests)
◎ planning and supervising remedial teaching
◎ planning educational programmes for children and adolescents with special educational needs (including the visually impaired and autistic)
◎ advising parents and teachers how to deal with children and adolescents with behaviour problems and/or learning difficulties.

Occupational (work or organisational) psychology

Occupational psychologists are involved in the selection and training of individuals for jobs and vocational guidance, including administration of aptitude tests and tests of interest. (This overlaps with the work of those trained in *personnel management*.)

Health psychology

This is one of the newer fields of applied psychology.

Box 1.5 The breadth of health psychology

This involves the use of psychological principles to promote changes in people's attitudes, behaviour and thinking about health and illness. This may involve:

• the use of psychological theories and interventions to prevent damaging behaviours (such as smoking, drug abuse, poor diet) and to change health-related behaviour in community and workplace settings (see Chapter 10)

• promoting and protecting health by encouraging behaviours such as exercise, healthy diet, tooth brushing, health checks/self-examination

• health-related cognitions – investigating the processes that can explain, predict and change health and illness behaviours (see Chapter 4)

• processes influencing health care delivery – the nature and effects of communication between health care practitioners and patients, including interventions to improve communication, facilitate adherence (such as taking medication), prepare for stressful medical procedures, and so on (see Chapters 3 and 5)

• psychological aspects of illness – looking at the psychological impact of acute and chronic illness on individuals, families and carers (see Chapter 3).

(Based on BPS, 2004)

Health psychologists work in a variety of settings, such as hospitals, academic health research units, health authorities, and university departments. They may deal with problems identified by health care agencies, including NHS Trusts and health authorities, health professionals (such as GPs, nurses and rehabilitation therapists), and employers outside the health care system.

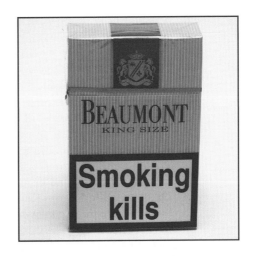

ASK YOURSELF ...
• What, if anything, has come as a surprise to you regarding what goes on in the name of 'psychology'?

THE LANGUAGE AND METHODS OF PSYCHOLOGY

As in all sciences, there's a special set of technical terms (jargon) to get used to, and this is generally accepted as an unavoidable feature of studying the subject. But over and above this jargon, psychologists use words that are familiar to us from everyday speech in a *technical way*, and it's in these instances that 'doing psychology' can become a little confusing.

Some examples of this are 'behaviour' and 'personality'. For a parent to tell a child to 'behave yourself' is meaningless to a psychologist's ears: behaving is something we're all doing all the time (even when we're asleep). Similarly, to say that someone 'has no personality' is meaningless because, as personality refers to what makes a person unique and different from others, you cannot help but have one!

Other terms that denote large portions of the research of experimental psychology, such as memory, learning and intelligence, are **hypothetical constructs** – that is, they don't refer to anything that can be directly observed but to something which can only be *inferred* from observable behaviour (see above, page 3). They're necessary for explaining the behaviour being observed, but there's a danger of thinking of them as 'things' or 'entities' (**reification**), rather than as a way of trying to make sense of behaviour.

Another way in which psychologists try to make sense of something is by comparing it with something else using an **analogy**. Often something complex is compared with something more simple. Since the 1950s and the development of computer science, the *computer analogy* has become very popular as a way of trying to understand how the mind works. As we saw earlier, the language of computer science has permeated the cognitive view of human beings as information processors.

A **model** is a kind of *metaphor*, involving a single, fundamental idea or image; this makes it less complex than a **theory** (although sometimes the terms are used interchangeably). A theory is a complex set of inter-related statements that attempt to explain certain observed phenomena. But in practice, when we refer to a particular theory (for example, Freud's or Piaget's), we often include *description* as well. Thomas (1985) defines a theory as 'an explanation of how the facts fit together' and he likens a theory to a lens through which to view the subject matter, filtering out certain facts and giving a particular pattern to those it lets in.

A **hypothesis** is a testable statement about the relationship between two or more variables, usually derived from a model or theory.

A **variable** is anything that can have different values (i.e. that can 'vary'). Variables are of two main types: (i) **participant** (for example, personality, gender, age, cultural background, diet); and (ii) **situational** (for example, the type and difficulty of a task presented, task instructions, time of day, room temperature).

In a (true) **experiment**, the researcher *manipulates* (deliberately changes) one variable (the **independent variable/IV**) in order to see its influence on another (the **dependent variable/DV**). These correspond, roughly, to cause and effect. The former may be something such as stress, and the latter may be some aspect of behaviour or physiology (such as immune system function). While most true experiments are conducted under controlled conditions in the laboratory, they can also occur in real-life (*naturalistic*) settings. One example of the latter is the study of obedience among nurses (Hofling *et al.*, 1966 – see Key Study 13.2, page 245).

Most participant variables cannot be manipulated (an exception, among the examples given here, being diet). Instead, participants are *selected* because they already possess these characteristics or already engage in certain activities. So, the IV occurs 'naturally' (without intervention by the researcher). An example is the study by Coffey *et al.* (1988) of the effects of different shift patterns on nurses' job performance (see Chapter 5, page 82). Such studies are sometimes referred to as 'pseudo-experiments'.

In a **correlational study**, two or more variables are measured to see how they are *related*. Neither is manipulated and neither can logically be thought of as the cause of the other. An example is the study of stress and illness, where stress is defined in terms of life changes, using instruments such as the Social Readjustment Rating Scale (Holmes and Rahe, 1967 – see Chapter 5, pages 83–86).

Formal vs informal psychology

Legge (1975) and others distinguish between *formal* and *informal psychology* (or professional versus amateur, scientific versus non-scientific).

Our common sense, intuitive or 'natural' understanding is unsystematic and doesn't constitute a body of knowledge. This makes it very difficult to 'check' an individual's 'theory' about human nature, as does the fact that each individual has to learn from his/her own experience. So part of the aim of formal psychology is to provide such a systematic body of knowledge.

Yet it could be argued that informal psychology *does* provide a 'body of knowledge' in the form of proverbs or sayings or folk wisdom, handed down from generation to generation (for example, 'Birds of a feather flock together', 'Too many cooks spoil the broth' and 'Don't cross your bridges before you come to them'). While these may contain at least a grain of truth, for each one there's another proverb that states the opposite ('Opposites attract', 'Many hands make light work' and 'Time and tide wait for no man' or 'Nothing ventured, nothing gained').

However, formal psychology may help us reconcile these contradictory statements. For example, there's evidence to support both proverbs in the first pair (see Gross, 2005). Formal psychology tries to identify the conditions under which each statement applies, and they *appear* contradictory if we assume that only one or the other can be true! In this way, scientific psychology throws light on our everyday, informal understanding, rather than negating or invalidating it.

Legge (1975) believes that most psychological research should indeed be aimed at demonstrations of 'what we know already', but that it should also aim to go one step further. Only the methods of science, he believes, can provide us with the public, communicable body of knowledge that we're seeking. According to Allport (1947), the

ASK YOURSELF ...
- What do you understand by the term science?
- What makes a science different from non-science?
- Are there different kinds of science and, if so, what do they have in common?

aim of science is 'understanding, prediction and control above the levels achieved by unaided common sense', and this is meant to apply to psychology as much as to the natural sciences.

WHAT DO WE MEAN BY 'SCIENCE'?

Asking this question is a necessary first step for considering the appropriateness of attempting to scientifically study human behaviour.

THE MAJOR FEATURES OF SCIENCE

Most psychologists and philosophers of science would probably agree that for a discipline to be called a science, it must possess certain characteristics. These are summarised in Box 1.6 and Figure 1.2.

> **Box 1.6 The major features of science**
>
> - **A definable subject matter:** this changed from conscious human thought to human and non-human behaviour, then to cognitive processes, within psychology's first 80 years as a separate discipline.
> - **Theory construction:** this represents an attempt to *explain* observed phenomena, such as Watson's attempt to account for (almost all) human and non-human behaviour in terms of classical conditioning, and Skinner's subsequent attempt to do the same with operant conditioning (see Chapter 2).
> - **Hypothesis testing:** this involves making specific *predictions* about behaviour under certain conditions (for example, predicting that by combining the sight of a rat with the sound of a hammer crashing down on a steel bar just behind his head, a small child will learn to fear the rat, as in Watson and Rayner's (1920) study of 'Little Albert' – see Gross, 2005).
> - **Empirical methods:** these are used to collect *data* (*evidence*) relevant to the hypothesis being tested.

WHAT IS 'SCIENTIFIC METHOD'?

The account given in Box 1.6 and Figure 1.2 of what constitutes a science is non-controversial. However, it fails to tell us how the *scientific process* takes place, the sequence of 'events' involved (such as where the theory comes from in the first place and how it's related to observation of the subject matter), or the exact relationship between theory construction, hypothesis testing and data collection.

Collectively, these 'events' and relationships are referred to as (the) *scientific method*. Table 1.1 summarises some common beliefs about both science and scientific method, together with some alternative views.

THE SCIENTIFIC STUDY OF HUMAN BEHAVIOUR

THE SOCIAL NATURE OF SCIENCE: THE PROBLEM OF OBJECTIVITY

'Doing science' is part of human behaviour. When psychologists study what people do, they're engaging in some of the very same behaviours they're trying to understand (such

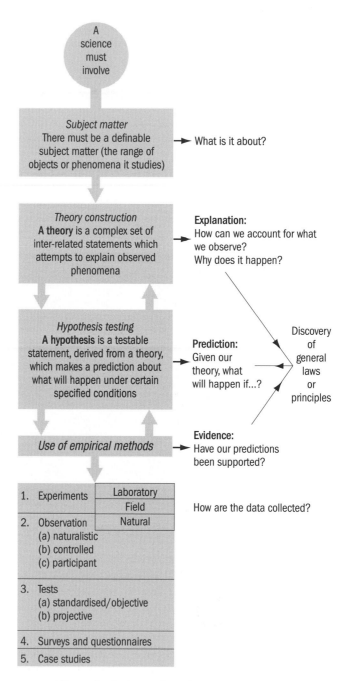

Figure 1.2 A summary of the major features of a science

as thinking, perceiving, problem-solving and explaining). This is what's meant by the statement that psychologists are part of their own subject matter, which makes it even more difficult for them to be objective than other scientists.

Table 1.1 Some common beliefs and alternative views about 'science' and 'scientific method'

Common beliefs	Alternative views
λ Scientific discovery begins with simple, unbiased, unprejudiced observation: the scientist simply 'samples' the world without any preconceptions, expectations or predetermined theories.	λ There's no such thing as 'unbiased' or 'unprejudiced' observation. Observation is always selective, interpretative, prestructured and directed: we must have at least some idea of what we're looking for, otherwise we cannot know when we've found it. Goldberg (2000) cites a philosophy professor who asserted that what we call 'data' (that which is given) should more accurately be called 'capta' (that which is taken).
ν From the resulting sensory evidence ('data'/sense-data), generalised statements of fact will take shape: we gradually build up a picture of what the world is like based on a number of separate 'samples'.	ν 'Data' don't constitute 'facts': evidence usually implies measurements, numbers and recordings, which need to be interpreted in the light of a theory. Facts don't exist objectively and cannot be discovered through 'pure observation'. 'Fact' = Data + Theory (Deese, 1972).
σ The essential feature of scientific activity is the use of empirical methods, through which the sensory evidence is gathered: what distinguishes science from non-science is performing experiments, etc.	σ Despite the central role of data collection, data alone don't make a science. Theory is just as crucial, because without it data have no meaning (see point above).
τ The truth about the world (the objective nature of things, what the world is 'really like') can be established through properly controlled experiments and other ways of collecting 'facts': science can tell us about reality as it is independent of the scientist or the activity of observing it.	τ Scientific theory and research reflect the biases, prejudices, values and assumptions of the individual scientist, as well as of the scientific community s/he belongs to. Science *isn't* value-free (see Gross, 2005).
υ Science involves the steady accumulation of knowledge: each generation of scientists adds to the discoveries of previous generations.	υ Science involves an endless succession of long, peaceful periods ('normal science') and 'scientific revolutions' (Kuhn, 1962 – see Table 2.1, page 38).
	ι Science has a warm, human, exciting, argumentative, creative 'face' (Collins, 1994).

(Based on Medawar, 1963; Popper, 1972)

According to Richards (1996):

> Whereas in orthodox sciences there is always some external object of enquiry – rocks, electrons, DNA, chemicals – existing essentially unchanging in the non-human world (even if never finally knowable 'as it really is' beyond human conceptions), this is not so for psychology. 'Doing psychology' is the human activity of studying human activity; it is human psychology examining itself – and what it produces by way of new theories, ideas and beliefs about itself is also part of our psychology!

Knowable 'as it really is' refers to objectivity, and Richards is claiming that it may be impossible for any scientist to achieve complete objectivity. One reason for this relates to the social nature of scientific activity. As Rose (1997) says:

> How biologists, or any scientists, perceive the world is not the result of simply holding a true reflecting mirror up to nature: it is shaped by the history of our subject, by dominant social expectations and by the patterns of research funding.

Does this mean that 'the truth' exists only 'by agreement'? Does science not tell us what things are 'really' like, but only what scientists happen to believe is the truth at any particular time?

According to Richardson (1991), science is a very *social* business. Research must be qualified and quantified to enable others to replicate it, and in this way the procedures, instruments and measures become standardised, so that scientists anywhere in the world can check the truth of reported observations and findings. This implies the need for universally agreed conventions for reporting these observations and findings.

However, even if there are widely accepted ways of 'doing science', 'good science' doesn't necessarily mean 'good psychology'. Is it valid to study human behaviour and experience as part of the natural world, or is a different kind of approach needed altogether? After all, it isn't just psychologists who observe, experiment and theorise (Heather, 1976).

The psychology experiment as a social situation

To regard empirical research in general, and the experiment in particular, as objective involves two related assumptions:

1. researchers influence the participant's behaviour (the outcome of the experiment) only to the extent that they decide what hypothesis to test, how the variables are to be operationalised (defined in a way that allows them to be measured), what design to use (for example, randomly allocating each participant to one experimental condition or testing every participant under each condition), and so on.
2. the only factors influencing the participant's performance are the objectively defined variables manipulated by the experimenter.

EXPERIMENTERS ARE PEOPLE TOO: THE PROBLEM OF EXPERIMENTER BIAS

> **Box 1.7 Some examples of experimenter bias**
>
> - According to Valentine (1992), experimenter bias has been demonstrated in a variety of experiments, including reaction time, animal learning, verbal conditioning, personality assessment, person perception, learning and ability, as well as in everyday life situations.
> - What these experiments consistently show is that if one group of experimenters has one hypothesis about what it expects to find and another group has the opposite hypothesis, *both* groups will obtain results that support their respective hypotheses. The results *aren't* due to the mishandling of data by biased experimenters, the experimenters' bias somehow creates a changed environment, in which participants actually behave differently.

ASK YOURSELF ...
- Try to formulate some arguments against these two assumptions.

- What do the experimenter and participant bring with them to the experimental situation that isn't directly related to the experiment, and how may this (and other factors) influence what goes on in the experimental situation (see Gross, 2005)?

- When experimenters were informed that rats learning mazes had been specially bred for this ability ('maze bright'), they obtained better learning from their rats than did experimenters who believed their rats were 'maze dull' (Rosenthal and Fode, 1963; Rosenthal and Lawson, 1964). In fact, both groups of rats were drawn from the same population and were *randomly* allocated to the 'bright' or 'dull' condition. The crucial point is that the 'bright' rats did actually learn faster. The experimenters' expectations in some way concretely changed the situation, although how this happened is far less clear.

- In a natural classroom situation, children whose teachers told them they'd show academic 'promise' during the next academic year showed significantly greater IQ gains than children for whom such predictions weren't made (although this latter group also made substantial improvements). In fact, the children were *randomly* allocated to the two conditions. But the teachers' expectations actually produced the predicted improvements in the 'academic promise' group, demonstrating a *self-fulfilling prophecy* (Rosenthal and Jacobson, 1968).

(Based on Valentine, 1992; Weisstein, 1993)

PARTICIPANTS ARE PSYCHOLOGISTS TOO: DEMAND CHARACTERISTICS

Instead of seeing the person being studied as a passive responder to whom things are done ('subject'), Orne (1962) stresses what the person *does*, implying a far more *active* role. Participants' performance in an experiment could be thought of as a form of *problem-solving behaviour*. At some level, they see the task as working out the true purpose of the experiment and responding in a way that will support the hypothesis being tested.

In this context, the cues that convey the experimental hypothesis to participants represent important influences on their behaviour, and the sum total of those cues are called the *demand characteristics* of the experimental situation. These cues include all explicit and implicit communications during the actual experiment (Orne, 1962). This tendency to identify the demand characteristics is related to the tendency to play the role of a 'good' (or 'bad') experimental participant.

KEY STUDY 1.1: The lengths that some people will go to to please the experimenter (Orne, 1962)

- Orne points out that if people are asked to do five push-ups as a favour, they'll ask 'Why?', but if the request comes from an experimenter, they'll ask 'Where?'

- Orne reports an experiment in which people were asked to add up sheets of random numbers, then tear them into at least 32 pieces. Five and a half hours later, they were still doing it, and the experimenter had to tell them to stop!

- This demonstrates very clearly the strong tendency of people to want to please the experimenter and not to 'upset the experiment'. It's mainly in this sense that Orne sees the experiment as a social situation, in which the people involved play different but complementary roles. In order for this interaction to proceed fairly smoothly, each must have some idea of what the other expects of him or her.

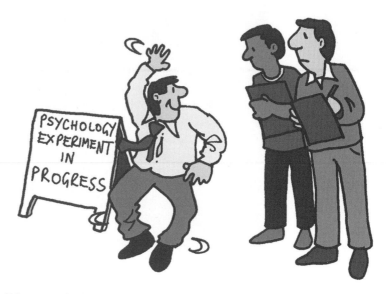

What we only do for the sake of science

The expectations referred to in Key Study 1.1 are part of the culturally shared understandings of what science in general, and psychology in particular, involves and without which the experiment couldn't 'happen' (Moghaddam *et al.*, 1993). So, not only is the experiment a social situation, but science itself is a *culture-related phenomenon*. This represents another respect in which science cannot claim complete objectivity.

THE PROBLEM OF REPRESENTATIVENESS

Traditional, mainstream experimental psychology adopts a *nomothetic* ('law–like') approach. This involves generalisation from limited samples of participants to 'people in general', as part of the attempt to establish general 'laws' or principles of behaviour (see Figure 1.2 and Chapter 6).

Despite the fact that Asch's experiments were carried out in the early 1950s, very little has changed as far as participant samples are concerned. In American psychology at least, the typical participant is a psychology undergraduate, who's obliged to take part in a certain number of studies as a course requirement, and who receives 'course credits' for doing so (Krupat and Garonzik, 1994).

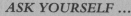

ASK YOURSELF ...

- The photograph below captures a fairly typical scene as far as participant characteristics in mainstream psychological research are concerned. In this photograph, which depicts one of Asch's famous conformity experiments (see Chapter 12, page 221), what are the most apparent characteristics of the experimental participants, and how are they similar to/different from those of Asch (who's pictured furthest right)?

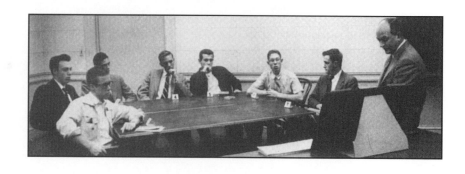

Mainstream British and American psychology has implicitly equated 'human being' with 'member of western culture'. Despite the fact that the vast majority of research participants are members of western societies, the resulting findings and theories have been applied to 'human beings', as if culture made no difference (they are 'culture-bound and culture-blind', according to Sinha, 1997). This *Anglocentric* or *Eurocentric bias* (a form of *ethnocentrism*) is matched by the *androcentric* or *masculinist bias* (a form of *sexism*), according to which the behaviours and experiences of men are taken as the standard against which women are judged (see Gross, 2005).

In both cases, while the bias remains implicit and goes unrecognised (and is reinforced by psychology's claim to be objective and value-free), research findings are taken as providing us with an objective, scientifically valid account of what 'women/people in general are like'. Once we realise that scientists, like all human beings, have prejudices, biases and values, their research and theories begin to look less objective, reliable and valid than they did before.

THE PROBLEM OF ARTIFICIALITY

Criticisms of traditional empirical methods (especially the laboratory experiment) have focused on their *artificiality*, including the often unusual and bizarre tasks that people are asked to perform in the name of science (see Key Study 1.1). Yet we cannot be sure that the way people behave in the laboratory is an accurate indication of how they're likely to behave outside it (Heather, 1976).

What makes the laboratory experiment such an unnatural and artificial situation is the fact that it's almost totally structured by one 'participant' – the experimenter. This relates to *power differences* between experimenters and their 'subjects', which is as much an *ethical* as a practical issue (see Gross, 2005).

Traditionally, participants have been referred to as 'subjects', implying something less than a person, a dehumanised and depersonalised 'object'. According to Heather (1976), it's a small step from reducing the person to a mere thing or object (or experimental 'subject') to seeing people as machines or machine-like ('mechanism' = 'machine-ism' = mechanistic view of people). This way of thinking about people is reflected in the popular definition of psychology as the study of 'what makes people tick' (see above).

THE PROBLEM OF INTERNAL VERSUS EXTERNAL VALIDITY

If the experimental setting (and task) is seen as similar or relevant enough to everyday situations to allow us to generalise the results, we say that the study has high *external* or *ecological validity*. But what about *internal validity*? Modelling itself on natural science, psychology attempts to overcome the problem of the complexity of human behaviour by using experimental control. This involves isolating an IV and ensuring that *extraneous variables* (variables other than the IV likely to affect the DV) don't affect the outcome (see Coolican, 2004). But this begs the crucial question: *how do we know when all the relevant extraneous variables have been controlled?*

Box 1.8 Some difficulties with the notion of experimental control

- While it's relatively easy to control the more obvious situational *variables* (see above), this is more difficult with *participant variables* (again see above), either for practical reasons (such as the availability of these groups) or because it isn't always obvious exactly what the relevant variables are. Ultimately, it's down to the experimenter's judgement and intuition: what s/he believes it is important (and possible) to control (Deese, 1972).

- If judgement and intuition are involved, then control and objectivity are matters of degree, whether in psychology or physics (see Table 1.1).

- It's the *variability/heterogeneity* of human beings that makes them so much more difficult to study than, say, chemicals. Chemists don't usually have to worry about how two samples of a particular chemical might be different from each other, but psychologists need to allow for *individual differences* between participants.

- We cannot just assume that the IV (or 'stimulus' or 'input') is identical for every participant, definable in some objective way, independent of the participant, and exerting a standard effect on everyone.

- Complete control would mean that the IV alone was responsible for the DV, so that experimenter bias and the effect of demand characteristics were irrelevant. But even if complete control were possible (even if we could guarantee the *internal validity* of the experiment), a fundamental dilemma would remain. The greater the degree of control over the experimental situation, the more different it becomes from real-life situations (the more artificial it gets and the lower its *external validity*).

In order to discover the relationships between variables (necessary for understanding human behaviour in natural, real-life situations), psychologists must 'bring' the behaviour into a specially created environment (the laboratory), where the relevant variables can be controlled in a way that's impossible in naturally occurring settings. However, in doing so, psychologists have constructed an artificial environment and the resulting behaviour is similarly artificial – it's no longer the behaviour they were trying to understand!

CONCLUSIONS

During the course of its life as a separate discipline, definitions of psychology have changed quite fundamentally, reflecting the influence of different theoretical approaches. Initially through the influence of behaviourism, psychology has taken the natural sciences as its model (*scientism*). In this chapter we've highlighted some of the major implications of adopting methods of investigating the natural world and applying them to the study of human behaviour and experience. In doing this, we've also examined what are fast becoming outdated and inaccurate views about the nature of science. Ultimately, whatever a particular science may claim to have discovered about the phenomena it studies, scientific activity remains just one more aspect of human behaviour.

CHAPTER SUMMARY

◎ Early psychologists, such as Wundt, attempted to study the mind through **introspection** under controlled conditions, aiming to analyse conscious thought into its basic elements (**structuralism**).

◎ Watson rejected introspectionism's **subjectivity** and replaced it with **behaviourism**. Only by regarding people as complex animals, using the methods of natural science and studying observable behaviour, could psychology become a true science.

◎ **Gestalt psychologists** criticised both structuralism and behaviourism, advocating that 'the whole is greater than the sum of its parts'. Freud's **psychoanalytic theory** was another major alternative to behaviourism.

◎ **Cognitive psychologists** see people as **information processors**, based on the **computer analogy**. Cognitive processes, such as perception and memory, are an acceptable part of psychology's subject matter.

◎ **Academic** psychologists are mainly concerned with conducting **research** (**pure** or **applied**), which may focus on underlying **processes/mechanisms** or on the **person**.

◎ The **process approach** consists of **physiological**, **cognitive** and **comparative** **psychology**, while the **person approach** covers **developmental** and **social psychology** and **individual differences**.

◎ Most **applied psychologists** work in **clinical**, **counselling**, **forensic**, **educational** or **occupational** psychology. Newer fields include **health** and **sport** psychology.

◎ A distinction is commonly made between **informal/common-sense** and **formal/scientific psychology**. The latter aims to go beyond common-sense understanding and to provide a public, communicable body of knowledge.

◎ A **science** must possess a **definable subject matter**, involve **theory construction** and **hypothesis testing**, and use **empirical methods** for **data collection**. However, these characteristics fail to describe the **scientific process** or **scientific method**.

◎ Science is a very **social** activity and consensus among the scientific community is paramount. This detracts from psychology's claim (or that of any other science) to **objectivity**.

◎ Environmental changes are somehow produced by experimenters' expectations (**experimenter bias**), and **demand characteristics** influence participants' behaviours by helping to convey the experimental hypothesis. The experiment is a social situation and science itself is **culture-related**.

◎ The **artificiality** of laboratory experiments is largely due to their being totally structured by experimenters. Also, the higher an experiment's **internal validity**, the lower its **external validity** becomes.

THEORETICAL APPROACHES 2

INTRODUCTION AND OVERVIEW

Different psychologists make different assumptions about what particular aspects of a person are worthy of study, and this helps to determine an underlying model or image of what people are like. In turn, this model or image determines a view of psychological normality, the nature of development, preferred methods of study, the major cause(s) of abnormality, and the preferred methods and goals of treatment.

An approach is a perspective that isn't as clearly outlined as a theory. As we shall see, all the major approaches include two or more distinguishable theories but, within an approach, they share certain basic principles and assumptions that give them a distinct 'flavour' or identity. The focus here is on the *behaviourist*, *psychodynamic*, *humanistic* and *social constructionist* approaches (see Gross, 2005, for a discussion of the cognitive and evolutionary approaches).

THE BEHAVIOURIST APPROACH

BASIC PRINCIPLES AND ASSUMPTIONS

As we saw in Chapter 1, Watson (1913) revolutionised psychology by rejecting the introspectionist approach and advocating the study of observable behaviour. Only by modelling itself on the natural sciences could psychology legitimately call itself a science. Watson was seeking to transform the very subject matter of psychology (from 'mind' to 'behaviour') and this is often called *methodological behaviourism*. According to Skinner (1987): '"Methodological" behaviourists often accept the existence of feelings and states of mind, but do not deal with them because they are not public and hence statements about them are not subject to confirmation by more than one person.'

In this sense, what was revolutionary when Watson (1913) first delivered his 'behaviourist manifesto' (see Box 2.1) has become almost taken-for-granted, 'orthodox' psychology. It could be argued that all psychologists are methodological behaviourists (Blackman, 1980). Belief in the importance of empirical methods, especially the experiment, as a way of collecting data about humans (and non-humans) that can be quantified and statistically analysed is a major feature of *mainstream psychology* (see Gross, 2005).

Box 2.1 Watson's (1913) 'behaviourist manifesto'

Watson's article, 'Psychology as the behaviourist views it', is often referred to as the 'behaviourist manifesto', a charter for a truly scientific psychology. Three features of this 'manifesto' deserve special mention.

1. Psychology must be purely *objective*, excluding all subjective data or interpretations in terms of conscious experience. This redefines psychology as the 'science of behaviour' (rather than the 'science of mental life').

2. The goals of psychology should be to *predict* and *control* behaviour (as opposed to describing and explaining conscious mental states), a goal later endorsed by Skinner's *radical behaviourism* (see text below).

3. There's no fundamental (*qualitative*) distinction between human and non-human behaviour. If, as Darwin had shown, humans evolved from more simple species, then it follows that human behaviour is simply a more complex form of the behaviour of other species (the difference is merely *quantitative* – one of degree). Consequently, rats, cats, dogs and pigeons became the major source of psychological data. Since 'psychological' now meant 'behaviour' rather than 'consciousness', non-humans that were convenient to study, and whose environments could easily be controlled, could replace people as experimental subjects.

(Based on Fancher, 1979; Watson, 1913)

In contrast to methodological behaviourists:

> 'Radical' behaviourists … recognise the role of private events (accessible in varying degrees to self-observation and physiological research), but contend that so-called mental activities are metaphors or explanatory fictions and that behaviour attributed to them can be more effectively explained in other ways. (Skinner, 1987)

For Skinner, these more effective explanations of behaviour come in the form of the *principles of reinforcement* derived from his experimental work with rats and pigeons (see Box 2.2). What's 'radical' about Skinner's *radical behaviourism* is the claim that feelings, sensations and other private events cannot be used to explain behaviour but are to *be explained* in an analysis of behaviour. Methodological behaviourism proposes to *ignore* such inner states (they're *inaccessible*), but Skinner *rejects* them as variables that can explain behaviour (they're *irrelevant*) and argues that they can be translated into the language of reinforcement theory (Garrett, 1996).

According to Nye (2000), Skinner's ideas are also radical because he applied the same type of analysis to covert behaviour (thoughts and feelings) occurring 'within the skin' as he did to overt, publicly observable behaviours. He stressed the importance of identifying *functional relations* (cause-and-effect connections) between environmental conditions and behaviours.

Given this important distinction between methodological and radical behaviourism, we need to consider some principles and assumptions that apply to behaviourism in general.

Box 2.2 Basic principles and assumptions made by the behaviourist approach

- Behaviourists emphasise the role of environmental factors in influencing behaviour, to the near exclusion of innate or inherited factors. This amounts essentially to a focus on *learning*. The key form of learning is *conditioning*, either *classical*, which formed the basis of Watson's behaviourism, or *operant*, which is at the centre of Skinner's radical behaviourism.

- *Classical conditioning* is also known as *Pavlovian*, after Pavlov, the Russian physiologist, who famously discovered that dogs learn to salivate at anything that has become associated with food. For example, if a bell is rung (the conditioned stimulus/CS) repeatedly just before the dog is given food (the unconditioned stimulus/UCS), the dog will eventually salivate when it hears the bell (without food having to be given). Salivating to food is an unconditioned (i.e. unlearned) response/UCR, but it becomes a conditioned response/CR to the bell. In both cases, salivation is an *automatic* response (hence, this form of learning is also known as *respondent* conditioning). The learner is responding *passively* to environmental events.

- *Operant conditioning* is also known as *instrumental* conditioning. This denotes the fact that the animal's behaviour is instrumental in producing certain *consequences*. In Skinner's experiments with rats, for example, they had to press a lever in order to receive a *positive reinforcement* (a food pellet) or a *negative reinforcement* (the switching off of an electric shock), or lever pressing would result in an electric shock (*punishment*). Reinforcement (positive or negative) makes the behaviour that produced it *more likely* to be repeated, while punishment makes it *less likely* to be repeated. Here, the learner is *actively* influencing what happens to it by manipulating its environment.

- Behaviourism is often referred to as 'S–R' psychology ('S' standing for 'stimulus' and 'R' for 'response'). However, classical and operant conditioning define the stimulus and response relationship in fundamentally different ways. Only in classical conditioning is the stimulus seen as triggering a response in a predictable, automatic way, and this is what's conveyed by 'S–R' psychology.

- Both types of conditioning are forms of *associative learning*, whereby associations or connections are formed between stimuli and responses that didn't exist before learning took place.

- The mechanisms proposed by a theory should be as simple as possible. Behaviourists stress the use of *operational definitions* (defining concepts in terms of observable, measurable events).

- The aim of a science of behaviour is to *predict* and *control* behaviour (see Box 2.1).

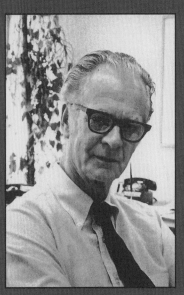

B.F. Skinner (1904–1990)

THEORETICAL CONTRIBUTIONS

Behaviourism made a massive contribution to psychology, at least up to the 1950s, and explanations of behaviour in conditioning terms recur throughout the subject (see Gross, 2005). For example, apart from learning and conditioning, imagery as a form of organisation in memory and as a memory aid is based on the principle of association, and the interference theory of forgetting is largely couched in stimulus–response terms. Language, moral and gender development have all been explained in terms of conditioning, and some influential theories of the formation and maintenance of relationships focus on the concept of reinforcement. The behaviourist approach also offers one of the major models of abnormal behaviour.

Theorists and researchers critical of the original, 'orthodox' theories have modified and built on them, making a huge contribution in the process. Noteworthy examples are Tolman's (1948) *cognitive behaviourism* and Bandura's (1971) *social learning theory* (renamed *social cognitive theory* in 1989).

PRACTICAL CONTRIBUTIONS

Methodological behaviourism, with its emphasis on experimentation, operational definitions and the measurement of observable events, has been a major influence on the practice of scientific psychology in general (what Skinner, 1974, called the 'science of behaviour'). This is quite unrelated to any views about the nature and role of mental events. Other, more 'tangible', contributions include:

◎ *behaviour therapy* and *behaviour modification* (based on classical and operant conditioning respectively) as major approaches to the treatment of abnormal behaviour (see Gross, 2005) and one of the main tools in the clinical psychologist's 'kit bag' (see Box 1.4, pages 8–9)

◎ *behavioural neuroscience*, an interdisciplinary field of study, using behavioural techniques to understand brain function and neuroscientific techniques to throw light on behavioural processes; while many believe that behaviour can be explained by (*reduced* to) brain processes, the evidence shows that each is dependent on the other (Leslie, 2002)

◎ *behavioural pharmacology*, which involves the use of *schedules/contingencies of reinforcement* to assess the behavioural effects of new drugs that modify brain activity (schedules of reinforcement refer to how often and regularly/predictably reinforcements are given following some desired behaviour); most importantly, the research has illustrated how many behavioural effects of drugs are determined as much by the current behaviour and reinforcement contingencies as by the effects of the drug on the brain (Leslie, 2002; see also Chapter 7)

◎ *biofeedback* as a non-medical treatment for stress-related symptoms, derived from attempts to change rats' autonomic physiological functions through the use of operant techniques (see Chapter 5).

AN EVALUATION OF BEHAVIOURISM

Both general and specific criticisms occur in the particular topic areas where behaviourist explanations have been proposed.

Skinner's claim that human behaviour can be predicted and controlled in the same way as the behaviour of non-humans is usually accepted only by other behaviour

---

ASK YOURSELF ...

• Try to think of examples of your work (including patients' and colleagues' behaviour, as well as your own) where behaviourist principles (such as reinforcement) and assumptions might help explain what happens.

ASK YOURSELF ...
• Do you agree with Skinner's claim that thoughts and other 'covert behaviours' don't *explain* our behaviour (because they cannot *determine* what we do)?

analysts. Possessing language allows us to communicate with each other and to think about 'things' that have never been observed (and may not even exist), including rules, laws and principles (Garrett, 1996). While these can only be expressed in or thought about in words, much of our behaviour is governed by them. According to Garrett, when this happens 'behaviour is now shaped by what goes on inside their [people's] heads … and not simply by what goes on in the external environment'. So, what people *think* is among the important variables determining what they do and say – the very *opposite* of what Skinner's radical behaviourism claims.

Behaviour analysts recognise the limitations of their approach. For example, Leslie (2002) admits that 'operant conditioning cannot provide a complete account of psychology from a behavioural perspective, even in principle'. Similarly, O'Donohue and Ferguson (2001) acknowledge that the science of behaviour cannot account for creativity, as in music, literature and science.

THE PSYCHODYNAMIC APPROACH

The term 'psychodynamic' denotes the active forces within the personality that motivate behaviour, and the inner causes of behaviour (in particular the *unconscious conflict* between the different structures that compose the whole personality). While Freud's was the original psychodynamic theory, the approach includes all those theories based on his ideas, such as those of Jung (1964), Adler (1927) and Erikson (1950). Freud's *psychoanalytic theory* is psychodynamic, but the psychodynamic theories of Adler, Jung and Erikson aren't psychoanalytic. So the two terms *aren't* synonymous. However, because of their enormous influence, Freud's ideas will be emphasised in the rest of this section.

BASIC PRINCIPLES AND ASSUMPTIONS

Freud's concepts are closely interwoven, making it difficult to know where a description of them should begin (Jacobs, 1992). Fortunately, Freud himself stressed the acceptance of certain key theories as essential to the practice of *psychoanalysis*, the form of psychotherapy he pioneered and from which most others are derived (see page 29).

> **Box 2.3 The major principles and assumptions of psychoanalytic theory**
>
> • Much of our behaviour is determined by unconscious thoughts, wishes, memories, and so on. What we're consciously aware of at any one time represents the tip of an iceberg: most of our thoughts and ideas are either not accessible at that moment (*pre-conscious*) or are totally inaccessible (*unconscious*). These unconscious thoughts and ideas can become conscious through the use of special techniques, such as *free association*, *dream interpretation* and *transference* – the cornerstones of psychoanalysis.
>
> • Much of what's unconscious has been made so through *repression*, whereby threatening or unpleasant experiences are 'forgotten'. They become inaccessible, locked away from our conscious awareness. This is a major form of *ego defence* (see Chapter 6). Freud singled

out repression as a special cornerstone 'on which the whole structure of psychoanalysis rests. It is the most essential part of it' (Freud, 1914). Repression is closely related to *resistance*, interpretation of which is another key technique used in psychoanalysis.

- According to the theory of *infantile sexuality*, the sexual instinct or drive is active from birth and develops through a series of five *psychosexual stages*. The most important of these is the *phallic stage* (spanning the ages 3–5/6), during which all children experience the *Oedipus complex*. This refers to the 'family romance', which in the case of boys refers to their 'falling in love' with their mother and becoming jealous of their father, whom they also fear will punish them through castration (see Gross, 2005).

- Freud used the German word *Trieb*, which translates as 'drive', rather than *Instinkt*, which was meant to imply that experience played a crucial role in determining the 'fate' of sexual (and aggressive) energy.

- Related to infantile sexuality is the general *impact of early experience* on later personality (see Chapter 14). According to Freud (1949):

  > It seems that the neuroses are only acquired during early childhood (up to the age of six), even though their symptoms may not make their appearance until much later … the child is psychologically father of the man and … the events of its first years are of paramount importance for its whole subsequent life.

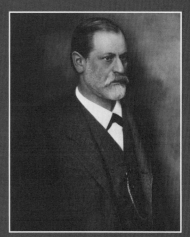

Sigmund Freud (1856–1939)

THEORETICAL CONTRIBUTIONS

As with behaviourist accounts of conditioning, many of Freud's ideas and concepts have become part of the vocabulary of mainstream psychology. You don't have to be a 'Freudian' to use concepts such as 'repression', 'unconscious', and so on, and many of the vast number of studies of different aspects of the theory have been conducted by critics hoping to discredit it (such as Eysenck, 1985; Eysenck and Wilson, 1973).

Like behaviourist theories, Freud's can also be found throughout psychology as a whole. His contribution is extremely rich and diverse, offering theories of motivation, dreams, and the relationship between sleep and dreams, moral and gender development, aggression, abnormality and forgetting (see Gross, 2005). Psychoanalytic theory also influenced Adorno *et al.*'s (1950) theory of the authoritarian personality (a major account of prejudice: see Chapter 11).

Finally, and as noted earlier, Freud's theories have stimulated the development of alternative theories, often resulting from the rejection of some of his fundamental principles and assumptions, but reflecting his influence enough for them to be described as psychodynamic.

ASK YOURSELF ...
- Repeat the exercise suggested for the behaviourist approach (see page 26).

Some major alternative psychodynamic theories

◎ *Ego psychology*, promoted by Freud's daughter, Anna, focused on the mechanisms used by the *ego* (the rational, decision-making part of the personality) to deal with the world, especially the ego defence mechanisms. Freud, by contrast, stressed the influence of the *id*'s innate drives (especially sexuality and aggression) and is often described as an instinct theorist (but see the fourth point in Box 2.3). (The id represents the infantile, pleasure-seeking part of the personality.) The ego, as well as the id, originates in basic human inheritance and has its own developmental course. It uses neutralised (non-sexual) energy, which makes possible an interest in objects and activities that aren't necessarily related to underlying sexual and aggressive drives.

◎ Erik Erikson, trained by Anna Freud as a child psychoanalyst, also stressed the importance of the ego, as well as the influence of social and cultural factors on individual development. He pioneered the *lifespan approach* to development, proposing eight *psychosocial stages*, in contrast with Freud's five psychosexual stages that end with physical maturity (see Chapters 17–20).

◎ Two of Freud's original 'disciples', Carl Jung and Alfred Adler, broke ranks with Freud and formed their own 'schools' (*analytical psychology* and *individual psychology* respectively). Jung attached relatively little importance to childhood experiences (and the associated personal unconscious) but considerable importance to the *collective* (or *racial*) *unconscious*, which stems from the evolutionary history of human beings as a whole (see Gross, 2005).

◎ Like Jung, Adler rejected Freud's emphasis on sexuality, stressing instead the *will to power* or *striving for superiority*, which he saw as an attempt to overcome feelings of inferiority faced by all children as they grow up. He also shared Jung's view of the person as an *indivisible unity* or whole, and Erikson's emphasis on the *social* nature of human beings.

◎ The *object relations school* (the 'British school') was greatly influenced by Melanie Klein's (1932) emphasis on the infant's earliest (pre-Oedipal) relationships with its mother. It places far less emphasis on the role of instincts and more on the *relationship with particular love objects* (especially the mother), seeing early relationships as crucial for later patterns of relationships with others. Fairbairn (1952), for example, saw the aim of the libido as *object-seeking* (as opposed to pleasure-seeking), and this was extended by Bowlby (1969) in his *attachment theory* (see Chapter 14).

PRACTICAL CONTRIBUTIONS

The current psychotherapy scene is highly diverse, with only a minority using Freudian techniques, but, as Fancher (1996) points out:

> Most modern therapists use techniques that were developed either by Freud and his followers or by dissidents in explicit reaction against his theories. Freud remains a dominating figure, for or against whom virtually all therapists feel compelled to take a stand.

Both Rogers, the major humanistic therapist (see below), and Wolpe, who developed *systematic desensitisation* (a major form of behaviour therapy), were originally trained in Freudian techniques. Perls, the founder of *Gestalt therapy*, Ellis, the founder of *rational emotive therapy* (RET), and Berne, who devised *transactional analysis* (TA), were also trained psychoanalysts.

Even Freud's fiercest critics concede his influence, not just within world psychiatry but in philosophy, literary criticism, history, theology, sociology, and art and literature generally. Freudian terminology is commonly used in conversations between therapists well beyond Freudian circles, and his influence is brought daily to therapy sessions as part of the cultural background and experience of nearly every client (Jacobs, 1992).

Many mental health practitioners (including psychotherapists, counsellors and social workers), although not formally trained as psychoanalysts, have incorporated elements of Freudian thought and technique into their approaches to helping their patients (Nye, 2000).

AN EVALUATION OF THE PSYCHODYNAMIC APPROACH

◎ A criticism repeatedly made of Freudian (and other psychodynamic) theories is that they're unscientific because they're *unfalsifiable* (incapable of being disproved). For example, if the Freudian prediction that 'dependent' men will prefer big-breasted women is confirmed, then the theory is supported. However, if such men actually prefer small-breasted women (Scodel, 1957), Freudians can use the concept of *reaction formation* (an ego defence mechanism – see Table 6.3 on pages 116–117) to argue that an unconscious fixation with big breasts may manifest itself as a conscious preference for the opposite – a clear case of 'heads I win, tails you lose' (Eysenck, 1985; Popper, 1959).

◎ However, it's probably a mistake to see reaction formation as typical of Freudian theory as a whole. According to Kline (1984, 1989), for example, the theory comprises a collection of hypotheses, some of which are more easily tested than others, some of which are more central to the theory than others, and some of which have more supporting evidence than others. Also, different parts of the theory have been tested using different methods (see Gvon, 2005).

◎ According to Zeldow (1995), the history of science reveals that those theories that are the richest in explanatory power have proved the most difficult to test empirically. For example, Einstein's general theory of relativity is still untestable. Eysenck, Popper and others have criticised psychoanalytic theory for being untestable. But even if this were true:

> … the same thing could (and should) be said about any psychological hypotheses involving complex phenomena and worthy of being tested … psychoanalytic theories have inspired more empirical research in the social and behavioural sciences than any other group of theories … (Zeldow, 1995)

◎ Freud's theory provides methods and concepts that enable us to interpret and 'unpack' underlying *meanings* (it has great *hermeneutic strength*). Popper's and Eysenck's criticism above helps to underline the fact that these meanings (both conscious and unconscious) cannot be measured in any precise way. Freud offers a way of understanding that's different from theories that are easily testable, and it may actually be *more* appropriate for capturing the nature of human experience and action (Stevens, 1995; see also Chapter 1). According to Fancher (1996): 'His ideas about repression, the importance of early experience and sexuality, and the inaccessibility of much of human nature to ordinary conscious introspection have become part of the standard Western intellectual currency.'

◎ Reason (2000) believes it's time to re-acknowledge Freud's greatness as a psychologist. Like James, he had a rare gift for describing and analysing the phenomenology of mental life. Perhaps Freud's greatest contribution was in recognising that apparent trivia we now commonly call 'Freudian slips' are 'windows on the mind'.

THE HUMANISTIC APPROACH

BASIC PRINCIPLES AND ASSUMPTIONS

As we noted earlier, Rogers, a leading humanistic psychologist (and therapist), was trained as a psychoanalyst. Although the term 'humanistic psychology' was coined by Cohen (1958), a British psychologist, this approach emerged mainly in the USA during the 1950s. Maslow (1968), in particular, gave wide currency to the term 'humanistic' in America, calling it a 'third force' (the other two being behaviourism and Freudianism). However, Maslow didn't reject these approaches but hoped to unify them, thus integrating both subjective and objective, the private and public aspects of the person, and providing a complete, holistic psychology.

Box 2.4 Some basic principles and assumptions of the humanistic approach

- Both the psychoanalytic and behaviourist approaches are *deterministic*. People are driven by forces beyond their control, either unconscious forces from within (Freud) or reinforcements from without (Skinner). Humanistic psychologists believe in free will and people's ability to choose how they act.

- A truly scientific psychology must treat its subject matter as fully human, which means acknowledging individuals as interpreters of themselves and their world. Behaviour, therefore, must be understood in terms of the individual's *subjective experience*, from the perspective of the actor (a *phenomenological approach*, which explains why this is sometimes called the 'humanistic-phenomenological' approach). This contrasts with the positivist approach of the natural sciences, which tries to study people from the position of a detached observer. Only the individual can explain the meaning of a particular behaviour and is the 'expert' – not the investigator or therapist.

- Maslow argued that Freud supplied the 'sick half' of psychology, through his belief in the inevitability of conflict, neurosis, innate self-destructiveness, and so on, while he (and Rogers) stressed the 'healthy half'. Maslow saw *self-actualisation* at the peak of a hierarchy of needs (see below and Chapter 6), while Rogers talked about the *actualising tendency*, an intrinsic property of life, reflecting the desire to grow, develop and enhance our capacities. A fully functioning person is the ideal of growth. Personality development naturally moves towards healthy growth, unless it's blocked by external factors, and should be considered the norm.

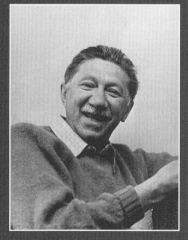

- Maslow's contacts with Wertheimer and other Gestalt psychologists (see Chapter 1) led him to stress the importance of understanding the *whole person*, rather than separate 'bits' of behaviour.

(Based on Glassman, 1995)

Abraham H. Maslow (1908–1970)

THEORETICAL CONTRIBUTIONS

Maslow's *hierarchy of needs* (see Chapter 6, pages 112–114) distinguishes between motives shared by both humans and non-humans and those that are uniquely human, and can be seen as an extension of the psychodynamic approach. Freud's id would represent physiological needs (at the hierarchy's base), Horney (a major critic of the male bias in Freud's theory) focused on the need for safety and love (corresponding to the next two levels), and Adler (see above) stressed esteem needs (at the fourth level). Maslow added self-actualisation to the peak of the hierarchy (Glassman, 1995).

According to Rogers (1951), while awareness of being alive is the most basic of human experiences, we each fundamentally live in a world of our own creation and have a unique perception of the world (the *phenomenal field*). It's our *perception* of external reality that shapes our lives (*not* external reality itself). Within our phenomenal field, the most significant element is our sense of *self*, 'an organised consistent gestalt, constantly in the process of forming and reforming' (Rogers, 1959; see also Chapter 6). This view contrasts with those of many other self theorists, who see it as a central, unchanging core of personality (see Chapter 16).

PRACTICAL CONTRIBUTIONS

ASK YOURSELF ...
• Repeat the exercise as for the behaviourist and psychodynamic approaches.

By far the most significant practical influence of any humanistic psychologist is Rogers' *client-* (or *person-) centred therapy* (see Gross, 2005). Originally (in the 1950s) it was called 'client-centred' (CCT), but since the mid-1970s it's been known as 'person–centred' therapy (PCT): 'psychotherapy is the releasing of an already existing capacity in a potentially competent individual' (Rogers, 1959).

The change in name was meant to reflect more strongly that the person, in his/her full complexity, is the centre of focus. Also, Rogers wanted to convey that his assumptions were meant to apply broadly to almost all aspects of human behaviour – not just to therapeutic settings. For example, he saw many parallels between therapists and teachers – they're both 'facilitators' of an atmosphere of freedom and support for individual pursuits. According to Nye (2000):

> A wide range of individuals – psychotherapists, counsellors, social workers, clergy and others – have been influenced by Rogers' assumptions that, if one can be a careful and accurate listener, while showing acceptance and honesty, one can be of help to troubled persons.

Nurses can be added to this list, especially in relation to their use of therapeutic conversation (see Chapter 3, pages 44–47).

Rogers helped develop research designs that enable objective measurement of the self-concept and ideal self, and their relationship over the course of therapy (see Chapter 16), as well as methodologies for exploring the importance of therapist qualities. These innovations continue to influence therapeutic practice, and many therapists are now concerned that their work should be subjected to research scrutiny.

By emphasising the therapist's personal qualities, Rogers opened up psychotherapy to psychologists and contributed to the development of therapy provided by non-medically qualified therapists (*lay therapy*). This is especially significant in the USA, where (until recently) psychoanalysts had to be psychiatrists (medically qualified). Rogers originally used the term 'counselling' as a strategy for silencing psychiatrists who objected to psychologists practising 'psychotherapy'. In the UK, the outcome of Rogers' campaign has been the evolution of a counselling profession whose practitioners are drawn from a wide variety of disciplines, with neither psychiatrists nor psychologists dominating. Counselling skills are used in a variety of settings throughout education, the health professions, social work, industry and commerce, the armed services and international organisations (Thorne, 1992).

AN EVALUATION OF THE HUMANISTIC APPROACH

◎ According to Wilson *et al.* (1996), the humanistic approach isn't an elaborate or comprehensive theory of personality, but should be seen as a set of uniquely personal theories of living created by humane people optimistic about human potential. It has wide appeal to those who seek an alternative to the more mechanistic, deterministic theories.

◎ Like Freud's theory, many of its concepts are difficult to test empirically (such as self-actualisation) and it cannot account for the origins of personality. Since it describes but doesn't explain personality, it's subject to the *nominal fallacy* (Carlson and Buskist, 1997) and so cannot really be called a theory.

◎ Nevertheless, for all its shortcomings, the humanistic approach represents a counterbalance to the psychodynamic (especially Freud) and the behaviourist approaches, and has helped to bring the 'person' back into psychology. Crucially, it recognises that people help determine their own behaviour and aren't simply slaves to environmental contingencies or to their past. The self, personal responsibility and agency, choice and free will are now legitimate issues for psychological investigation.

THE SOCIAL CONSTRUCTIONIST APPROACH

BASIC PRINCIPLES AND ASSUMPTIONS

Social constructionism (SC) has played a central role in the various challenges that have been made to mainstream, academic psychology during the last 30 years or so. The emergence of SC is usually dated from Gergen's (1973) paper 'Social psychology as history'. In this, he argued that all knowledge, including psychological knowledge, is historically and culturally specific, and that we therefore must extend our inquiries beyond the individual into social, political and economic realms for a proper understanding of the evolution of present-day psychology and social life. Since the only constant feature of social life is that it is continually *changing*, psychology in general – and social psychology in particular – becomes a form of *historical undertaking*: all we can ever do is try to understand and account for how the world appears to be *at the present time*.

The paper was written at the time of 'the crisis in social psychology'. Starting in the late 1960s and early 1970s, some social psychologists were becoming increasingly concerned that the 'voice' of ordinary people was being omitted from social psychological research. By concentrating on *decontextualised* laboratory behaviour, it was ignoring the real-world contexts that give human action its meaning. Several books were published, each proposing an alternative to positivist science and focusing on the accounts of ordinary people (e.g. Harré and Secord, 1972). These concerns are clearly seen today in SC.

While there's no single definition of SC that would be accepted by all those who might be included under its umbrella, we could categorise as social constructionist any approach that is based on one or more of the following key attitudes (as proposed by Gergen, 1985). Burr (2003) suggests we might think of these as 'things you would absolutely have to believe in order to be a social constructionist'.

◎ *A critical stance towards taken-for-granted knowledge*: our observations of the world don't reveal in any simple way the true nature of the world, and conventional knowledge isn't based on objective, unbiased 'sampling' of the world. The categories with which we understand the world don't necessarily correspond to natural or 'real' categories/distinctions. Belief in such natural categories is called *essentialism*, so social constructionists are *anti-essentialism*.

◎ *Historical and cultural specificity*: how we commonly understand the world, and the categories and concepts we use, are historically and culturally *relative*. Not only are they specific to particular cultures and historical periods, they're seen as products of that culture and history, and this must include the knowledge generated by the social sciences. The theories and explanations of psychology thus become time- and culture-bound and cannot be taken as once-and-for-all descriptions of human nature: 'The disciplines of psychology and social psychology can therefore no longer be aimed at discovering the "true" nature of people and social life ...' (Burr, 2003).

CRITICAL DISCUSSION 2.1 Transcultural and cross-cultural psychology, and the universalist assumption

• If knowledge is culturally created, then we shouldn't assume that our ways of understanding are necessarily any better (closer to 'the truth') than other ways. Yet this is precisely what mainstream (social) psychology has done. According to Much (1995), a new (*trans*)*cultural psychology* has emerged in North America (e.g. Bruner, 1990; Cole, 1990; Shweder, 1990) as an attempt to overcome the bias of *ethnocentrism* that has too often limited the scope of understanding in the social sciences (see Gross, 2005).

• Shweder (1990) makes the crucial distinction between *cultural psychology* and *cross-cultural psychology* (C-CP), which is a branch of experimental social, cognitive and personality psychology.

(a) Most of what's been known as 'cross-cultural' psychology has presupposed the categories and models that have been based on (mostly experimental) research with (limited samples of) Euro-American populations. It has mostly either 'tested the hypothesis' or 'validated the instrument' in other cultures or 'measured' the social and psychological characteristics of members of other cultures with the methods and standards of western populations, usually assumed as a valid universal norm.

(b) The new 'cultural psychology' rejects this *universalist* model (Much, 1995). It's become almost a 'standing joke' that experimental (social) psychology is really the psychology of the American undergraduate/psychology major. Apart from their accessibility, the argument commonly assumed to justify the practice of studying mostly student behaviour is based upon a sweeping and gratuitous universalist assumption: since we're all human, we're all fundamentally alike in significant psychological functions, and

> cultural/social contexts of diversity don't affect the important 'deep' or 'hardwired' structures of the mind. The corollary of this assumption is that the categories and standards developed on western European/North American populations are suitable for 'measuring', understanding and evaluating the characteristics of other populations.
>
> • By contrast, a genuinely transcultural psychology – 'the interplay between the individual and society and [symbolic] culture' (Kakar, 1982, quoted in Much, 1995) – would base its categories, discriminations and generalisations upon empirical knowledge of the fullest possible range of existing human forms of life, without privileging one form as the norm or standard for evaluation.'

◎ *Knowledge is sustained by social processes*: our current accepted way of understanding the world ('truth') doesn't reflect the world as it really is (*objective reality*), but is constructed by people through their everyday interactions. Social interaction of all kinds, and particularly language, is of central importance for social constructionists: it's other people, both past and present, who are the sources of knowledge.

> ... We are born into a world where the conceptual frameworks and categories used by the people of our culture already exist ... Concepts and categories are acquired by each person as they develop the use of language and are thus reproduced every day by everyone who shares a culture and language. This means that the way a person thinks, the very categories and concepts that provide a framework of meaning for them, are provided by the language that they use. Language therefore is a necessary pre-condition for thought as we know it ... (Burr, 2003)

By giving a central role to *social interactions* and seeing these as actively producing taken-for-granted knowledge of the world, it follows that language itself is more than simply a way of expressing our thoughts and feelings (as typically assumed by mainstream psychology). When people talk to each other, they (help to) *construct* the world, such that language use is a form of action (it has a '*performative*' role).

◎ *Knowledge and social action go together*: these 'negotiated' understandings could take a wide variety of forms, so that there are many possible 'social constructions' of the world. But each different construction also brings with it, or invites, a different kind of action: how we account for a particular behaviour (what caused it) will dictate how we react to and treat the person whose behaviour it is (see Chapter 9).

Mainstream psychology looks for explanations of social phenomena *inside* the person – for example, by hypothesising the existence of attitudes, motives, cognitions, and so on (*individualism*). This can also be seen as *reductionist*. Social constructionists reject this view: explanations are to be found neither inside the individual psyche nor in social structures or institutions (as advocated by sociologists), but in the *interactive processes* that take place routinely between people. For Burr (2003), 'Knowledge is therefore seen not as something that a person has or doesn't have, but as something that people do together ...'.

THEORETICAL CONTRIBUTIONS AND AN EVALUATION OF SOCIAL CONSTRUCTIONISM

Social constructionism and social representation theory

◎ According to *social representation theory* (SRT), people come to understand their social world by way of images and social representations (SRs) shared by members of a social group. These representations act like a map that makes a baffling or novel terrain familiar and passable, thereby providing evaluations of good and bad areas. Attitudes are secondary phenomena, underpinned by SRs. SRT tries to provide a historical account of people's understanding of the world (Potter, 1996).

◎ During the 1950s, the French psychologist, Moscovici, conducted one of the classic pieces of research on SRs. He was interested in how the ideas/concepts of psychoanalytic theory could be absorbed within a culture (post-Second World War France), through women's magazines, church publications and interviews. He concluded that psychoanalytic theory had trickled down from the analytic couch and learned journals into both 'high' culture and popular common sense: people 'think' with psychoanalytic concepts, without it seeming as if they are doing anything theoretical at all. But rather than the general population of Paris being conversant with/conversing with psychoanalytic theory in all its complexities, they were working with a simplified image of it, with some concepts having a wide currency (such as repression) and others not (such as libido) (Potter, 1996).

◎ SRT is a *constructionist* theory: instead of portraying people as simply perceiving (or misperceiving) their social worlds, it regards these worlds as constructed, and an SR is a device for doing this construction. It allows someone to make sense of something potentially unfamiliar and to evaluate it. For Moscovici, all thought and understanding is based on the working of SRs, each of which consists of a mixture of concepts, ideas and images; these are both in people's minds and circulating in society.

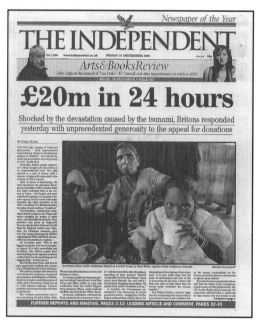

The power of the media to circulate social representations by capturing the 'national mood'

CONCLUSIONS: CAN PSYCHOLOGY BE A SCIENCE IF PSYCHOLOGISTS CANNOT AGREE WHAT PSYCHOLOGY IS?

As we saw in Chapter 1, definitions of psychology have changed during its lifetime, largely reflecting the influence and contributions of its major theoretical approaches or orientations. In this chapter, we've seen that each approach rests upon a different image of what people are like. Freud's 'tension-reducing person', Skinner's 'environmentally controlled person' and Rogers' 'growth-motivated person' really are quite different from each other (Nye, 2000). SC's image of the person is rather less concrete and more elusive: what people are like and what they do is *relative* to their culture, historical period, and so on.

However, we've also noted some important similarities between different approaches, such as the deterministic nature of Freud's and Skinner's theories. Each approach has something of value to contribute to our understanding of ourselves – even if it is only to reject the particular explanation it offers. The diversity of approaches reflects the complexity of the subject matter, so, usually, there's room for a diversity of explanations.

These different conceptualisations of the person in turn determine what's considered worthy of investigation, as well as the methods of study that can and should be used to investigate it. Consequently, different approaches can be seen as self-contained disciplines, as well as different facets of the same discipline (Kline, 1988; Kuhn, 1962).

As Table 2.1 shows, Kuhn (and others) believe that psychology is still in a state (or stage) of *prescience*. Whether psychology has, or has ever had, a paradigm, continues to be hotly debated.

Table 2.1 Stages in the development of a science (σ) and their application to psychology (ν)

σ   *Prescience:* A majority of those working in a particular discipline don't yet share a common or global perspective (*paradigm*), and there are several schools of thought or theoretical orientations.

ν   Like Kuhn (1962), Joynson (1980) and Boden (1980) argue that psychology is *preparadigmatic*. Kline (1988) sees its various approaches as involving different paradigms.

σ   *Normal science:* A paradigm has emerged, dictating the kind of research that's carried out and providing a framework for interpreting results. The details of the theory are filled in and workers explore its limits. Disagreements can usually be resolved within the limits allowed by the paradigm.

ν   According to Valentine (1992), *behaviourism* comes as close as anything could to a paradigm. It provides: (a) a clear definition of the subject matter (behaviour as opposed to 'the mind'); (b) fundamental assumptions, in the form of the central role of learning (especially conditioning), and the analysis of behaviour into stimulus–response units, which allow prediction and control; (c) a methodology, with the controlled experiment at its core.

Table 2.1 *continued*

σ *Revolution:* A point is reached in most established sciences where the conflicting evidence becomes so overwhelming that the old paradigm has to be abandoned and is replaced by a new one (*paradigm shift*). For example, Newtonian physics was replaced by Einstein's theory of relativity. When this paradigm shift occurs, there's a return to *normal science*.

ν Palermo (1971) and LeFrancois (1983) argue that psychology has already undergone several paradigm shifts. The first paradigm was *structuralism*, represented by Wundt's introspectionism. This was replaced by Watson's *behaviourism*. Finally, *cognitive psychology* largely replaced behaviourism, based on the computer analogy and the concept of information processing (see Chapter 1). Glassman (1995) disagrees, claiming that there's never been a complete reorganisation of the discipline, as has happened in physics.

CHAPTER SUMMARY

◎ Different theoretical **approaches/perspectives** are based on different models/images of the nature of human beings.

◎ **Methodological behaviourism** focuses on what can be quantified and observed by different researchers. Skinner's **radical behaviourism** regards mental processes as both **inaccessible** and **irrelevant** for explaining behaviour.

◎ The **behaviourist approach** stresses the role of environmental influences (**learning**), especially **classical** and **operant conditioning**. Psychology's aim is to **predict** and **control** behaviour.

◎ Tolman's **cognitive behaviourism** and Bandura's **social learning/social cognitive theory** represent modifications of 'orthodox' learning (conditioning) theory.

◎ Methodological behaviourism has influenced the practice of scientific psychology in general. Other practical contributions include **behaviour therapy** and **modification**, **behavioural neuroscience** and **pharmacology**, and **biofeedback**.

◎ The **psychodynamic approach** is based on Freud's **psychoanalytic theory**. Central aspects are the **unconscious** (especially **repression**), **infantile sexuality** and the impact of **early experience**.

◎ Freud's ideas have become part of **mainstream psychology**, contributing to our understanding of motivation, sleep and dreams, forgetting, attachment, aggression and abnormality.

◎ Major modifications/alternatives to Freudian theory include **ego psychology**, Erikson's **psychosocial theory** and the **object relations school**.

◎ All forms of **psychotherapy** stem directly or indirectly from **psychoanalysis**. Many trained psychoanalysts have been responsible for developing radically different therapeutic approaches, including Rogers, Perls and Wolpe.

◎ Maslow called the **humanistic approach** the 'third force' in psychology. It believes in free will, adopts a **phenomenological perspective**, and stresses the **positive** aspects of human personality.

◎ Rogers was a prolific researcher into the effectiveness of his **client/person-centred therapy**, opened up psychotherapy to psychologists and other non-medically qualified practitioners, and created a counselling profession that operates within a wide diversity of settings.

◎ One of the goals of **social constructionism** (SC) is to correct the tendency of mainstream psychology to **decontextualise** behaviour. Related to this is the **universalist assumption**, which is challenged by **(trans)cultural** (as distinct from **cross-cultural**) **psychology**. **Social representation theory** (SRT) is a social constructionist theory.

◎ Different **theoretical approaches** can be seen as self-contained disciplines, making psychology **pre-paradigmatic** and so still in a stage of **prescience**.

◎ Only when a discipline possesses a **paradigm** has it reached the stage of **normal science**, after which **paradigm shifts** result in **revolution** (and a return to normal science).

PSYCHOLOGICAL ASPECTS OF ILLNESS

3

INTRODUCTION AND OVERVIEW

According to Ogden (2004), health psychology represents one of several challenges that were made during the twentieth century to the *biomedical model*. This maintains that:

◎ diseases either come from outside the body and invade it, causing internal physical changes, or originate as internal involuntary physical changes; such diseases can be caused by chemical imbalances, bacteria, viruses or genetic predisposition

◎ individuals aren't responsible for their illnesses, which arise from biological changes beyond their control; people who are ill are victims

◎ treatment should consist of vaccination, surgery, chemotherapy or radiotherapy, all of which aim to change the physical state of the body

◎ responsibility for treatment rests with the medical profession

◎ health and illness are qualitatively different – you're either healthy or ill, and there's no continuum between the two

◎ mind and body function independently of each other; the abstract mind relates to feelings and thoughts, and is incapable of influencing physical matter

◎ illness may have psychological consequences, but *not* psychological causes.

In opposition to these ideas, health psychology maintains that human beings should be seen as complex systems. Illness is often caused by a combination of biological (e.g. viruses), psychological (e.g. behaviours and beliefs) and social (e.g. employment) factors. These assumptions reflect the *biopsychosocial model* of health and illness (Engel, 1977, 1980).

According to Stroebe (2000), the biopsychosocial model reflects fundamental changes in the nature of illness, causes of death and overall life expectancy during the twentieth century. The influence of non-biological factors (for example, improvements in medical treatment and significant changes in lifestyle) in major causes of death such as cardiovascular disease and cancer is incompatible with the biomedical model. By conceptualising disease in purely biological terms, the model has little to offer the *prevention* of chronic diseases through efforts to change people's health beliefs, attitudes and behaviour.

Similarly, the biomedical model, by ignoring the role of psychological and socio-cultural factors, is unable to explain:

◎ how pre-operative psychological preparation (including anxiety reduction) can affect wound healing and recovery rate

◎ the relationship between patients' perception of symptoms and symptom control

◎ why patients sometimes don't comply with treatment (see Chapter 13)

◎ how the attitudes towards their illness can affect its course and prognosis in patients with chronic illnesses (such as HIV/AIDS, cancer, obesity and coronary heart disease), and

◎ the enormous diversity in patients' experience/tolerance of pain.

In all these cases, the relationship between the patient and the nurse (or doctor, physiotherapist, etc.) also plays a crucial role.

From my diary (1): Year 1/Community/District Nurse

My first visit to a patient with Sally, my mentor in this placement, was to Maisie, a pale, thin woman of 68, who'd had a hysterectomy three weeks previously. Sally explained that visiting patients in their homes means we are their guests; it also gives us an ideal opportunity to explore the biopsychosocial model of health care.

Maisie's wound was still oozing and, while she was dressing it, Sally asked her if she was eating properly as she seemed to have lost weight. Maisie admitted she'd lost 'a few pounds' since her operation and that she didn't have much of an appetite. When Sally suggested that might be the reason her wound wasn't healing, Maisie looked upset and shook her head. I felt in the way, so tried to busy myself putting things away as Sally sat on the bed, took Maisie's hand in hers and asked gently if she was worried about anything. Maisie began to cry, but although Sally waited patiently, said nothing more. Sally then asked me if I'd mind waiting in the car, so I said goodbye to Maisie and left.

WHAT IS HEALTH PSYCHOLOGY?

Maes and van Elderen (1998) define health psychology as:

> … a sub-discipline of psychology which addresses the relationship between psychological processes and behaviour on the one hand and health and illness on the other hand … however … health psychologists are more interested in 'normal' everyday-life behaviour and 'normal' psychological processes in relation to health and illness than in psycho-pathology or abnormal behaviour …

However, Turpin and Slade (1998) believe that health psychology is an *extension* of clinical psychology (see Chapter 2), focusing specifically on people with physical health problems and their associated psychological needs. They advocate the biopsychosocial model (see Figure 3.1).

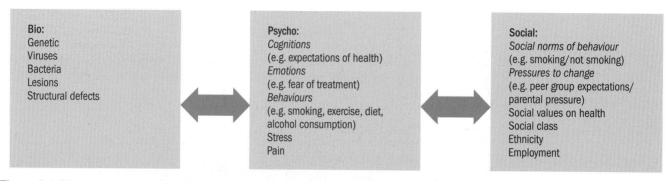

Bio:
Genetic
Viruses
Bacteria
Lesions
Structural defects

Psycho:
Cognitions
(e.g. expectations of health)
Emotions
(e.g. fear of treatment)
Behaviours
(e.g. smoking, exercise, diet, alcohol consumption)
Stress
Pain

Social:
Social norms of behaviour
(e.g. smoking/not smoking)
Pressures to change
(e.g. peer group expectations/
parental pressure)
Social values on health
Social class
Ethnicity
Employment

Figure 3.1 The biopsychosocial model of health and illness (adapted from Ogden, Open University Press, 2000)

THE MEANING OF PSYCHOLOGICAL CARE

ASK YOURSELF ...
- In what ways do you care for your patients?
- What do you understand by the term 'psychological care'?
- Why might patients need this as much as they need physical care?

According to Nichols (2005):

> ... Despite 20 years of major expansion and research in psychology – and in particular health psychology – the average-patient test will almost always reveal our failure to develop psychological care as part of the thinking, culture and routines of general hospitals and health centres.

The 'average-patient test' involves visiting your local hospital, picking a ward at random, going with the clinical nurse manager to the third bed on the left or right, and asking 'Who is handling this patient's psychological care and how is it going?'

Despite nursing becoming more psychologically minded during the 1990s via Project 2000, publications encouraging the introduction of psychological approaches into health care, and psychologists producing specific local provisions, such as some stroke, intensive care or cancer units, 'psychological care is still not a common provision in hospitals' (Nichols, 2005). This neglect of psychological care has real – and serious – clinical consequences.

It was obvious Maisie was upset but I had no idea why. Sally was clearly concerned for her emotional state and I sensed I was 'in the way' of Maisie talking about it. I was relieved not to have to deal with it, yet felt a bit resentful when asked to leave.

ASK YOURSELF ...
- List some of the common psychological responses to illness and injury displayed by patients.

Nichols includes shock and even post-traumatic stress disorder, confusion and distress, loss of self-worth, lowered personal control and a collapse into dependency. Apart from these responses being highly undesirable in themselves, they can also undermine medical efforts and interfere with rehabilitation. For example, Hemingway and Marmot (1999) found that the probability of cardiac patients suffering a second heart attack increased if they were in 'emotional disarray' and lacked support. Nichols believes this is exactly what psychological care is about – monitoring for signs of such responses and intervening with basic care techniques or referral to psychological treatment. Such referral represents the link between Levels 2 and 3 in a model of psychological care (Nichols, 2003), like that shown in Table 3.1.

Table 3.1 The components of psychological care (Nichols, 2003)

Level 1 (awareness)	**Awareness of psychological issues** Patient–centred listening Patient–centred communication Awareness of the patient's psychological state and relevant action
Level 2 (intervention)	**Monitoring the patient's psychological state with records kept** Informational and educational care Emotional care Counselling care Support/advocacy/referral
Level 3 (therapy)	**Psychological therapy**

Well, at least I achieved the first bit of Level 1 this morning – I recognised Maisie's distress. Sally immediately followed it up by sitting down and attending to Maisie.

Nurses, therapists, medical staff (and anyone else involved in the patient's care) can all play a part under the guidance of psychologists (Nichols, 2005).

Interestingly, a recent survey of 354 physiotherapists, chiropractors and osteopaths found that at least 10 per cent continued long-term treatment with patients, even after three months or more without demonstrable improvement. Follow-up interviews with a sample of these physical therapy practitioners revealed that many see it as their responsibility to provide psychological support and health advice to patients. Despite international guidelines for the treatment of lower back pain in primary care recommending that patients be referred back to their GP in the absence of any improvement, many of the interviewees were unhappy to discharge patients and were uncertain about what would happen to them once they'd left their care (The Psychologist, 2006).

SKILLED COMMUNICATION, PSYCHOLOGICAL SAFETY AND THERAPEUTIC CONVERSATION

What Nichols' model calls 'patient-centred listening' and 'patient-centred communication' seems to correspond with 'skilled communication' (Minardi and Riley, 1988) and 'therapeutic conversation' (Burnard, 1987).

According to Minardi and Riley, the standard of care delivered to patients depends on the quality of the relationships that individual nurses build with them. A prerequisite for the development of such relationships beyond the merely 'social' level is that both participants feel safe enough to openly discuss their feelings. However, most nurses have experienced a patient who consistently under-reports either physical or psychological discomfort. Equally, many nurses hide a variety of feelings under a mask of willing cooperation, in interaction with both patients and colleagues.

This mutual reluctance to express true feelings may reflect perception of the other person as a threat. In order to reduce this threat, and to ensure a free-flowing discussion, it's necessary to provide a degree of *psychological safety* for each other.

When Sally got back, she apologised for excluding me, but explained that Maisie wouldn't have said anything while I was there; she knew her well as she'd nursed her husband who'd died of cancer a year ago. I understand now that Sally had established a relationship with her patient that was 'psychologically safe' and which I, a stranger, was compromising.

Egan (1977) suggests that the provision of understanding, support and encouragement enables another person to feel secure enough to disclose important emotional concerns. This would involve an individual being listened to, being allowed to speak without interruption, and receiving feedback that shows they have been understood. It requires recognition of the person's beliefs, values, needs and wishes without judging that person: 'It would appear, therefore, that the provision of psychological safety centres around the ability to communicate to an individual that their beliefs, values, needs and wishes are recognised and understood in an open and non-judgemental way' (Minardi and Riley, 1988).

Agreeing with Nichols (2005) above, Minardi and Riley argue that, in most nursing situations, the 'recovery of health' involves meeting individuals' emotional

ASK YOURSELF ...
- What do you understand by the term 'psychological safety'?

- With what kinds of communication skills might you show a patient (or colleague) that you understand and support them?

needs as much as meeting their physical needs. Such strategies are also a vital part of nurses' relationships with one another: '... the perception of a degree of psychological safety which allows a full and free expression of the concerns and anxieties which may exist in our professional relationships is essential to our work' (Minardi and Riley, 1988).

Psychological safety can be enhanced by what Burnard (1987) calls 'therapeutic conversations'.

Box 3.1 Five components of the therapeutic conversation (based on Burnard, 1987)

- **Emphasis on the here-and-now:** Many people find the present painful to live in, while the past, however inaccurate our recollection, feels more comfortable. But it's more therapeutic if the nurse stays with the patient's moment-to-moment phenomenology and notes his/her changing verbal and non-verbal cues as they occur (see Chapter 8). This requires concentration, close awareness of subtle changes and the ability to 'stay awake' and remain focused on the patient.

- **Focus on feelings:** The nurse uses reflection and empathy-building to convey that s/he understands what the patient is feeling. This helps the patient to confront the feelings as they occur, rather than having a theoretical debate about *why* the patient is feeling this way. This focus on feelings requires training in basic counselling techniques.

- **Empathic understanding:** This involves attempting to enter the other person's frame of reference or way of looking at the world – that is, to see things from *their* perspective, rather than our own (see Chapter 15, pages 282–283 and 287–288). By understanding the patient's belief and value system, we can better appreciate why they are experiencing this set of feelings at this time. This too requires training.

- **A non-prescriptive approach:** To be prescriptive is to make suggestions or offer opinions about what the patient should do. It's usually more appropriate in a health care setting to help the patient to make his/her own decisions and draw his/her own conclusions.

- **The patient should remain the central focus:** While in ordinary social conversation there's a to-and-fro between the two speakers, in the therapeutic conversation the patient is 'telling the story' while the nurse is essentially *listening* (albeit *actively* listening – Watts, 1986). This is another skill that can be developed – through experiencing what it's like to be *heard*.

Sally was concerned with Maisie's immediate distress. I didn't hear the exchange between them, but it must have been skilled as Sally discovered a great deal. Maisie was getting 'indigestion' pain after meals, and to avoid it had resorted to not eating. She was convinced she had cancer of the stomach, the cause of her husband's death, but had been afraid to complain of the pain and have her suspicions confirmed.

Another answer to the question 'What do we mean by psychological care?' is offered by Bassett (2002) in a study focusing on the lived and expressed experiences of 15 qualified nurses and six nursing students (two from each year of a three-year Advanced Diploma in Nursing programme).

ASK YOURSELF …

• Which of the major theoretical approaches discussed in Chapter 2 is most closely related to the various communication skills described above? (See also Chapter 6 and Gross, 2005.)

ASK YOURSELF …

• What do you consider to be some of the strengths and weaknesses of Bassett's study? (For example, how confident can we be about the themes applying to nurses in general, was the sample size adequate, and what other methods could be used to explore nurses' perceptions of care?)

KEY STUDY 3.1 Nurses' and students' perceptions of care (Bassett, 2002)

The participants were interviewed about their understanding of the phenomenon of care and caring. Transcriptions from the taped interviews were read to develop a 'feeling' for them and to make sense of them. Statements were then categorised according to their perceived meanings and arranged into five main themes, as follows.

1. **Encouraging autonomy:** This relates to *patient empowerment*, wanting to allay patients' fears and anxieties by giving them greater control over their care.

2. **Giving of oneself:** 'Caring, it can be argued, is the essence of giving of oneself' (Bassett, 2002). Nurses give to patients in terms of time, energy and effort. They spend time learning skills and gaining knowledge, both as students and throughout their nursing careers. But to simply provide mechanical care may not be enough in their eyes – providing care without *genuineness* isn't adequate.

3. **Taking risks:** This theme comprises the sub-categories 'taking risks', 'getting a buzz' and 'challenge'. Taking risks in nursing isn't about putting patients at risk, but refers to testing the boundaries of accepted care, moving from the defined boundaries, and developing new and innovative ways of caring for patients. Sometimes, it may be necessary to *disobey* a doctor's orders if this is in the patient's best interests (see Chapter 13) or to take a stand against colleagues' interpretations of normal nursing procedures or protocols. For students, this means 'standing up' for patients when they feel the care was less than the patient deserved.

4. **Supporting care:** Certain supporting factors are essential to ensure that care can be delivered effectively. These are managerial, organisational and psychological support systems.

5. **Emotional labour:** This theme was unique to the student participants and seemed to reflect the fact that learning to nurse can constitute an emotional assault. It describes the often difficult things that nurses are expected to do in their daily work, causing them to experience sadness and emotional trauma. If unresolved or buried, these responses may lead nurses to leave nursing or not develop the caring attributes necessary for quality nursing care (see Chapter 5, page 87).

This study raises a daunting number of issues, but even in my first nursing experience, and in a small way, it did help me understand the 'emotional labour' bit. Just seeing Maisie's tears this morning made me feel uncomfortable; Sally had cared for her husband until he died at home, which must have been so much more difficult. I also had to acknowledge a feeling of rejection when Sally (wisely) asked me to leave.

The final theme in Bassett's study can be seen as related to the concept of *emotional intelligence*: 'a type of social intelligence that involves the ability to monitor one's own and others' emotions, to discriminate among them, and to use the information to guide one's thinking and actions' (Salovey and Mayer, 1990, in Evans and Allen, 2002).

People who are able to manage their own feelings well while reading and dealing with other people's emotions are particularly suited to the caring professions. So it's surprising that most nurse education programmes fail to embrace this aspect of training (Evans and Allen, 2002).

Evans and Allen cite the work of Sims and Lindberg (1978), who argue that 'negative self-concepts are barriers to the effective independent functioning vital to the successful performance of professional roles'. This is reflected in the notion of the *wounded healer* (Clarkson, 1997, in Evans and Allen, 2002): if you are a passive person, you'll be a passive nurse. According to Evans and Allen: 'Self-awareness is an important part of nursing. The key to self-knowledge lies in intrapersonal intelligence … If they [students] are able to deal with their own feelings well, they will be able to deal with others confidently, competently and safely.'

This explains why we have to acknowledge our feelings in the reflective writing we do (Gibbs, 1988, in Jasper, 2003). Recognising my own emotional discomfort is the first step to acknowledging the need to find a way to deal with such situations. Sally didn't seem upset, presumably because she knew what to do. As we drove back, she explained she had reassured Maisie, but was referring her to the GP for investigations to exclude cancer. This is the support, advocacy and, in this case, medical referral in Level 2 of Nichols' model (see Table 3.1).

PSYCHOSOCIAL ASPECTS OF SURGERY AND OTHER TREATMENTS

For many people, patients and relatives alike, hospitals and other health care settings can be unpleasant, frightening, even bewildering places. Those environments within a hospital that are designed to help those with the most life-threatening conditions are also likely to evoke the most extreme negative reactions – in both patients and staff. These 'extreme' environments include coronary care units (CCUs), cancer wards/units, intensive care units (ICUs) and Accident and Emergency (A&E) departments.

PRE-SURGICAL ANXIETY

Hospital admission is a stressor that produces severe anxiety in some form or another in 10–80 per cent of patients. Although medication is often used to manage pre-operative anxiety, many nurses believe that reassurance and listening to patients' concerns are more beneficial. However, research suggests that nurses generally play a minor part in patients' psychological care, and the nurse–patient relationship on most surgical wards is task-related, short and to the point, with therapeutic discussion almost non-existent (Toogood, 1999).

Severe anxiety can affect a patient's ability to assimilate and retain information, while moderate anxiety can produce increased adrenaline and cortisol levels, inhibiting wound healing (Pediani, 1992; Toogood, 1999). It can also cause electrolyte imbalance and harm the body's immune response, leading to increased risk of wound infections (see Chapter 5).

So not just poor nutrition, but Maisie's anxiety about her condition could be delaying her wound healing.

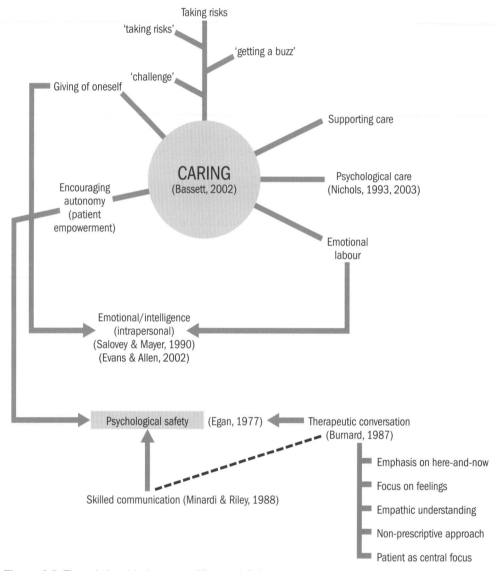

Figure 3.2 The relationship between different definitions and components of care

Personality (see Chapter 6), health status, age (see Chapters 15 and 19), cultural background and family role may all affect anxiety. Also, surgery that produces a change in body image (such as mastectomy, hysterectomy or amputation) may have greater psychological impact (see Chapter 16).

Information-giving

It's widely acknowledged that understanding helps reduce anxiety. If a situation cannot be interpreted, it cannot be dealt with and the individual experiences helplessness and

ASK YOURSELF ...
- What sorts of factors are likely to affect a pre-operative patient's anxiety level?

ASK YOURSELF ...
- What non-medical methods could be used to reduce patients' pre-operative anxiety?

anxiety (Lazarus and Averill, 1978; see Chapter 5). However, just giving information, though beneficial, isn't enough. Even assuming the patient is able to understand the information sent before admission, it can actually increase stress (Salmon, 1993, in Toogood, 1999). What's needed is a careful assessment of a patient's needs and appropriate care. Nurses must bear in mind that patients' levels of intelligence and understanding vary, and that one answer may not suit the needs of any two patients (Toogood, 1999).

Boore (1978, in Pediani, 1992) compared a group of 'informed' patients with an 'uninformed' group, both groups receiving the same amount of 'nurse time' prior to surgery. The former had lower levels of steroids in their urine, suggesting that information allows patients to interpret and understand their surroundings and helps them to anticipate the events usually occurring in the post-operative period. This minimises feelings of helplessness and so lowers anxiety. Other studies have found that good psychological preparation can lead to earlier discharge from hospital, less need for analgesia, lower incidence of urinary retention and lower pulse rate and blood pressure (Pediani, 1992).

What these studies suggest is that 'good wound care is not just a matter of physical administration of dressings; it involves the need to prepare the patient psychologically' (Pediani, 1992).

Panda *et al.* (1996, in Toogood, 1999) suggest that patients value information from doctors most. But, in reality, nurses offer an emotional support service and are often required to fill in the gaps left by doctors, interpreting medical information that patients don't understand, so providing them with clear, detailed and logical explanations.

Is interpreting medical information an aspect of advocacy? Although Maisie would have been given a pre-operative examination and information, she no doubt needed reassurance about her operation and her stay in hospital.

CORONARY CARE UNITS (CCUs)

Admission to a CCU is a stressful experience for both patients and relatives. Vetter *et al.* (1977, in Lowe, 1989) found that patients with myocardial infarction (heart attack) who expressed extreme emotional upset often suffered complications related to poor prognosis. Consistent with this finding, arrthymias and further ischaemia are related to catacholamine production and the increased coaguability of the blood (Carruthers, 1969, in Lowe, 1989). This demonstrates the importance of alleviating anxiety – not to do so may prove fatal (see Chapter 5).

North (1988) points out that in some cardiac surgery units patients may be invited to meet others who have recently undergone coronary bypass surgery and who are now recovering. This policy is supported by an American study by Kulik and Mahler (1989), who found that patients waiting for this surgery preferred to share a room with someone who had already had it, rather than another patient waiting for the same operation. The preference seemed to be motivated by the need for information about the stress-inducing situation (see above and Chapter 5).

CANCER WARDS/UNITS

Approximately 25 per cent of patients receiving anti-cancer chemotherapy experience anticipatory nausea and vomiting (ANV), which is also referred to as *psychogenic emesis* (nausea and vomiting caused by psychological factors). ANV is a conditioned response, acquired when anything that becomes associated with chemotherapy-induced emesis becomes capable of triggering it on its own (see Figure 3.3). This may include the mere sight of the hospital, the sign for the cancer ward/unit, an alcohol swab, a white coat – or even a nurse! The process involved is classical conditioning and involves three steps or stages (see Chapter 2, page 25).

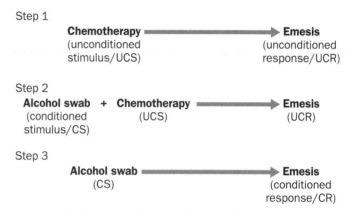

Figure 3.3 The steps involved in classically conditioned ANV

This explanation is supported by the finding that patients don't develop ANV unless they have first experienced post-treatment emesis (Weddington *et al.*, 1984, in Banks, 1991).

Sally told me that Maisie's distress and anxiety about her husband's inability to keep food down in the later stages of his illness (UCS) led to her needing to take antacids for her own 'indigestion pain' (UCR). Although the anxiety about her husband has now gone, she could be left with the association of food (CS) and pain (CR). Of course, there could be many other causes.

Many non-pharmacological approaches have been used to try to control the emesis associated with chemotherapy, with varying degrees of success. One of the most effective *behavioural* techniques is *systematic desensitisation* (SD). The patient is first taught progressive relaxation techniques and is then asked to list those stimuli that trigger emesis, from the least to the most likely. Beginning with the least likely, and while in a relaxed state, the patient is asked to concentrate on each stimulus in the list for 20 seconds, then to imagine the stimulus fading away and dissolving. The aim is for the patient to be able to confront the actual stimulus without experiencing ANV. This method has been particularly effective when used with children and adolescents receiving chemotherapy (Zeltzer *et al.*, 1984, in Banks, 1991).

INTENSIVE CARE UNITS (ICUs)

According to Calne (1994), some adult patients in ICU undergo a process of *dehumanisation*.

ASK YOURSELF ...
- What do you understand by the term dehumanisation?
- What is it about ICUs that you think brings about this condition?

> **Box 3.2 Dehumanisation and self-identity**
>
> • The term is sometimes used to refer to situations where an individual loses his/her human identity and becomes (or is perceived as) machine- or animal-like.
>
> • It can include the restriction or denial of attributes that contribute to an individual's self-identity and personality, leading to a loss of 'humanness'.
>
> • According to Goffman (1971), there are two fundamental ways of expressing self-identity: (a) 'narrow' communication (direct communication through talking or body language); and (b) 'broad' communication – a wide range of actions and activities, including how an individual gives an impression of self-identity through physical appearance or dress, which may signal social status or social role (see Chapter 16). We create impressions of our self-identity by using these tactics (see Chapter 8).

Typically, dehumanised patients have developed multiple organ failure and have been in ICU for a long time. They are always intubated and unable to communicate verbally, are mostly unresponsive and require complex technical monitoring. According to Calne (1994), the key factors that affect critically ill patients' freedom of self-expression are:

◎ reduced ability to communicate
◎ the distracting nature of the technical equipment
◎ altered physical appearance
◎ lack of personal belongings.

Critically ill patients often experience restricted self-identity because they're unable to communicate verbally or non-verbally. They are dependent on the nurse's ability to interpret the fragmentary clues (such as change in the sound of the ventilator or in displayed patterns on their chart), which reveal their real fears and desires (Ashworth, 1990, in Calne, 1994). Similarly, a sudden rise in heart rate, or a previously settled patient becoming agitated, would lead most nurses to infer that the patient is in pain, uncomfortable or frightened. At the same time, technical equipment can be a source of distraction, diverting attention away from the patient (Ashworth, 1980, in Calne, 1994).

Changes in a critically ill patient's physical appearance can occur as a result of drug therapies, surgical interventions and altered physiology. These changes may include surgical wounds, extensive oedema, jaundice, anaemia, exaggerated skin loss, bruising from clotting disorders, and loss of body mass. Their physical appearance may be so radically altered that even relatives don't immediately recognise the patient.

Calne (1994) cites several studies showing that ICU nurses may actually distance themselves, both psychologically and physically, from critically ill patients. They may protect themselves from emotional involvement with patients who are 'unlikely to survive'. Patients' physical appearance can be a source of stress for ICU staff and non-task–related/non-invasive interaction is often limited.

This is a situation where the patient would depend heavily on the nurse to be an advocate. It's also an example of difficult emotional labour, where health professionals must sort out their own feelings in order to help patients and relatives.

> **ASK YOURSELF ...**
> • Take each of Calne's four factors in turn and consider (a) how they might affect the patient's self-identity, and (b) how they are perceived by both nurses and relatives.

Sensory overload and sensory deprivation

According to Glide (1994), patients in ICUs experience both sensory overload and sensory deprivation. Noise levels are excessive and there's evidence that long-term exposure to high noise levels leads to increased tension and anxiety.

The most significant form of sensory deprivation patients experience appears to be lack of human touch. Although ICU patients are often exposed to physical touch, this is mostly associated with technical intervention (task-related/invasive interaction) rather than personal, comforting physical contact. Clearly, relatives can help to provide touch, but nurses can also help to reduce the sensory deprivation by allowing patients to wear glasses, hearing aids or dentures if at all possible. These also sustain the patient's dignity and ability to communicate.

Significantly, it was when Sally took Maisie's hand that she allowed her feelings to show. Her husband's death had changed her social circumstances too; no doubt she missed his caring presence.

ACCIDENT AND EMERGENCY (A&E)

According to Hole (1998), advances in technology and treatment have increased the chances of surviving once-fatal injuries. However, the full impact of the trauma and surgery comes after the physiological effects have passed. While surgery may produce a marked cosmetic benefit to the injury, the medical staff may focus more on the cosmetic, functional progress than the patient's emotional state.

Since the severely injured patient loses much more than their health, a psychological approach is vital for preventing 'detrimental attitude formation, extreme psychopathology and various other treatment-related problems' (Badenhorst, 1990, in Hole, 1998). The injured person experiences three traumatic events: (a) the injury itself; (b) the medical intervention to limit or rectify the anatomical and physiological effects; and (c) the road back to 'normality' (Hole, 1998). According to Kübler-Ross (1969), where a changed body image occurs, a bereavement takes place. The person grieves for the loss of the 'old' self and learns to live with the 'new'. This process may become stuck at one or other stage (see Chapters 16 and 20).

Relatives of the severely injured person need to be included in their care and treatment. They too are victims of the traumatic event (Brown, 1991, in Hole, 1998). Family members are crucial in the patient's reintegration into society, and they also need help to reintegrate.

However, it's not just relatives who need support. Nursing trauma patients can be harrowing. They are often young people with devastating and sometimes disfiguring injuries, whose lives have suddenly been thrown off course and who longer have any idea what their future holds. Faced with trauma patients and their traumatised relatives,

> 'nurses have the normal human reactions of shock, horror, pity, sometimes even revulsion. But they have to overcome these feelings if they are to nurse the patient effectively' (Fursland, 1998).

I'm glad I don't have to face these situations now – or I might give up! It makes me realise how much there is to learn about psychological, as well as physical, care before I can cope with all this.

Nurses might also feel guilty about being healthy and able-bodied in the face of the appalling injuries of their patients (a form of survivor guilt?). The grief reactions of seriously injured patients will include anger, which may be directed (displaced – see Chapter 6) at nurses. They may be left feeling rejected and unsure how to respond.

PSYCHOSOCIAL ASPECTS OF CHRONIC ILLNESS

Rather than being seen as a passive response to biomedical factors, chronic illnesses (such as HIV/AIDS, cancer, coronary heart disease/CHD and obesity) are better understood in terms of a complex interaction between physiological and psychological processes (Ogden, 2004). Health psychology has studied HIV, for example, in terms of attitudes towards HIV, changing these attitudes and examining predictors of behaviour (see Chapter 10).

HIV/AIDS

According to Hedge (1995):

> ... the uncertainty attached to the course of disease [HIV] and its poor prognosis frequently cause intense emotional reactions, even in those who are clinically well and asymptomatic. Good care addresses an individual's quality of life as well as its length: it aims to help people live with HIV infection rather than simply wait to die from it ...

As the number of people infected with HIV continues to rise, it's essential for all health carers to have some knowledge of the psychological and social implications of the disease.

Psychological and emotional impact of an HIV diagnosis

Although people with HIV infection and AIDS develop mental health problems common to other life-threatening illnesses, they may experience psychological disorders that are specifically related to:

◎ uncertainty surrounding disease progression and outcomes, the distressing nature of the symptoms themselves, and the knowledge that HIV is potentially fatal; related disorders include acute stress reactions (see Chapter 5), adjustment disorders, functional psychoses (such as depression and schizophreniform disorders – see Gross, 2005), and suicidal ideas and attempts

◎ the direct effects of the virus (Firn and Norman, 1995); these include a dementia-type illness characterised by progressive cognitive and/or motor impairment, which may be accompanied by behavioural disturbances.

Some of these reactions are related to the stigma associated with the disease, and anti-gay (and anti-drug user) prejudice and discrimination (see Chapter 11). This means that many people following a positive test result have to deal not only with the medical implications of the diagnosis but also with the potentially negative reactions of partners, friends, family and other social contacts. This is likely to exacerbate any existing mental health problems. Also, the continued spread of HIV and improved treatment prophylaxis, which ensures that people with HIV live longer, mean that the incidence of HIV-related mental health problems is likely to *increase* (Firn and Norman, 1995).

People with it are often perceived as having engaged in activities that may be proscribed by society and, by implication, as belonging to a stigmatised group (such as gay men and drug users). These beliefs are often expressed in the language of blame – and even nurses who've chosen to work in specialist wards caring for AIDS patients can

ASK YOURSELF ...
• In what ways might the concept of emotional intelligence (see above) be relevant to the quote from Fursland?

ASK YOURSELF ...
• In what ways do you think AIDS is potentially stigmatising?

have difficulties in viewing them completely non-judgementally (see Chapters 9 and 11).

Stigma adds a social dimension to this disease and highlights all aspects of the biopsychosocial approach to health and illness. However, even a seemingly simple wound dressing like Maisie's turned out to be a lesson in looking for all three components of the model.

PAIN

WHAT IS IT?

According to the International Association for the Study of Pain (IASP, 1986), pain is 'an unpleasant sensory and emotional experience associated with actual or potential tissue damage, or described in terms of such damage'. This definition indicates that pain is a subjective, personal experience involving both sensory (e.g. shooting, burning, aching) and emotional (e.g. frightening, annoying, sickening) qualities. Fear/anxiety can increase the perception of pain, and depression often accompanies chronic pain (Bradley, 1995).

While pain is a physiological *protective mechanism* for the body (Collins, 1994), this doesn't explain the pain *experience*, which includes both the pain sensation and certain autonomic responses and 'associated feeling states' (Zborowski, 1952). For example, understanding the physiology of pain cannot explain the acceptance of intense pain in torture or the strong emotional reactions of certain individuals to the slight sting of a hypodermic needle.

'Pure' pain is never detected as an isolated sensation. It's always accompanied by emotion and meaning, so that each pain is unique to the individual (O'Connell, 2000). Ultimately, the *subjective* nature of pain makes it difficult to find a satisfactory scientific definition. According to McCaffrey and Beebe (1994, in Howarth, 2002), pain is 'whatever the experiencing person says it is, existing whenever the experiencing person says it does'.

> **Box 3.3 Different types of pain**
>
> - **Acute pain** serves as a warning to tell people that something is wrong and to seek help. The problems causing the pain can usually be diagnosed and, if treated, will usually get rid of the pain. It is normally time-limited, so patients have an idea how long it's going to last, and it usually elicits sympathy in others.
> - **Chronic non-malignant pain (CNMP)** 'persists beyond the point at which healing would be expected to be complete or ... occurs in disease processes in which healing does not take place' (Clinical Standards Advisory Group, 2000, in Howarth, 2002). Unlike acute pain, it often serves no purpose. A diagnosis cannot always be given, which can be difficult for the patient to accept. The approach is to *manage* it, not to cure or remove it. Back pain constitutes a significant proportion of CNMP, but can be caused by whiplash injuries, arthritis, diabetic neuropathy and trigeminal neuralgia. It can also be secondary to other chronic conditions, such as multiple sclerosis and stroke.

- **Psychological pain** is a multifaceted experience that includes feelings of hopelessness, guilt, unresolved anger and fear of the unknown. It is often expressed in body language and physical symptoms (see Chapter 20).

- **Spiritual pain** – 'The realisation that life is likely to end soon may well give rise to feelings of the unfairness of what is happening, and at much of what has gone before, and above all a desolate feeling of meaninglessness' (Saunders, 1988, in Morrison, 1992). Spiritual pain is often now considered in relation to the care of the bereaved, but is just as relevant to terminally ill patients (again, see Chapter 20).

(Based on Howarth, 2002; Morrison, 1992; Sheahan, 1996)

Sally said that Maisie likened her pain to indigestion (a biological explanation), but O'Connell (2000) suggests there could be emotional elements as well – anxiety in case she had cancer, or the effects of her husband's illness and death.

PAIN AND INJURY

Pain without injury

The IASP definition above recognises that an individual *needn't* suffer actual tissue damage at a specific body site in order to perceive pain at that site, as in the 'phantom limb' phenomenon (see Gross, 2005). In describing treatment of phantom limb pain, Ramachandran and Blakeslee (1998) maintain that, 'pain is an *opinion* on the organism's state of health rather than a mere reflexive response to an injury. There is no direct hotline from pain receptors to "pain centres" in the brain'.

Two-thirds of amputees suffer pain in their phantom limb. Paraplegics sometimes complain that their legs make continuous cycling movements, which produces painful fatigue – despite the fact that their actual legs are lying immobile on the bed (Curtiss, 1999).

Phantom limb pain is one of several examples of how it's possible to experience pain in the absence of any physical damage/injury. Others include *neuralgia* (nerve pain) and *caucalgia* (a burning pain that often follows a severe wound, such as stabbing), both of which develop *after* the wound/injury has healed. Tension headaches/migraines are surprisingly difficult to explain: the widely held account in terms of dilation of blood vessels has been discredited in the light of research showing that dilation is more likely to be the *result* than the cause (Melzack and Wall, 1988).

According to Munro (2000), 4.7 per cent of the UK population suffer from fibromyalgia/chronic widespread pain (CWP) (or chronic musculoskeletal pain of no identifiable origin). This often 'overlaps' with other syndromes, such as irritable bowel, temperomandibular disorder and tension headache, and is definitely associated with psychiatric disturbance and hypochondriacal anxieties about health (Bass, in Munro, 2000). As yet, there's no convincing medical explanation.

Maisie's pain has now become as interesting a nursing problem as her wound, and perhaps more complicated.

Injury without pain

People with *congenital analgesia* are incapable of feeling pain (a potentially life-threatening disorder), while those with *episodic analgesia* experience pain only minutes or even hours after the injury has occurred. This can sometimes be *life-saving*, as when soldiers suffer horrific injuries but suffer little/no pain while waiting for medical attention (e.g. Beecher, 1956). Similarly, Melzack *et al.* (1982, in Curtiss, 1999) found that of 138 accident patients in A&E departments, 37 per cent reported not feeling any pain at the time of the injury (embarrassment seemed to be the most relevant emotion!). Most reported pain within an hour of the injury – but in some cases this was delayed by up to nine hours.

FACTORS INFLUENCING THE EXPERIENCE AND PERCEPTION OF PAIN

Pain as a cultural phenomenon

Zborowski (1952) describes the culturally determined attitudes towards different types of pain:

◎ *pain expectancy* refers to the anticipation of pain as being unavoidable in a given situation (such as childbirth, sport or battle)

◎ *pain acceptance* is the willingness to experience pain, which is manifested mostly as the inevitable component of culturally accepted experiences (such as initiation rites and medical treatment).

So, labour pain is expected as part of childbirth, but in most western cultures it's not accepted (and various steps are taken to keep it to a minimum), while in others (such as Poland) it's both expected and accepted (and little or nothing is done to relieve it).

A patient's cultural background is one of the factors influencing the inferences a nurse makes about his/her physical pain and psychological distress (Davitz *et al.*, 1977). But, equally, nurses' own cultural background can affect the kind of judgements they make about patients' suffering. For example, if nurses from Anglo-Saxon or Germanic backgrounds (the majority of the American sample in Davitz *et al.*'s study) tend to minimise physical pain and psychological distress, how do these beliefs affect relationships with patients from another culture? They conclude by saying that recognising cultural differences regarding beliefs about suffering can prevent a great deal of misunderstanding and misperceptions, and lead to more effective, sensitive patient care.

My own experience of childbirth didn't include having the epidural, which was offered several times. At the time I didn't analyse why, but think now it was cultural: my Asian grandmother's influence is still powerful within the family perhaps?

Cognitive aspects of pain

Expectancy and acceptance are as much cognitive as emotional dimensions of pain. Trusting the doctor's ability to ease your suffering (whether this takes the form of a cure or merely the relief of pain and suffering) represents part of the *cognitive appraisal* aspect of pain – that is, the belief that the illness/symptoms are controllable. If we *attribute* our symptoms to something that's controllable, this should make us feel more optimistic (see Chapter 5). The *meaning* of our illness may be a crucial factor in how we react to it, including any associated pain (see Chapter 4).

If patients are allowed to perform necessary painful procedures on themselves (such as debridement of dead skin in severe burn cases), they tend to find the pain is *reduced* compared with the same procedure performed by a nurse (Melzack and Wall, 1991). This suggests the role of *control* in influencing the patient's level of anxiety, which, in turn, affects subjective pain (see below and Chapter 5).

I see now both control and meaning influenced my decision. I anticipated and prepared for the pain of childbirth and was confident I could manage it. I also saw the pain as purposeful, whereas Maisie probably sees her pain as having a sinister outcome. I didn't recognise it as a 'cognitive perspective' at the time!

Individual differences

People's pain thresholds (the lowest stimulus value reported as painful) clearly differ (although the reasons are much less clear – Starr, 1995). Post-operative pain is influenced by anxiety, neuroticism and extroversion (Taenzer *et al.*, 1986, in Starr, 1995; see also Chapter 6).

TREATING PAIN

Several methods and techniques used in the treatment of stress are also used for treating (mainly chronic) pain (see Chapter 5). Bradley (1995) groups these behavioural treatments into three major kinds.

1. **Contingency management:** this is a form of *behaviour modification* (see Chapter 2 and Gross, 2005).
2. **Self-management/cognitive behaviour treatment:** this refers to multiple treatments, such as learning coping skills, progressive muscle relaxation training, practice in communicating effectively with family and health care providers, and providing positive reinforcement for displaying coping behaviour. Patients are encouraged to take responsibility for managing their pain and to attribute their success to their own efforts.
3. **Biofeedback:** this involves giving patients information (via monitors or buzzers) about certain autonomic functions (such as blood pressure, heart rate and muscle tension), enabling them to bring these functions under voluntary control.

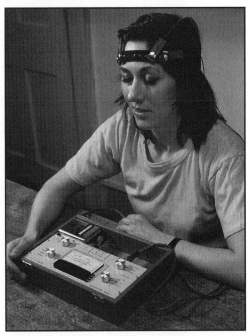

Biofeedback

KEY STUDY 3.2 Giving birth the EMG way (Duchene, 1990)

- Duchene used electromyograph (EMG) biofeedback to reduce the *acute* pain associated with childbirth among 40 first-time mothers. This measures muscle tension.

- They were randomly assigned to the experimental or control group, the former attending six weekly training sessions and loaned biofeedback machines for practice at home. The feedback was provided through both sound and a visual monitor, based on the tension of the abdominal muscles, which the women focused on relaxing when they felt a pain or contraction.

- All the women were monitored for pain perception, starting at admission, and then at various points during labour, again at delivery and once more 24 hours after delivery (to recall the overall pain intensity).

- While 14 of the 20 control group women requested and had epidurals for pain relief, only eight of the experimental group did so (a significant difference). The experimental group's labours were also significantly shorter.

This helps explain my experience. I attended relaxation classes regularly, although not with biofeedback, and became good at relaxing at will.

CRITICAL DISCUSSION 3.1 Do children feel pain?

- According to Hodges (1998), one widely held myth maintains that children don't feel pain with the same intensity as adults; another that narcotic analgesia shouldn't be administered to young children because they'll become addicted. As a consequence, many young patients are left to suffer needlessly.

- The fear of addiction is also relevant to pain management in adults. But less than 1 per cent of all patients become addicted to opiates and children are no more at risk than adults. Also, 'addiction' is not the same as 'dependence' (see Chapter 7).

- Nurses play a central role in assessing when and how much analgesia is required. Hodges cites a number of studies which show that nurses often wrongly perceive and underestimate a child's pain compared with the child's own rating.

- McCaffery and Beebe (1989, in Hodges, 1998) argue that children aren't more tolerant of pain, they just use distraction techniques more effectively than adults. A Royal College of Surgeons report (1990, in Hodges, 1998) also concluded that children's pain, although different, 'is no less severe than adults'.

- Poor pain control can also result from the difficulties of assessing pain in children. Their ability to understand and describe their pain depends on several factors, including their age, cognitive and linguistic ability (see Chapter 15), neurological development, experience, personality, and family and cultural beliefs (Ramsay, 1995, in Hodges, 1998).

- Another barrier to adequate pain relief is the reluctance of medical and nursing staff to use painful intramuscular injections to deliver analgesics. A major alternative is *patient-controlled analgesia* (PCA), which is suitable for children over the age of four or five (Hodges, 1998).

The idea that children don't feel as much pain as adults seems irrational, and the idea that nurses underestimate pain is worrying. Ramsay's (1995, in Hodges, 1998) observation about children's difficulty in communicating seems to explain some of the problem.

Multidisciplinary pain management clinics

These are found in most large teaching hospitals and district general hospitals. The clinics comprise a variety of health care professionals (doctors, nurses, clinical psychologists/psychiatrists, physiotherapists, pharmacists and occupational therapists), who will assess the patient and offer expert help in pain management.

Treatment is wide-ranging and may include improving physical and lifestyle functioning by, for example, improving muscle tone, self-esteem and self-efficacy (the belief that we can act effectively and control events that influence our life (Bandura, 1977, 1986) – see Chapter 5), or reducing boredom and inappropriate pain behaviours (such as being 'rewarded' for 'being in pain'). These are all designed to reduce reliance on drugs.

The treatment of pain seems to encompass most of the psychological approaches described in Chapter 2: biological, cognitive, humanistic and behaviourist.

The experience of my visit to Maisie has shown me the importance of the 'psychological aspect' of care. I need to be more sensitive to the emotional needs of patients and to develop some of Sally's skill in responding to them.

CHAPTER SUMMARY

◎ Underlying **health psychology** is the **biopsychosocial model**, which is the major alternative to the **biomedical model**. Only the former is compatible with the influence of non-biological factors on major causes of death and can aid the prevention of chronic diseases.

◎ Poor **psychological care** can have detrimental effects on patients' physical health. Common psychological responses to illness and injury (including shock, distress and loss of self-worth) can undermine medical treatment and interfere with rehabilitation.

◎ A major aspect of psychological care is providing **psychological safety**. This can be achieved through **therapeutic conversations** that comprise **focus on the here-and-now**, **emphasis on feelings**, **empathic understanding** and a **non-prescriptive approach**, and **focus on the patient**.

◎ Care and caring can also be defined in terms of **encouraging autonomy, giving of oneself, taking risks, supporting care** and **emotional labour**. The last of these is similar to the concept of **emotional (intrapersonal) intelligence**.

◎ **Pre-surgical anxiety**, which can harm the immune system causing increased risk of wound infections, can be reduced through **information giving**, provided this is tailored to the individual patient's needs. Nurses often help patients interpret information given to them by doctors.

◎ **Systematic desensitisation/SD** is one of the most effective non-pharmacological techniques used to control **anticipatory nausea and vomiting (ANV)/psychogenic emesis**.

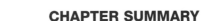

◎ Some adult patients in intensive care units/ICUs undergo a process of **dehumanisation**. They also experience both **sensory overload** and **deprivation**.

◎ Nursing trauma patients can be harrowing, especially when young victims are involved, and nurses may feel guilty about being healthy and able-bodied.

◎ The mental health problems of people with HIV/AIDS are both common to those with other life-threatening conditions and related to the stigmatising nature of the disease.

◎ **Pain** is a subjective experience involving both sensory and emotional qualities. This makes it difficult to define objectively. It can take many forms, including **acute**, **chronic non-malignant/CNMP**, **psychological** and **spiritual**.

◎ Pain can occur in the absence of actual tissue damage, as demonstrated in phantom limb pain, **neuralgia** and **caucalgia**, but injury can also occur without pain, as in **congenital** and **episodic analgesia**, and many trauma patients.

◎ Pain can also be thought of as a **cultural phenomenon**, with **cognitive** dimensions (such as **pain expectancy** and **acceptance**, **cognitive appraisal** and pain **attribution**).

◎ **Treatment** of pain can be conducted through **contingency management**, **self-management/cognitive behaviour treatment**, **biofeedback** and **multi-disciplinary pain clinics**.

SOCIAL COGNITION AND HEALTH BEHAVIOUR

4

INTRODUCTION AND OVERVIEW

According to the biomedical model, *disease* is a deviation from a measurable biological norm. This view, which still dominates medical thinking and practice, is based on several invalid assumptions. Most importantly, the *specificity assumption* maintains that understanding of an illness is greater if it can be defined at a more specific biochemical level. According to Maes and van Elderen (1998), traditional medicine is more focused on disease than on health: 'It would be more appropriate to call our health care systems "disease care systems", as the primary aim is to treat or cure people with various diseases rather than to promote health or prevent disease …'

By contrast with the biomedical model's *reactive* attitude towards *illness*, the biopsychosocial model underlying health psychology adopts a more *proactive* attitude towards *health*. Many definitions of health have been proposed since the 1940s, mostly in terms of the *absence* of disease, dysfunction, pain, suffering and discomfort. Also, in opposition to the biomedical model's reductionist view, the biopsychosocial model adopts a *holistic* approach – that is, the *person as a whole* needs to be taken into account. It maintains that both '*micro-level*' (small-scale causes, such as chemical imbalances) and '*macro-level*' (large-scale causes, such as the extent of available social support) processes interact to determine someone's health status.

Health beliefs are important determinants of health behaviour. Understanding why people do or don't practise behaviours to protect their health can be assisted by the study of *models/theories of health behaviour*, such as:

◎ the Health Belief Model (HBM)
◎ the Theory of Reasoned Action (TRA)
◎ the Theory of Planned Behaviour (TPB)
◎ Protection Motivation Theory (PMT), and
◎ the Health Action Process Approach (HAPA).

According to Ogden (2004), these various models/theories are often referred to, collectively, as *social cognition models*, because they regard cognitions as being shared by individuals within the same society (see Chapter 2). But Ogden prefers to distinguish between:

◎ social cognition models (such as TRA and TPB), which aim to account for social behaviour in general and are much broader than health models, and
◎ cognition models (such as HBM, PMT and HAPA), which are specifically *health models*.

From my diary (2): *Year 1/Community/District Nurse*

My second visit with Sally, my mentor, was to Diana who is 42, grossly obese, has hypertension and a pressure sore that needs dressing. She lives alone following her divorce some years ago and is a smoker; she's had several attacks of bronchitis. My first reaction when I saw her was shock; she was so overweight I don't know how she managed to walk, although Sally had said she could. As she's over 25 stone, she has a special bariatric wheelchair, reclining chair and toilet, and has also had a special shower room installed.

Sally went through Diana's medical history for my benefit: medications, diet, etc. She showed me how to take Diana's blood pressure (BP). I managed it at my second attempt, and then Sally attended to her dressing. I tried to chat in a friendly way to Diana and asked how her diet was going. She became very despondent and told us that yesterday a friend had brought her some chocolate biscuits and Diana had eaten the lot. She said she knew she was hopeless, but couldn't resist them. Although I felt disapproving, I was sorry for her then, but later when we were discussing Diana's chesty cough I was off again – thinking, well, it's all her own fault for smoking.

ASK YOURSELF ...

• What do you understand by the terms 'health' and 'illness'?

• Are you healthy if you're not ill, or is health a more positive state than this?

DEFINING HEALTH AND ILLNESS

HEALTH BELIEFS

According to Holland and Hogg (2001), the concept of health is broad and complex, with a wide range of meanings. Health beliefs (HBs) are ideas or conceptualisations about health and illness derived from the prevailing worldview and, like the culture which determines that worldview, they may change over time. For example, despite the link with skin cancer, sunbathing/suntans are still associated with health and well-being (Holland and Hogg, 2001). Like health behaviour, HBs may be *health-damaging* as well as *health-promoting* (sunbathing again).

Box 4.1 Defining health and illness

- According to the World Health Organization (WHO, 1947), *health* is 'a complete state of physical, mental, and social well-being and not merely the absence of disease or infirmity'.

- *Disease* (which reflects the medical approach) is a 'state of the body characterised by deviations from the norm or measurable biological or somatic variables' (Maes and van Elderen, 1998).

- *Illness* is 'the state of being ill, implying that illness is a more psychological concept, which is closely related to one's own perception of a health problem (e.g. pain)' (Maes and van Elderen, 1998). Subjective psychological symptoms, such as anxiety, also play a substantial role in the construction of illness. Similarly, although illness is usually associated with evidence of medical abnormality, 'it also incorporates aspects of the individual's wider functioning, self-perceptions and behaviours, and requires consideration of social context and societal norms' (Turpin and Slade, 1998).

- The concepts of health and illness incorporate physical, psychological and social aspects, reflecting the biopsychosocial model.

Diana's weight and BP deviate from the norm, but she doesn't seem to consider herself ill. However, I certainly don't consider her healthy. Her hypertension and intermittent bronchitis are probably the result of her health-damaging behaviour.

According to Ogden (2004), for most people in the West being healthy is the norm and beliefs about being ill exist in the context of beliefs about being healthy (for example, illness means not being healthy or feeling different from normal). Healthiness is most people's normal state and represents the backdrop to their beliefs about being ill. Most people define health *positively* (not just as the absence of illness).

Lau (1995) found that young, healthy adults described 'being healthy' in terms of several dimensions:

◎ *physiological/physical* (for example, good condition/has energy)
◎ *psychological* (happy, energetic, feeling good)
◎ *behavioural* (eating and sleeping properly)
◎ *future consequences* (live longer)
◎ *the absence of* (not sick, no disease, no symptoms).

Diana doesn't meet any of these criteria, which is sad because she could be healthy if she changed her lifestyle. However, this would mean changing her health beliefs and behaviour.

HEALTH BELIEFS IN NURSING PRACTICE

According to Holland and Hogg (2001), conflicting HBs can leave both nurses and patients feeling frustrated and failing to understand each other. Ultimately, this may cause the patient to abandon or ignore health care services (see Chapter 13). They quote Spector (1996), who maintains that:

> We have to find a way of caring for the client that matches the client's perception of the health problem and its treatment ... for the health care provider, the needs most difficult to meet are those of people whose belief systems are most different from the 'mainstream' health care provider culture.

Nurses enter the profession with ideas about health and illness that are unique and that have been shaped by their ethnic and cultural background. They then bring those beliefs to the health arena, hospital wards, community and therapeutic settings, influencing nursing practice in the prevention and treatment of illness. These beliefs may change as nurses integrate with their professional colleagues and absorb the beliefs, values and attitudes of the nursing culture. This is reflected in nursing language, such as 'doing the obs', 'off duty', 'doing the cares', 'doing the backs' and 'handover'. As with all cultures, the nursing culture may become 'hidden', because nursing practices become the norm ('second nature'). Unless nurses are aware of this, a gap may develop between the nurse/other health care providers and the recipient (Holland and Hogg, 2001).

Health beliefs also change over time within the same culture. Most of the expressions above reflect a traditional approach to care, based on the biomedical model. My beliefs are already being changed by knowledge of the biopsychosocial model in nursing. However, reviewing our visit (at length), I confessed to Sally that I found it difficult to feel sympathetic towards Diana as I felt her condition was partly self-inflicted. She agreed that Diana's behaviour was frustrating sometimes, but said that we must care for her as she is, not as we want her to be or think she ought to be.

> **Box 4.2 Three categories/systems of health beliefs (Holland and Hogg, 2001)**
>
> 1. **HBs based on biomedicine:** This, of course, corresponds to the biomedical model, which was developed in and dominates the health systems of North America and western Europe. It has been exported all over the world. Diseases are caused by *pathogens* (bacteria/viruses) entering the body, or by biochemical changes in the body due to conditions or events (such as wear and tear, accidents, nutritional deficiencies, the ageing process, injury, stress, smoking and alcohol). The body is a complex machine, whose various parts function together to ensure health. Health practitioners are highly educated, powerful and respected specialists, whose position and power are upheld by the law. In general, they concentrate on treating just the diseased/injured body part, with mind and body being seen as two separate entities (see Chapter 3): 'Biomedicine may be regarded as an attacking force, and militaristic terminology such as "battling cancer", "fighting disease", or "winning the war against germs" is commonly used …'.
>
> 2. **HBs based on personality (or magico-religious) systems:** Illness is caused by: (a) the active intervention of a sensate agent, possibly a supernatural force (such as God or some other deity); (b) non-humans (such as ghosts, ancestors or evil spirits); or (c) human beings, witches or sorcerers. These are all forces beyond the individual's control, but illness may be punishment for some misdeed. The 'evil eye' as a cause of illness or distress is accepted in Europe, the Middle East, North Africa, Central and South America. An Indian Muslim woman who, according to a biomedical perspective, might have been diagnosed with post-natal depression and treated with antidepressants, believed that her low mood, insomnia and leg pains were caused by the 'Jinns' (malevolent spirits that cause ill health). The Imam at her local mosque performed the appropriate ceremony and she returned to 'normal' health.
>
> 3. **HBs in naturalistic systems:** Naturalism (or *holism*) dates back to the ancient civilisations of Greece, India and China. They explain illness in personal and systemic terms. Health is the balance between elements (such as heat and cold) in the body. Human life is only one aspect of nature and is part of the natural cosmos. Any disturbance or imbalance causes illness, disease or misfortune. These beliefs form the basis of traditional health practices in many Asian countries (including China, Japan, Singapore, Taiwan and Korea), as well as South America, the Philippines, Iran and Pakistan.

CULTURE AND HEALTH

As Box 4.2 shows, health beliefs differ between cultures. Culture represents one of the 'macro-level' processes referred to above. *Cross-cultural health psychology* (Berry, 1994) involves two related domains:

1. the earlier, more established study of how cultural factors influence various aspects of health
2. the more recent and very active study of the health of individuals and groups as they settle into and adapt to new cultural circumstances, through migration, and of their persistence over generations as ethnic groups.

Box 4.3 Health, disease and illness as cultural concepts

- Many studies have shown that the very concepts of health and disease are defined differently across cultures. While 'disease' may be rooted in pathological biological processes (common to all), 'illness' is now widely recognised as a culturally influenced subjective experience of suffering and discomfort (Berry, 1998; see Box 4.1).

- Recognising certain conditions as either healthy or as a disease is also linked to culture. For example, trance is seen as an important curing (health-seeking) mechanism in some cultures, but may be classified as a sign of psychiatric disorder in others. Similarly, how a condition is expressed is also linked to cultural norms, as in the tendency to express psychological problems *somatically* (in the form of bodily symptoms) in some cultures (e.g. Chinese) more than in others (see Gross, 2005).

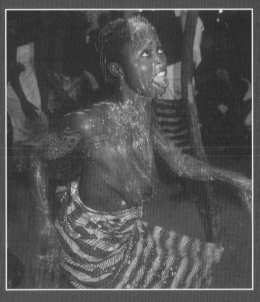

A Minah medium of the violent God Jagli, who induces trances and wild dances

- Disease and disability are highly variable. Cultural factors (such as diet, substance abuse and social relationships within the family) contribute to the prevalence of diseases including heart disease, cancer and schizophrenia (Berry, 1998).

At this time, in western culture, obesity is well defined. Diana has a body mass index of >30, which categorises her as high-risk obese; we know this contributes to her diseases.

Acculturation

Cross-cultural psychologists believe that there's a complex pattern of continuity and change in how people who've developed in one cultural context behave when they move to and live in a new cultural context. This process of adaptation to the new ('host') culture is called *acculturation*. With increasing acculturation (the longer immigrants live in the host country), health status 'migrates' to the national norm (Berry, 1998).

For example, coronary heart disease among Polish immigrants to Canada increased (their rates were initially lower), while for immigrants from Australia and New Zealand the reverse was true. Immigrants from 26 out of 29 countries shifted their rates towards those of the Canadian-born population. Similar patterns have been found for stomach and intestinal cancer among immigrants to the USA (Berry, 1998).

One possibility is exposure to widely shared risk factors in the physical environment (e.g. climate, pollution, pathogens), over which there is little choice. Alternatively, it could be due to choosing to pursue assimilation (or possible integration) as the way to acculturate. This may expose immigrants to *cultural* risk factors, such as diet, lifestyle and substance abuse. This 'behavioural shift' interpretation would be supported if health status both improved *and* declined relative to national norms. However, the main evidence points to a *decline*, supporting the 'acculturative stress' (or even 'psychopathology') interpretation – that is, the very process of acculturation may involve risk factors that can reduce health status. This explanation is supported by evidence that stress can lower resistance to disease, such as hypertension and diabetes (Berry, 1998; see also Chapter 5).

Diana says she smokes 'to calm her nerves', which indicates she's stressed. But smoking also exacerbates her hypertension and bronchitis.

ILLNESS COGNITIONS

In the same study described above, Lau (1995) asked participants 'What does it mean to be sick?' Responses revealed several dimensions:
◎ *not feeling normal* ('I don't feel right')
◎ *consequences of illness* ('I can't do what I normally do')
◎ *timeline* (how long the symptoms last), and
◎ *absence of health* (not being healthy).

These dimensions have been described within the context of *illness cognitions* (illness beliefs or representations), a patient's own implicit common-sense beliefs about their illness (Leventhal *et al.*, 1980, 1997). These provide patients with a framework for coping with and understanding their illness, telling them what to look out for if they're becoming ill. Based on interviews with adults who were chronically ill, recently diagnosed with cancer or healthy, Leventhal *et al.* identified five cognitive dimensions of these beliefs (overlapping with those found by Lau: see above).

1. **Identity:** the label given to the illness (medical diagnosis) and the symptoms experienced.
2. **Perceived cause:** may be biological (virus/lesion) or psychosocial (stress/health-related behaviour).
3. **Timeline:** beliefs about how long the illness will last (acute/short term or chronic/long term).
4. **Consequences:** may be physical (pain/lack of mobility), emotional (loss of social contact/loneliness), or some combination of these.
5. **Curability and controllability:** can it be treated/cured? How controllable is it – either by themselves or powerful others (e.g. doctors)?

Diana has developed identifiable 'diseases': hypertension and chronic bronchitis. I'm not sure how she perceives their cause; does she realise that over-eating and smoking is a factor in both? Sally said Diana watched a great deal of TV; she doesn't go out as, apart

ASK YOURSELF ...
● How could you explain such findings?
● What is it about living in a different cultural situation that can increase or decrease your chances of developing life-threatening diseases?

from her reduced mobility, she doesn't like people staring at her. I got the impression she accepts her obesity as being irreversible and something she 'can't help'.

Health locus of control (HLoC) refers to an individual's belief as to whether their health:
◎ is controllable by them (e.g. 'I'm directly responsible for my health')
◎ is in the hands of fate (e.g. 'Whether I'm well or not is a matter of luck')
◎ is under the control of powerful others (e.g. 'I can only do what my doctor tells me to do').

The first example describes someone with an *internal* HLoC, while the second and third describe an *external* HLoC (see Chapter 5).

Diana does see herself as a victim: it wasn't her fault she started comfort eating and smoking! She felt guilty at 'breaking her diet' and 'disobeying' her doctor's and dietician's advice. She's clearly an external HLoC person.

Coping with illness

According to Leventhal *et al.*'s (1997) *self-regulatory model of illness cognitions*, people go through the following three stages of 'problem-solving' when faced with their own illness.

1. **Interpretation** involves making sense of the illness, giving meaning to symptoms or a doctor's diagnosis by accessing their illness cognitions. This is likely to be accompanied by changes in emotional state (such as anxiety), and any coping strategies have to relate to both illness cognitions and the emotional state.

2. **Coping** involves dealing with the illness in order to regain a state of equilibrium. This can take the form of either (a) approach coping (such as taking pills, going to the doctor, resting, talking to friends about the anxiety), or (b) avoidance coping (such as denial or wishful thinking – see Chapter 5).

3. **Appraisal** involves evaluating the effectiveness of the coping strategies and deciding whether to continue with this strategy or opt for an alternative.

Most of Diana's coping strategies are avoidance ones; the only positive thing she attempts is a reducing diet, and that isn't consistent or successful.

Coping with a diagnosis

According to Shontz (1975, in Ogden, 2004), based on observations of hospital patients, people go through a series of stages following diagnosis of a chronic illness (see Box 4.4).

> **Box 4.4 Stages of coping with a diagnosis (Shontz, 1975, in Ogden, 2004)**
>
> • **Shock:** stunned, bewildered, behaving in an automatic way, with feelings of detachment.
>
> • **Encounter reaction:** disorganised thinking, and feelings of loss, grief, helplessness and despair.
>
> • **Retreat:** denial of the problem and its implications, retreat into the self. This is only a temporary stage, as denial cannot last for ever. It represents a launchpad for a gradual reorientation towards reality.

Shontz's model focuses on the *immediate* changes following a diagnosis, suggesting that the desired outcome of any coping process is to face up to reality and that reality orientation is an adaptive coping mechanism (Ogden, 2004).

At the same time, we shouldn't underestimate the impact that diagnosis can have, both in the short and long term – especially when a life-threatening disease is involved. Indeed, according to Moos and Schaefer's (1984) *crisis theory*, physical illness can be considered a crisis, a turning point in the individual's life, which produces certain inevitable changes.

ASK YOURSELF ...
• What do you think some of these changes might be?

◎ Change in identity: e.g. 'breadwinner ' to 'person with illness'/'patient'.
◎ Change in location: e.g. becoming bedridden or hospitalised.
◎ Change in role: e.g. from independent adult to passive dependant.
◎ Change in social support: e.g. isolation from friends and family.
◎ Changes to 'the future': e.g. a future involving children, career or travel can become uncertain.

Diana's obesity, hypertension and bronchitis developed gradually following her divorce; she worked in a school canteen until she became too unfit for work. Now she's housebound, dependent, comparatively isolated and has no plans for the future.

Crisis theory is meant to account for the impact of *any* form of disruption to an individual's established personal and social identity. A good example of such disruption is bereavement, and the changes described above are consistent with the concept of the *assumptive world:* 'everything that we assume to be true on the basis of our previous experience … the internal model of the world that we are constantly matching against incoming sensory data in order to orient ourselves, recognise what is happening, and plan our behaviour accordingly' (Parkes, 1993).

Like the loss of a loved one through death (see Chapter 20), being diagnosed with a serious illness represents a *psychosocial transition* that threatens the patient's assumptive world. However, according to crisis theory, psychological systems are driven to the maintenance of homeostasis or equilibrium (in the same way as physical systems). Any crisis is self-limiting, as the individual will find a way of returning to a stable state: people are self-regulators.

While this may be true in general terms, there are often factors specific to illness, such as unpredictability, lack of clear information/ambiguity (especially about cause, seriousness and prognosis), the need for quick decisions (e.g. regarding treatment options and what to tell people) and limited prior experience ('I've never had cancer before, what should I do next?') (Ogden, 2004).

For Diana, her divorce triggered a psychosocial transition; could overeating and smoking have been her way of attempting to recover her psychological equilibrium?

ILLNESS AND HEALTH PSYCHOLOGY

According to the biopsychosocial model:
◎ individuals aren't just passive victims, but are responsible for taking their medication, changing their beliefs and behaviour
◎ health and illness exist on a continuum – people aren't *either* healthy *or* ill, but progress along the continuum, in both directions
◎ psychological factors contribute to the *aetiology* (causation) of illness – they're not just consequences of illness.

ASK YOURSELF ...

• Can you think of examples of where your being ill was (partly) caused by psychological factors *and* where your illness affected you psychologically?

All these apply to Diana – she seems to perceive herself as a victim. However, given the motivation, she could reverse the 'direction' of her condition by changing her behaviour.

According to Ogden (2000, 2004), health psychology aims to:

◎ *evaluate* the role of behaviour in the aetiology of illness, such as the link between smoking, CHD, cholesterol level, lack of exercise, high blood pressure and stress (see Chapter 5)

◎ *predict* unhealthy behaviours – for example, smoking, alcohol consumption and high-fat diets are related to beliefs, and beliefs about health and illness can be used to predict behaviour (see above, below, and Chapter 7)

◎ *understand* the role of psychological factors in the experience of illness – for example, understanding the psychological consequences of illness could help to alleviate pain, nausea, vomiting, anxiety and depression (see Chapter 3)

◎ *evaluate* the role of psychological factors in the treatment of illness (see Chapter 3).

These aims are put into practice by:

◎ *promoting* health behaviour, such as changing beliefs and behaviour (see Chapter 10)

◎ *preventing* illness – for example, by training health professionals to improve communication skills and to carry out interventions that may help prevent illness (see Chapter 13).

All these factors relate to Diana but, as Sally said, although we understand the reasons she behaves as she does, the problem is how to help her change her beliefs and behaviour. Diana has had the help of a physiotherapist, dietician, occupational therapist and social services, all to no avail.

MODELS OF HEALTH BEHAVIOUR

As we saw in the Introduction and Overview, Ogden (2004) distinguishes between cognition models, which are specifically *health* models, and social cognition models, which are general accounts of cognitions shared by individuals within a particular society.

A fundamentally important question for health psychology is why people adopt – or don't adopt – particular health-related behaviours. Models of health behaviour try to answer this question, and most of those discussed below belong to the family of *expectancy-value models* (Stroebe, 2000). These assume that decisions between different courses of action are based on two types of cognition:

1. *subjective probabilities* that a given action will produce a set of expected outcomes
2. *evaluation* of action outcomes.

Individuals will choose from among various alternative courses of action the one most likely to produce positive consequences and avoid negative ones. Different models differ in terms of the *types* of beliefs and attitudes that should be used in predicting a particular class of behaviour. They are rational reasoning models, which assume that individuals consciously deliberate about the likely consequences of behavioural alternatives available to them before engaging in action.

THEORY OF REASONED ACTION (TRA)

ASK YOURSELF ...

• Do you agree with this view of people as rationally/consciously choosing health behaviours?

• How would you explain your own behaviours in relation to diet, smoking, alcohol, exercise, and so on?

This has been used extensively to examine predictions of behaviour and was central to the debate within social psychology regarding the relationship between attitudes and behaviour (see Chapter 10). TRA assumes that behaviour is a function of the *intention* to perform that behaviour (Ajzen and Fishbein, 1970; Fishbein, 1967; Fishbein and Ajzen, 1975). A behavioural intention is determined by:

◎ a person's *attitude* to the behaviour, which is determined by (a) beliefs about the outcome of the behaviour, and (b) evaluation of the expected outcome

◎ *subjective norms* – a person's beliefs about the desirability of carrying out a certain health behaviour in the social group, society and culture s/he belongs to.

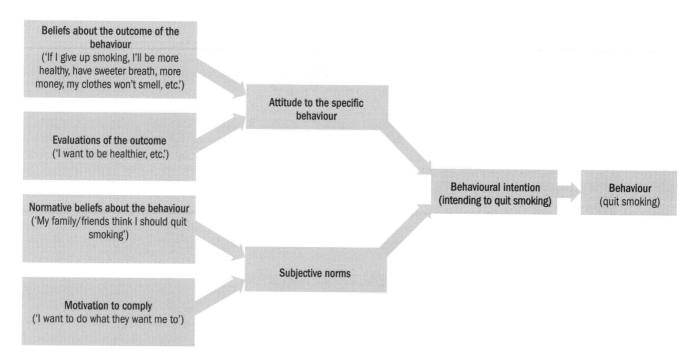

Figure 4.1 Main components of the theory of reasoned action (adapted from Penny, 1996; Maes & van Elderen, 1998)

Diana knew she should stick to her diet and believed it would make her healthier. She was depressed that she'd 'failed again', as she put it. So why couldn't she succeed?

Evaluation of TRA

TRA has successfully predicted a wide range of behaviours, including blood donation, smoking marijuana, dental hygiene and family planning. However, attitudes and behaviour are only *weakly* related: people don't always do what they say they intend to (see Chapter 10). The model doesn't consider people's past behaviour, despite evidence that this is a good predictor of future behaviour. Nor does it account for people's irrational decisions (Penny, 1996). Similarly, Maes and Elderen (1998) argue that, 'The assumption that behaviour is a function of intentions … limits the applicability … of the model to volitional behaviour, that is, to behaviours that are perceived to be under personal control …'.

A purely cognitive approach like TRA doesn't help us understand why Diana ate the biscuits on impulse; or allow for the fact that people act on feelings as well as reason.

THEORY OF PLANNED BEHAVIOUR (TPB)

This represents a modification of TRA. It reflects the influence of Bandura's (1977, 1986) concept of *self-efficacy* – our belief that we can act effectively and exercise some control over events that influence our lives. Ajzen (1991) added the concept of self-efficacy to TRA, claiming that control beliefs are important determinants of *perceived behavioural control*. This is crucial for understanding motivation: if, for example, you think you're unable to quit smoking, you probably won't try. Perceived behavioural control can have a *direct* effect on behaviour, bypassing behavioural intentions.

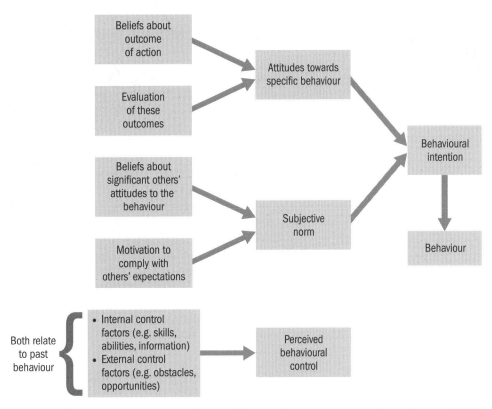

Figure 4.2 Main components of the Theory of Planned Behaviour (adapted from Ogden, 2004)

Diana described herself as 'hopeless', which indicated a lack of perceived behavioural control. She's defeated before she starts.

Evaluation of TPB

According to Walker *et al.* (2004), TPB is currently the most popular and widely used social cognition model in health psychology. It has been used to assess a variety of health-related behaviours. For example, Brubaker and Wickersham (1990) examined its different components in relation to testicular self-examination: attitude, subjective norm and behavioural control (measured as self-efficacy) all correlated with the behavioural intention. Schifter and Ajzen (1985) found that weight loss was predicted by the model's components, especially perceived behavioural control. TPB (like TRA) has the advantage over HBM (see below) of including a degree of irrationality (in the form of evaluations), and it attempts to address the problem of social and environmental factors (normative beliefs). The extra 'ingredient' of perceived behavioural control provides a role for past behaviour. For example, if you've tried several times in the past to quit smoking, you're less likely to believe you can do so successfully in the future and, therefore, you're less likely to intend to try (Ogden, 2000; Penny, 1996).

This sounds more realistic, if more complicated. It shows Diana needs to believe in her ability to succeed, which her past failures undermine. But it still doesn't explain why she fails – or how we can help her change.

HEALTH BELIEF MODEL (HBM)

This was originally developed by social psychologists working in the US Public Health Service (Becker, 1974; Janz and Becker, 1984). They wanted to understand why people failed to make use of disease prevention and screening tests for early detection of diseases not associated with clear-cut symptoms (at least in the early stages). It was later also applied to patients' responses to symptoms and compliance with/adherence to prescribed medication among acutely and chronically ill patients. More recently, it has been used to predict a wide range of health-related behaviours (Ogden, 2004).

HBM assumes that the likelihood that people will engage in a particular health behaviour is a function of:
◎ the extent to which they believe they're *susceptible* to the associated disease
◎ their perception of the *severity of the consequences* of getting the disease.
Together, these determine the *perceived threat* of the disease. Given the threat, people then consider whether or not the action will bring benefits that outweigh the costs associated with the action. In addition, *cues to action* increase the likelihood that the action will be adopted; these might include advice from others, a health problem or mass-media campaigns. Other important concepts include *general health motivation* (the individual's readiness to be concerned about health matters) and *perceived control* (for example, 'I'm confident I can give up smoking' – Becker and Rosenstock, 1987, see Figure 4.4).

The idea of cost is important in Diana's case; she may well consider food and cigarettes the most pleasurable things in her life. Her motivation would have to be very high to overcome their loss and I think her perceived behavioural control isn't high.

Evaluation of HBM

It allows for demographic variables – such as age and gender – and psychological characteristics – such as ways of coping with stress and locus of control (see above and Chapter 5) – that might affect health beliefs (Forshaw, 2002). For example, young women are likely to engage in dieting behaviour. So 'the HBM covers most, if not all, of the factors which, on the face of it, should be relevant in determining if a person engages in a particular behaviour …' (Forshaw, 2002).

There's considerable evidence supporting the HBM's predictions, in relation to a wide range of behaviours. Dietary compliance, safe sex, having vaccinations, having regular dental checks, participation in regular exercise programmes – all are related to people's perception of their susceptibility to the related health problem, their belief that the problem is severe and their perception that the benefits of preventative action

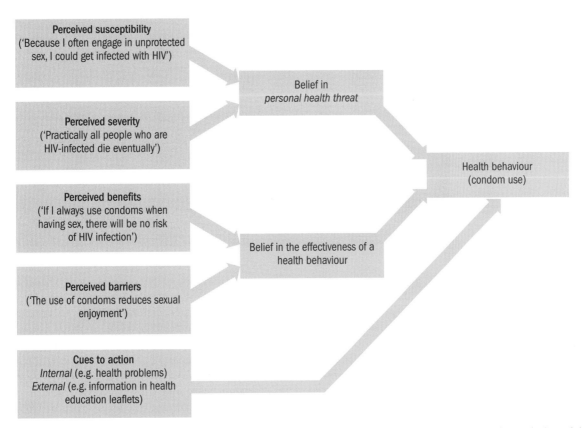

Figure 4.3 Main components of the health belief model (adapted from Stroebe, 2000, reproduced with kind permission of the Open University Press/McGraw-Hill publishing company)

outweigh the costs (e.g. Becker, 1974; Becker and Rosenstock, 1984; Becker *et al.*, 1977).

However, there's also conflicting evidence. For example, Janz and Becker (1984) found that healthy behavioural intentions are related to *low* perceived seriousness (not high as the model predicts). Also, several studies have suggested an association between *low* susceptibility (not high) and healthy behaviour (Ogden, 2004).

This seems opposed to common sense! Perhaps it's because it's more to do with cost–benefit factors than with perceived threat?

HBM has also been criticised for assuming that people's behaviour is governed by rational decision-making processes, ignoring emotional factors, such as fear and anxiety, and overemphasising the individual. A factor that may explain the persistence of unhealthy behaviours is people's inaccurate perceptions of risk and susceptibility.

Box 4.5 Are we unrealistic optimists?

- Weinstein (1983, 1984) asked participants to examine a list of health problems and to state, 'Compared with other people of your age and sex, are your chances of getting [the problem] greater than, about the same, or less than theirs?' Most believed they were *less* likely, displaying what Weinstein called *unrealistic optimism*: not everyone can be less likely! Weinstein identified four cognitive factors contributing to unrealistic optimism:

1. lack of personal experience with the problem

2. belief that the problem is preventable by individual action

3. belief that, if the problem hasn't yet appeared, it won't appear in the future

4. belief that the problem is uncommon.

- This suggests that perception of one's own risk *isn't* a rational process. People show *selective focus*, ignoring their own risk-taking behaviour (for example, the times they've not used a condom) and concentrating primarily on their risk-reducing behaviour (the times they have).

- This is compounded by the tendency to ignore others' risk-reducing, and emphasise their own risk-taking, behaviour. These tendencies produce unrealistic optimism.

Perceptions of invulnerability

According to Ogden (2000), one of the most consistent findings to emerge from the research is the perception of personal invulnerability to HIV, in both heterosexual and homosexual populations. For example, Woodstock *et al.* (1992, in Ogden, 2000) interviewed 125 16–25 year olds about their sexual behaviour and examined how they evaluated their personal risk. Even though most acknowledged some degree of risk, some managed to dismiss it by claiming, 'it would show by now', 'it was in the past', 'AIDS wasn't around in those days', 'it's been blown out of proportion' and 'AIDS is a risk you take in living'. The themes of being run over by a bus and 'it couldn't happen to me' were also quite common. These are classic examples of people *rationalising* behaviour that conflicts with important aspects of self-concept (see Festinger's (1957) *cognitive dissonance theory* in Chapter 10). Most commonly, people denied they'd ever put themselves at risk.

While most models, such as HBM, TRA and TPB, emphasise people's rational decision-making, including their assessment of personal susceptibility to/being at risk from HIV:

> … many people do not appear to believe that they are themselves at risk, which is perhaps why they do not engage in self-protective behaviour, and even when some acknowledgement of risk is made, this is often dismissed and does not appear to relate to behaviour change. (Ogden, 2000)

Unrealistic optimism – the compelling sense that we are somehow less vulnerable to the kinds of problems others face ('it only happens to other people') – can be very hard to break down, thus undermining the extent to which we adopt health precautions (see Box 4.5). AIDS fits perfectly the profile of a risk for which most people tend to manifest unrealistic optimism (Harris and Middleton, 1995).

As Diana's illnesses are at present controlled by medication, she may not regard them as a threat, although Sally said they'd discussed the risk of heart attack. Diana probably believes it won't happen to her.

Unlike TRA and TPB, there's no explicit reference in HBM to behavioural *intention*. Instead, central beliefs and perceptions act directly on the likelihood of behaviour. But it's been shown that adding intention to HBM increases its level of predictability, so it's now typically added when testing it. However, this blurs the distinction between HBM and other models. According to Harris and Middleton (1995), the trend is towards the development of generic models of health behaviour that incorporate the best 'bits' of other models. HAPA is a good example of such a generic model (see below).

Protection Motivation Theory (Rogers, 1975, 1985; Schwarzer, 1992) is an extension of HBM to include *fear* as a motivating factor. Like HBM, it's a cognitive model, but unlike it, it proposes a motivation to protect oneself from danger. Once aroused, fear acts to promote, sustain and direct self-protective activity. Neither threat (HBM) nor fear (PMT) plays any role in TRA or TPB (Harris and Middleton, 1995).

A heart attack is a powerful cue to action! If she had one, would Diana then give up smoking?

HEALTH ACTION PROCESS APPROACH (HAPA)

Schwarzer (1992) criticised TPB for its lack of a *temporal* element – it doesn't describe either the order of the different beliefs or any direction of causality. Schwarzer attempted to address this issue in his HAPA. This explicitly brought together elements from TRA, TPB and HBM to form a generic model.

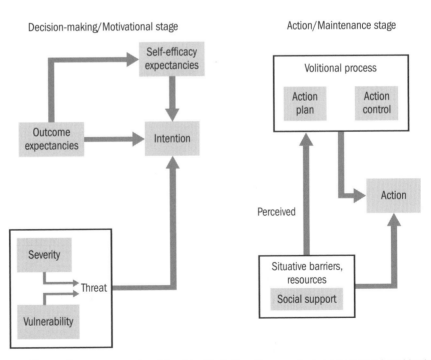

Figure 4.4 The major components of the Health Action Process Approach (based on Harris & Middleton, 1995; Schwarzer, 1992)

The *decision-making/motivational stage* is an attempt to identify the key general processes involved when people make up their minds about whether or not to adopt health precautions. The *action/maintenance stage* tries to identify the factors that determine how hard they try and how long they persist. This is lacking in the other models (Harris and Middleton, 1995).

The HAPA is a useful model. It encourages us to analyse Diana's problems from all aspects of her lifestyle and attitude: her thoughts, feelings and the different stages of her health behaviour. The barriers and social support elements are also important – in Diana's case her sister supports her attempts to diet but smokes with her. The 'friend' who brought chocolate biscuits is a barrier, not a support.

According to Schwarzer, self-efficacy is the most important factor, followed by outcome expectancy and threat. Consistent with this, he suggests they (especially threat) may exert most of their impact on intention indirectly. So, perceiving yourself as at risk of lung cancer may be more influential in producing your intention to give up smoking if it prompts you to think of ways in which you might increase your self-efficacy for quitting. It will be less influential if it contributes to an intention to quit that you feel will be difficult to carry through.

So if Diana said 'Smoking is killing me – instead of a cigarette I'll chew nicotine gum and ban smoking in the house', it would increase her self-efficacy; but if she decided to save her cigarette money for a holiday as soon as she'd got her weight down (a long-term reward), that wouldn't?

Evaluation of HAPA

Perhaps more than the other models, HAPA addresses the key issue of *behaviour change*. This represents one of the central difficulties people face when adopting healthier regimes. According to Schwarzer, the key to successful *action control* (the amount of effort invested and the degree to which people will persevere in the face of obstacles) is *self-reinforcement*. The rewards associated with old habits (e.g. smoking) are fairly immediate (see Chapter 7), while those associated with the new ones (not smoking) are more remote and less tangible – and in the short term less powerful. Just as you cannot be sure the smoking would have killed you, so you can quit and die of something equally unpleasant:

> … As a consequence, some people are ready to take risks with their health precisely because they construe this in terms of a gamble – they hope that they will be among the lucky few who will not get ill or believe that there are many other risks out of their control and that they might as well reap the benefits of their unhealthy habits in the meantime … (Harris and Middleton, 1995)

This means that change is more likely to be permanent if people focus on the short-term rewards of the change (e.g. feeling fitter). The rewards that have to be sacrificed are often *social*, but Schwarzer's distinction between *perceived* and *actual* social support is consistent with the reasonable assumption that how friends and family actually respond has some bearing on the final outcome ('action') (Harris and Middleton, 1995).

Schwarzer's claim that self-efficacy is consistently the best predictor of behavioural intentions and change for a variety of behaviours is supported by studies of the effective use of contraception, addicts' intentions to use clean needles, breast self-examination, quitting smoking, losing weight and exercising (Ogden, 2004). However, HAPA is subject to many of the limitations of all the models (see below).

What practical use are health belief models that don't facilitate behaviour change? HAPA includes planning strategies to maintain changed behaviour. And – back to behaviourism – includes rewarding oneself to compensate for loss of pleasure. This is balancing cost by benefit. But does it address the underlying causes of negative health behaviour? There must be some (unknown) reason why Diana's health-damaging behaviour is so resistant to change.

AN EVALUATION OF MODELS OF HEALTH BEHAVIOUR

A limitation shared by all the models is their failure to consistently predict behavioural intentions. Most seriously of all, they're unable to predict actual behaviour (the *intention–behaviour gap*). One response to these criticisms has been the concept of *implementation intentions* (Gollwitzer, 1993). Carrying out an intention involves the development of specific plans about what to do given a specific set of environmental conditions. These plans describe the 'what' and 'when' of a particular behaviour. There's some evidence that encouraging people to make implementation intentions can actually increase the correlation between intentions and behaviour for taking vitamin pills and performing breast self-examination (Ogden, 2000). Overall, though, current models are relatively poor predictors of actual behaviour (Turpin and Slade, 1998).

Implementation intentions allow a person to rehearse positive health choices, like the sessions at school where children practise saying 'no' to drugs or sexual advances.

The models are all very general, covering all kinds of health-related behaviours; it may simply be invalid to apply the same model to a whole range of behaviours and illnesses. It may be necessary to model specific behaviour, such as in response to the threat of AIDS (as in Catania *et al.*'s AIDS risk reduction model, 1990, in Harris and Middleton, 1995).

Forshaw (2002) points out that our models of health behaviour are *culturally relative:* we cannot just assume that they apply universally. He cites a study by Sissons Joshi (1995) of causal beliefs about insulin-dependent diabetes in England and India. Far more Indian diabetics believed that eating too much sweet food caused their diabetes (38 per cent compared with 6 per cent of the English sample).

Identifying 'causal belief' is part of understanding 'where patients are coming from', whatever their culture; we can't be sure about the cause of Diana's health-damaging behaviour. My initial feelings about Diana worried me; I felt guilty at being judgemental. I should have been more concerned for her feelings and less about mine, which got in the way of thinking about her health problem objectively.

I found the HAPA model particularly useful in identifying a wide range of factors that could be involved in Diana's health behaviour, and that makes me more sympathetic towards her. It also showed that adopting a biopsychosocial model reveals that health care is far more complex than it first appears and often, as in Diana's case, needs multi-disciplinary care.

CHAPTER SUMMARY

◎ The **biomedical model** adopts a reactive and reductionist approach to **disease**, while the **biopsychosocial model** adopts a more proactive and holistic approach towards **health**.

◎ **Health beliefs** (**HBs**) are important determinants of health behaviour and can be **health-damaging** as well as **health-promoting**. For most western people, being healthy is the norm and is defined in positive terms.

◎ While the concept of **disease** reflects the biomedical model, **illness** (like the concept of health) incorporates physical, psychological and social aspects, reflecting the biopsychosocial model.

◎ HBs vary across cultures, which represent **macro-level** influences on people's health status. Conflicting HBs can leave both nurses and patients feeling frustrated and failing to understand one another.

◎ HBs **based on biomedicine** dominate the health systems of North America and western Europe. Others are **based on personality (or magico-religious) systems** and **naturalistic systems** (holism).

◎ The migration of immigrants' health status to the host nation's norm through **acculturation** is best explained in terms of risk factors associated with adapting to the new culture ('acculturative stress').

◎ **Illness cognitions** provide patients with a framework/schema for coping with and understanding their illness. Five associated dimensions are **identity**, **perceived cause**, **timeline**, **consequences**, and **curability and controllability**.

◎ According to **crisis theory**, physical illness (especially if life-threatening) is a turning point that produces changes in **identity**, **location**, **role**, **social support** and **'the future'**. A similar concept is that of a **psychosocial transition**, which threatens the patient's assumptive world.

◎ **Social cognition models** can be divided into those that are specifically **health models** (Health Belief Model/HBM, Protection Motivation Theory/PMT, and **Health Action Process Approach/HAPA**) and those that aim to account for social behaviour in general (**Theory of Reasoned Action/TRA** and **Theory of Planned Behaviour/TPB**).

◎ Both types of model try to explain why people adopt/don't adopt particular health-related behaviours. These **expectancy–value models** assume that people choose between alternative courses of action, based on **subjective probabilities** and **evaluation** of action outcomes.

◎ All models fail to predict actual behaviour (the **intention–behaviour gap**) and they are also **culturally relative**.

◎ Most models emphasise people's rational decision-making and underestimate their **perception of personal invulnerability/unrealistic optimism**.

STRESS

5

INTRODUCTION AND OVERVIEW

According to Bartlett (1998):

> ... the notion that stress is bad for you and can make you ill has become a modern cultural truism. However, there is also a significant body of research evidence which lends support to this idea ... The study of stress must ... be central to ... health psychology which concerns, at its most basic level, the role of psychosocial processes in health and disease.

Definitions of stress fall into three categories (Bartlett, 1998; Goetsch and Fuller, 1995):

1. stress as a *stimulus*
2. stress as a *response*
3. stress as *interaction* between an organism and its environment.

In turn, this classification corresponds very closely to the three models of stress identified by Cox (1978):

1. the *engineering model*, which is mainly concerned with the question 'What causes stress?'
2. the *physiological model* – 'What are the effects of stress?', and
3. the *transactional model*, which is concerned with both these questions, plus 'How do we cope with stress?'

While stressors are faced by everyone (especially, perhaps, those living in constantly changing western cultures), some face greater demands than others. As a group, patients (both in and out of hospital) face sources of stress that they didn't have to deal with before becoming ill. Similarly, while all occupations are stressful, some are more stressful than others. Several studies have suggested that health workers experience more stress than comparable groups of non-health workers (Jones, 1995). In terms of Warr's (1987) *vitamin model*, which identifies several environmental factors that affect mental health, nurses and other health professionals are likely to suffer from organisational stressors that are common to many other occupations (such as lack of clarity, conflicting roles, work overload and lack of control). However, nurses often suffer additional stressors that are intrinsic to the job, such as providing terminal care, counselling bereaved parents, and dealing with disturbed and violent patients (see Chapter 3).

 From my diary (12): Year 2/Medical Ward – Night Duty

My first night duty. I was on a gastro-enterology ward with Adam, a Staff Nurse (and my mentor) on internal rotation from the ward, a 'bank' Staff Nurse and a Health Care Assistant (HCA) who works regular night duty on this ward.

At first I helped the HCA to settle patients and then worked with Adam. We were 'on take' and had two admissions before midnight; one (Mr Hendon) with a bleeding gastric ulcer. Before the HO arrived Mr Hendon had a massive haematemesis and went into hypovolaemic shock, which was very frightening. He needed oxygen, a blood transfusion, the naso-gastric tube and a urinary catheter. Adam appeared totally in control but I felt inadequate and overwhelmed. Adam suggested I take Mrs Hendon, who unfortunately witnessed the incident, to the day room. She asked me if her husband was going to die and, at the time, I was afraid he might. But I tried to calm her, made her some tea and said I'd get the HO to speak to her. After that, I mostly stayed with Adam, who suggested I do all the paperwork under his supervision.

Trying to do everything quietly made me more tense; surprisingly, some patients did sleep in spite of the disturbance. By 4 am, when things were quieter, I realised I felt sick, shivery and deathly tired. Adam said you got used to it; S/N said she didn't but she had two children and it was the only time she could work. The HCA seemed alert and cheerful, as if she was on day duty.

ASK YOURSELF ...

• What do you understand by the term 'stress'?

• Is the term used in different ways to refer to different things or processes?

• What makes you feel stressed, and how does it feel?

STRESS: WHAT IS IT?

MODELS OF STRESS

◎ The *engineering model* (Cox, 1978) sees external stresses giving rise to a stress reaction, or strain, in the individual. The stress is located in the stimulus characteristics of the environment: stress is what happens *to* a person (not what happens within a person). Up to a point, stress is inevitable and can be tolerated, and moderate levels may even be beneficial (*eustress*: Selye, 1956).

◎ The *physiological model* is primarily concerned with what happens *within* the person as a result of stress (the 'response' aspects of the engineering model), in particular the physiological changes.

The impetus for this view was Selye's (1956) definition of stress as 'the individual's psychophysiological response, mediated largely by the autonomic nervous system (ANS) and the endocrine system, to any demands made on the individual'. While a medical student, Selye noticed a general malaise or syndrome associated with 'being ill', regardless of the particular illness. The syndrome was characterised by: (i) a loss of appetite; (ii) an associated loss of weight and strength; (iii) loss of ambition; and (iv) a typical facial expression associated with illness.

Further examination of extreme cases revealed major physiological changes (confirmed by Cox, 1978). This non-specific response to illness reflected a distinct phenomenon, which Selye called the *General Adaptation Syndrome* (GAS: see below).

◎ The *transactional model* represents a blend of the first two models. It sees stress as arising from an interaction between people and their environment – in particular, when there's an imbalance between the person's perception of the demands being made of them by the situation and their ability to meet those demands. Because it's the person's *perception* of this mismatch between demand and ability that causes stress, the model allows for important *individual differences* in what produces stress and how much stress is experienced. There are also wide differences in how people attempt to cope with stress, psychologically and behaviourally.

For Mr Hendon and his wife, the engineering model would locate stress in his illness; for the nurses, in the demands of their job. The physiological model would be concerned with the changes happening in our bodies in response to external pressures and the transactional one with how we individually perceived and coped with them.

WHAT CAUSES STRESS?

The causes of stress don't exist objectively, and individuals differ in what they see as a stressor in the first place (Lazarus, 1966). So, in this section, we're really identifying *potential* stressors, the kinds of event or experience that most people are likely to find exceed their capacity to handle the demands that are involved.

Lazarus (1966) is offering a transactional explanation: that although Adam and I shared the same experience, Adam may not have perceived it as a stressor as he was capable of coping with the situation.

DISRUPTION OF CIRCADIAN RHYTHMS

The word 'circadian' ('about one day') describes a particular periodicity or rhythm of a number of physiological and behavioural functions, which can be seen in almost all living creatures. Many studies have shown that these rhythms persist if we suddenly reverse our activity pattern and sleep during the day and are active during the night. This indicates that these rhythms are internally controlled (*endogenous*).

However, our circadian rhythms are kept on their once-every-24-hours schedule by regular daily environmental (*exogenous*) cues called *zeitgebers* (German for 'time givers'). The most important zeitgeber is the daily cycle of light and dark. If we persist with our reversal of sleep and activity, the body's circadian rhythms will reverse (after a period of acclimatisation) and become synchronised to the new set of exogenous cues.

Individual differences and the effects of shift work

ASK YOURSELF ...
• What is it about the disruption of circadian rhythms that could account for the effects of shift work?

Some people take five to seven days to adjust, others take up to fourteen, and some may never achieve a complete reversal. But not all physiological functions reverse at the same time: body temperature usually reverses inside a week for most people, while the rhythms of adrenocortical hormone take much longer. During the changeover period, the body is in a state of *internal desynchronisation* (Aschoff, 1979). This is very stressful and shift workers often report experiencing insomnia, digestive problems, irritability, fatigue, even depression, when changing work shifts. In shift work, the zeitgebers stay the same, but workers are forced to adjust their natural sleep–wake cycles in order to meet the demands of changing work schedules (Pinel, 1993).

Body temperature is endogenously controlled, which explains why I felt shivery (when it naturally dropped) in the early hours of the morning. Night duty usually doesn't exceed seven nights, so presumably most night nurses are in a permanent state of internal desynchronisation.

> **KEY STUDY 5.1 Night nurses aren't all the same (Hawkins and Armstrong-Esther, 1978)**
>
> - Hawkins and Armstrong-Esther studied eleven nurses during the first seven nights of a period of night duty.
> - They found that performance was significantly impaired on the first night, but improved progressively on successive nights. However, body temperature hadn't fully adjusted to night working after seven nights.
> - There were significant differences between individual nurses, with some appearing relatively undisturbed by working nights and others never really adjusting at all.

This could explain why some nurses, like Adam and the HCA, seem less disturbed by night duty. Or perhaps those who regularly work night duties learn to ignore external cues. And patients who sleep through in spite of lights on all round them – is that a case of endogenous cues overcoming those exogenous zeitgebers?

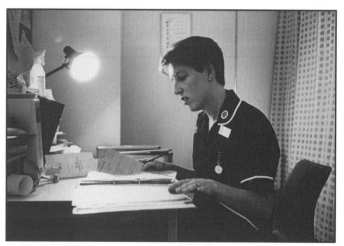

Night shift involves an enforced adjustment of sleep–wake cycles

ASK YOURSELF ...
- Which shifts do you think produced (a) the highest job performance and (b) the most job-related stress?

- Give your reasons.

Coffey *et al.* (1988) examined the influence of day, afternoon, night and rotating shifts on the job performance and job-related stress of 463 female nurses at five US hospitals.

Using a structured questionnaire, Coffey *et al.* found that job performance was highest for nurses on the day shift, followed by the night, afternoon and rotating shifts. Rotating shift nurses reported the highest job-related stress, followed by afternoon, day and night shift nurses. These results contrast with those of mainly male factory workers, where individuals are doing essentially the same type of work regardless of the shift. But the type of work carried out by nurses differs considerably depending on their particular shift. So, performance by shift may be affected by the social organisation of hospital work, as well as circadian rhythm synchronisation.

Rotating shift nurses may suffer the most stress and have the least successful job performance due to both the disturbance of circadian rhythms and the fact that they often work with different colleagues and patients on each shift. This may make it more difficult to establish working relationships. Although day shift nurses suffer the least from circadian rhythm disruption, they're responsible for the instrumental activities of supervising patient preparation for diagnostic testing, treatment and therapy. The pace is rapid and the nurse is interacting with a maximum number of colleagues, both nursing and non-nursing. This can all be very stressful (see below).

Conversely, the pace is slower and interaction with others considerably reduced on night shift, helping to reduce stress levels. Concentration is on the expressive activities of making patients comfortable, and ensuring rest and sleep. So, what about the afternoon shift? Circadian rhythm disruption is moderate, but nurses face the stress of both instrumental and expressive functions. They're responsible for continuing and monitoring the medical treatment initiated during the day shift, while at the same time dealing with the social and psychological aftermath of the medical regimen. This may account for their high stress levels (Coffey *et al.*, 1988).

According to Singer (in Brown, 1988), who compared rota systems in different countries, there's a very high error and accident rate among people working an early morning shift that follows a late afternoon/evening shift. This combination should be avoided at all costs. Yet a late followed by an early shift is the staple diet of the internal rotation duty pattern in the UK (Brown, 1988).

Working with different staff, the demands of technical activities and lack of control over activities were all sources of stress for me. From 11 pm to 4 am the pace was the same as on day duty! Although night duty disturbs circadian rhythm most, Coffey et al. (1988) found job performance still relatively high, so perhaps control is a significant factor. Adam said one good thing about night duty is that he feels more in charge of what he does.

Box 5.1 Singer's recommendations on rota systems (based on Brown, 1988)

- There should be no more than three nights in succession.
- The morning shift shouldn't begin too early (8 am is recommended).
- The shift change times should be flexible.
- The shift length should depend on the physical and mental workload. The night shift should be shorter than the day shift.
- Short intervals of time off between shifts (split shifts) should be avoided.
- There should be some free weekends, including at least two consecutive days off.
- The shift rota should be regular.
- The shift rota should move *forwards* (earlies, lates, nights, off) and not vice versa. (This is sympathetic to the body's running/internal clock.)
- Twelve-hour shifts cause least erosion of quality and quantity of sleep.

However beneficial, I think some of these would be difficult to organise in a hospital.

LIFE CHANGES: THE SRRS

Holmes and Rahe (1967) examined 5000 patient records and made a list of 43 life events, of varying seriousness, which seemed to cluster in the months preceding the onset of their illness. Out of this grew the *Social Readjustment Rating Scale* (SRRS). Several studies have shown that people who experience many significant life changes (a score of 300 life change units (LCUs) or over) are more susceptible to physical and mental illness than those with lower scores. The range of health problems includes sudden cardiac death, heart attacks (non-fatal), TB, diabetes, leukaemia, accidents and even athletics injuries.

Table 5.1 Selected items from the Social Readjustment Rating Scale

Rank	Life event	Mean value
1	Death of spouse	100
2	Divorce	73
3	Marital separation	65
4	Jail term	63
5	Death of close family member	63
6	Personal injury or illness	53
7	Marriage	50
8	Fired at work	47
9	Marital reconciliation	45
10	Retirement	45
11	Change in health of family member	44
12	Pregnancy	40
13	Sex difficulties	39
16	Change in financial state	38
17	Death of close friend	37
18	Change to different line of work	36
22	Change in responsibilities at work	29
23	Son or daughter leaving home	29
28	Change in living conditions	25
30	Trouble with boss	23
31	Change in work hours or conditions	20
32	Change in residence	20
38	Change in sleeping habits	16
41	Vacation	13
42	Christmas	12
43	Minor violations of the law	11

The amount of stress a person has experienced in a given period of time, say one year, is measured by the total number of life change units (LCUs). These units result from the addition of the values (shown in the right-hand column) associated with events the person has experienced during the target time period. The mean value (item weightings) was obtained empirically by telling 100 judges that 'marriage' had been assigned an arbitrary value of 500 and asking them to assign a number to each of the other events in terms of 'the intensity and length of time necessary to accommodate ... regardless of the desirability of the event relative to marriage'. The average of the numbers assigned each event was divided by 10 and the resulting value became the weighting of each life event.

(Reprinted from *Journal of Psychosomatic Research*, *11*, Holmes and Rahe, 1967, The Social Readjustment Rating Scale, pp. 213–218, © 1967, with permission from Elsevier).

Holmes and Rahe's engineering perspective is that change leads to stress leads to increased susceptibility to illness. Discovering (from Mrs Hendon) that both Mr Hendon's parents had recently died within three months of each other didn't help us care for him in this acute situation. However, Worden (1991) states that if the process of mourning is suppressed, grief can become a source of chronic stress. Encouraging Mr Hendon to articulate his feelings and making him aware of available bereavement counselling might help reduce future vulnerability.

Evaluation of the SRRS

◎ The SRRS assumes that *any* change, by definition, is stressful – that is, certain events are *inherently* stressful (stressful in themselves). But the *undesirable* aspects of events are at least as important as the fact that they change people's lives (Davison and Neale, 1994). A quick glance at Table 5.1 suggests that life changes have a largely *negative* feel about them (especially those in the top ten, which receive the highest LCU scores). So, the scale may be confusing 'change' and 'negativity'.

◎ Similarly, life changes may be stressful only if they're unexpected and, in this sense, uncontrollable. In other words, it may not be change as such that's stressful, but change we cannot prevent or reverse. Studies have shown that when people are asked to classify the undesirable life events on the SRRS as either 'controllable' or 'uncontrollable', only the latter are significantly correlated with subsequent onset of illness (Brown, 1986).

The need for control

According to Parkes (1993), the *psychosocial transitions* that are most dangerous to health are those that are sudden and allow little time for preparation. The sudden death of a relative from a heart attack, in an accident or as a result of crime are examples of the most stressful kinds of life changes (see Chapter 20).

Using Rotter's (1966) *Locus of Control Scale*, and devising a new scale (the *Life Events Scale*), Johnson and Sarason (1978) found that life events stress was more closely related to psychiatric symptoms (in particular, depression and anxiety) among people rated as high on *external* locus of control than among those rated as high on internal locus of control. In other words, people who believe that they don't have control over what happens to them are more vulnerable to the harmful effects of change than those who believe they do. This is related to Seligman's (1975) concept of *learned helplessness* (see Gross, 2005).

Acutely ill patients like Mr Hendon can't control events. Might a realisation of helplessness be more stressful for someone with an internal locus of control?

OCCUPATION-LINKED STRESSORS

Along with social work, teaching and the police force, nursing is identified as a high-stress occupation. A study by Borrill *et al.* (1996, in Carson *et al.*, 1997) of 11,000 NHS staff found nurses had the second-highest stress score among seven staff groups. We've already seen how shift work, although not unique to nurses, is an inherently stressful aspect of the job; this is common to all those working in the emergency services (police, fire, ambulance, emergency medical teams and mountain rescue). They also share routine encounters with death, tragedy and horror. They're required to deal with people in pain and distress, and handle dead bodies. They may also face personal danger and injury.

RESEARCH QUESTION

● Why is it a mistake to infer that life events *cause* illness?

● Is it possible that (some) life events are *caused by* illness?

● What kind of data are produced by studies that investigate the link between life events and illness?

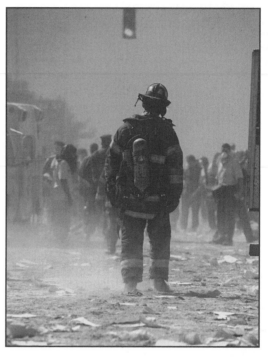

High stress levels, an occupational hazard for those working in the emergency services

CRITICAL DISCUSSION 5.1 It's tough at the bottom: student nurse stress (based on Snell, 1995)

- Nursing has never been an easy option, but nursing students have never had it so bad. The fallout from the 'revolution' in nursing is starting to take its toll – the hours are longer and the emotional demands greater than for most other students. While they used to be part of a close-knit community living in heavily subsidised nurses' accommodation, today's students face rocketing rents and increasing isolation; they often have to travel long distances to split-site colleges or community placements.

- While Project 2000 students were meant to be supernumerary, in practice this often didn't happen. Traditionally trained staff may expect more from the student than s/he can deliver. These job demands, together with the academic ones, plus the financial hardships (which might mean students having to work night shifts before going to college), all add up to very high stress levels.

- Rocketing stress levels mean students are more prone to problems with drugs and alcohol (see Chapter 7).

Apart from classes, I don't often meet up with my student cohort. We're encouraged to take responsibility for our own learning, which means we go to different placements most of the time.

The emotional labour of nursing

Intrinsic sources of stress (such as constantly having to deal with patients' pain, anxiety and death, as well as giving emotional support to patients' families) are made worse by the inadequate training received for handling such demands (Gaze, 1988). According to Mazhindu (1998), there's also been little research into the effects that emotional labour in nursing has on the quality of nursing practice and on nurses' personal lives.

The term 'emotional labour' was first used by Hochschild (1983) in her study of flight attendants, who are able to maintain a cool, calm, caring and comforting exterior despite working in often quite deplorable and emotionally draining conditions. Being friendly, kind, courteous and smiling are all part of the job (and have financial value for the airline), hence, 'labour' (rather than 'care'). Hochschild defined emotional labour as 'the induction or suppression of feeling in order to sustain an outward appearance that produces in others a sense of being cared for in a convivial safe place'.

ASK YOURSELF ...
- Try to identify the components of emotional labour involved in nursing (see Key Study 3.1, page 46).

I was aware I mustn't reveal my feelings to Mrs Hendon and don't think I did. Adam reacted calmly, reassuring Mr Hendon and his wife, and asked me to take her to the day room. He quietly said to ask S/N to page the 'on call' doctor and organise a unit of blood for Mr Hendon from the blood bank. Now I wonder if he was feeling as calm and confident as he looked! If not, he fooled me, along with the patient. But Hochschild (1983) argues it would cost him, emotionally.

ASK YOURSELF ...
- How much emotional labour do you consider you perform in your nursing role?

- Do you regard it as an inherent part of the job or is it something you do 'beyond the call of duty'?

- How does it affect you, compared with physical and technical work?

- How do you manage these effects?

Smith (1992, in Small, 1995) drew on Hochschild's work in her own study of student nurses' experiences of being socialised into nursing. She carried out her research on elderly care wards, an environment in which high-tech nursing tasks are few, but opportunities to listen to reminiscences (see Chapter 19), provide companionship and clip toenails are many. In such wards, 'the functioning hearing aid was just as much a lifeline to survival as the intravenous infusion to the post-operative patient in the acute surgical ward' (Smith, 1992, in Small, 1995).

However, while the demands of emotional work can be as tiring and hard as physical and technical labour, they're not so readily recognised and valued. Smith (1988, in Small, 1995) found that, on most general wards, sisters tended to encourage nurses to involve themselves in physical and technical activities rather than emotional care. This was relegated to the quiet periods of the day, after the 'real' work was completed.

*Emotional care isn't a separate thing, is it? By being in control, Adam was **behaviourally** reassuring Mr Hendon and his wife. And, on reflection, whatever I was thinking, I continued her care in the same way.*

ASK YOURSELF …

- Do you consider that certain types of nursing are inherently more stressful than others (such as CCUs, cancer wards/units, ICUs, A&E, or defined in terms of different patient groups, either through age or nature of illness; see Chapter 3)?

- Give your reasons. (Again, see Chapter 3.)

Stress related to different types of nursing work

Nurses in ICUs have to maintain high levels of concentration for long periods, are often emotionally drained by continuous close contact with a distressed and frightened family, and the process of dying may not follow a natural course: technology (such as ventilators) and drugs may prolong it (Fromant, 1988). Staff working in A&E are in the front line at times of major disasters, such as the 1989 Hillsborough disaster and the July 2005 London bombings. However well prepared they may be practically, nothing can prepare them for the emotional demands (Owen, 1990).

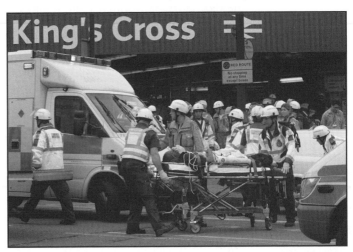

This is recognised; victims of disasters have counsellors; students like me have mentors. I did discuss Mr Hendon's bleed briefly with Adam before going off duty; I hadn't considered he too might need to talk about it.

Mental health nurses

O'Donnell (1996) reported the findings of a survey in which nurses were asked about 16 different stressors. Overall, most of these stressors were perceived as being more extensive among mental health nurses (MHNs) than in nursing as a whole. 'Violence' was found to be substantially more extensive than average, as were 'job insecurity', 'not involved in decision-making' and 'career uncertainty'.

According to Sullivan (1993, in Nolan *et al.*, 1995), there's a growing body of research evidence that nursing in general, and MHN in particular, is a stressful occupation. All those professionals working in mental health may be at greater risk of stress than their colleagues working in physical health care. For example, psychiatrists have the highest suicide rate among doctors. As MHN is often carried out against a background of risk-taking and uncertainty because of the volatile and potentially aggressive nature of some psychiatric patients, nurses will inevitably experience stress (Cahill *et al.*, 1991, in Nolan *et al.*, 1995).

According to Burnard *et al.* (2000), psychological distress, emotional exhaustion and increased alcohol consumption are just some of the consequences of increased workplace stressors among *community* MHNs (CMHNs). They see themselves as overworked, struggling with too much paperwork and administration, having too many clients, and having serious concerns about their client groups. As many as 20 per cent feel they have no job security. These are among the key findings of a survey into stress among CMHNs in Wales, the largest of its kind in the UK. It included nurses working in a wide range of both urban and rural settings. What the findings describe is *burnout*.

These relate to Warr's vitamin model of occupational stressors. Are things like the high patient turnover and all the changes in the NHS and in nurse education increasing stress levels?

CRITICAL DISCUSSION 5.2 Burnout and HIV

- Maslach and Jackson (1981) define burnout as a combination of emotional exhaustion, depersonalisation (see Chapter 3, page XX) and a reduced sense of personal accomplishment. Cherniss (1980, in Firth *et al.*, 1987) defines it simply as 'negative changes in work-related attitudes and behaviour in response to job stress'. It is an 'occupational hazard' for a variety of health care professionals, especially those caring for the terminally ill (Hedge, 1995).

- For example, those working with HIV patients have to deal with profound physical and mental deterioration, which induces in staff a sense of helplessness, frustration and inadequacy at being unable to cure. They also experience anxiety, depression, feeling overworked, fatigued, stressed out, a fear of death and a decreased interest in sex (Hortsman and McKusick, 1986, in Hedge, 1995).

- According to Hedge, many of the factors associated with burnout are experienced by workers in other fields (such as oncology and cystic fibrosis). But Bennett *et al.* (1991, in Hedge, 1995) found that the increased nurse–patient contact and emotional intensity of the work in HIV units increase stress levels. Nurses who identify closely with their patients will experience a grief reaction (see Chapter 20), but older, more experienced nurses are less likely to suffer from burnout. Perhaps they are better able to maintain professional boundaries in order to reduce emotional stress, while at the same time expressing warmth and empathy.

ASK YOURSELF ...
- How might the care patients receive be affected by nurse burnout?

- Try to identify some of the stressors experienced by patients coming into hospital and how these might be influenced by nurse stress.

I can see if nurses get to this stage they would leave. Which makes the understanding of occupational stress, its causes and management of vital importance surely? Later, I discussed it with Adam and he said he agreed with Bennett et al. (1991, in Hedge, 1995). Adam's term for professional detachment – which he emphasised didn't mean not caring – was 'arm's length nursing'. It's one step back from total emotional involvement, which might adversely affect competence and efficiency.

WHAT ARE THE EFFECTS OF STRESS?

HOW DOES STRESS MAKE US ILL?

The General Adaptation Syndrome (GAS)

According to Selye (1956), GAS represents the body's defence against stress. The body responds in the same way to any stressor, whether it's environmental or arises from within the body itself. GAS comprises three stages: the *alarm reaction*, *resistance* and *exhaustion*.

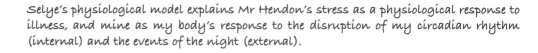

Selye's physiological model explains Mr Hendon's stress as a physiological response to illness, and mine as my body's response to the disruption of my circadian rhythm (internal) and the events of the night (external).

Alarm reaction

When a stimulus is perceived as a stressor, there's a brief, initial *shock phase*. Resistance to the stressor is lowered. But this is quickly followed by the *countershock* phase. The sympathetic branch of the ANS is activated, which, in turn, stimulates the *adrenal medulla* to secrete increased levels of adrenaline and noradrenaline (*catecholamines*).

These are associated with sympathetic changes, collectively referred to as the *fight-or-flight syndrome* (the individual's instinctive, biological preparation for confronting danger or escaping it). The catecholamines mimic sympathetic arousal ('*sympathomimetics*'), and noradrenaline is the transmitter at the synapses of the sympathetic branch of the ANS. Consequently, noradrenaline from the adrenals prolongs the action of noradrenaline released at synapses in the ANS. This prolongs sympathetic arousal after the stressor's removal. This is referred to as the *ANS-adrenal-medulla system* (or *sympatho-adrenomedullary axis*).

When Mr Hendon suddenly vomited a large amount of blood, I experienced a surge of panic and was aware of my heart racing. I wasn't thinking clearly at all.

Resistance

If the stressor isn't removed, there's a *decrease* in sympathetic activity, but an *increase* in output from the other part of the adrenal gland: the *adrenal cortex*. This is controlled by the amount of *adrenocorticotrophic hormone* (ACTH) in the blood. ACTH is released from the anterior pituitary (the 'master' endocrine gland) upon instructions from the hypothalamus. The adrenal cortex is essential for the maintenance of life and its removal results in death.

The effect of ACTH is to stimulate the adrenal cortex to release *corticosteroids* (or *adrenocorticoid hormones*), one group of which are the *glucocorticoid hormones* (chiefly, corticosterone, cortisol and hydrocortisone). These control and conserve the amount of glucose in the blood (*glucogenesis*), which helps to resist stress of all kinds. The glucocorticoids convert protein into glucose, make fats available for energy, increase blood flow and generally stimulate behavioural responsiveness. In this way, the *anterior pituitary-adrenal cortex system* (or *hypothalamic-pituitary-adrenal axis*) contributes to the fight-or-flight syndrome.

I rushed to find staff and then ran all the way to the blood bank. I realise now this was literally a 'flight' reaction.

Exhaustion

Once ACTH and corticosteroids are circulating in the bloodstream, they tend to inhibit the further release of ACTH from the pituitary. If the stressor is removed during the resistance stage, blood sugar levels will gradually return to normal. But when the stress situation continues, the pituitary-adrenal excitation will continue. The body's resources are now becoming depleted, the adrenals can no longer function properly, blood glucose levels drop and, in extreme cases, hypoglycaemia could result in death.

It's at this stage that *psychophysiological disorders* develop, including high blood pressure (hypertension), heart disease (coronary artery disease, CAD), coronary heart disease (CHD), asthma and peptic (stomach) ulcers. Selye called these the *diseases of adaptation*.

By the time I got back with the blood, I was calmer but still feeling shaky; this may have been due to 'using up' blood glucose.

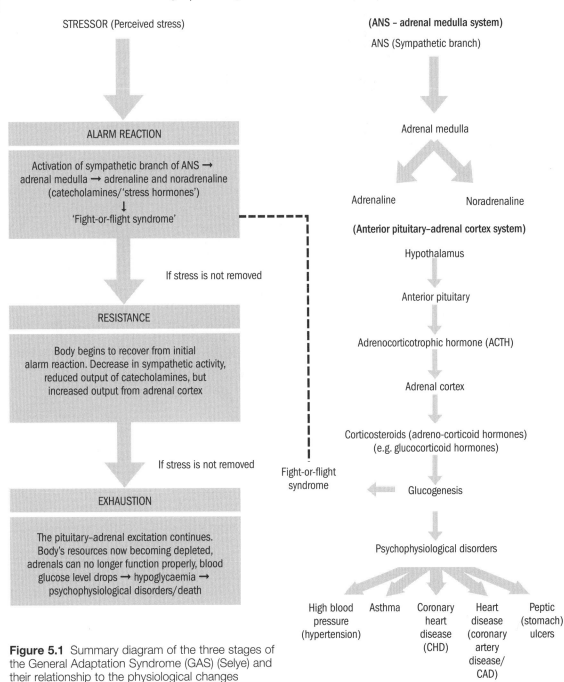

Figure 5.1 Summary diagram of the three stages of the General Adaptation Syndrome (GAS) (Selye) and their relationship to the physiological changes associated with (i) the ANS – adrenal medulla and (ii) anterior pituitary – adrenal cortex systems (Cannon)

Evaluation of GAS

Lazarus (1999) cites a study of patients dying from injury or disease. Post-mortem examination showed that those who remained unconscious had normal levels of corticosteroids, while the opposite was true for those who were conscious (presumably aware they were dying). Lazarus infers from this that 'some psychological awareness – akin to a conscious perception appraisal – of the psychological significance of what is happening may be necessary to produce the adrenal cortical changes of the GAS'.

Selye helped us understand how stressors affect the body. But in order to understand what makes a psychological event stressful, we must put the person into the equation. In effect, says Lazarus, 'it takes both the stressful stimulus conditions and a *vulnerable person* to generate a stress reaction'.

This is a good example of why we need to put the O (organism/person) between the S (stimulus) and R (response) (see Chapter 2). Adam's and my perception of, and ability to deal with, the 'same' situation were completely different.

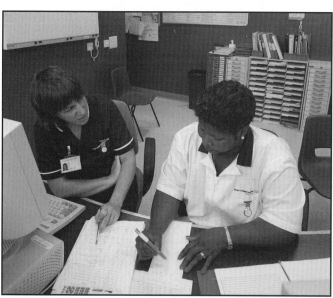

A modern stressor

◎ In the case of heart rate and blood pressure, chronic stress will involve repeated episodes of increases in heart rate and BP which, in turn, produce increases in plaque formation within the cardiovascular system.

◎ Stress also produces an increase in blood cholesterol levels, through the action of adrenaline and noradrenaline on the release of free fatty acids. This produces a clumping together of cholesterol particles, leading to clots in the blood and in the artery walls, and occlusion of the arteries. In turn, raised heart rate is related to a more rapid build-up of cholesterol on artery walls. High BP results in small lesions on the artery walls and cholesterol tends to get trapped in these lesions (Holmes, 1994).

Stress and the immune system

The immune system is a collection of billions of cells, which travel through the bloodstream and move in and out of tissues and organs, defending the body against invasion by foreign agents (such as bacteria, viruses and cancerous cells). These cells are produced mainly in the spleen, lymph nodes, thymus and bone marrow. The study of the effect of psychological factors on the immune system is called *psychoneuroimmunology* (PNI – see Ogden, 2004).

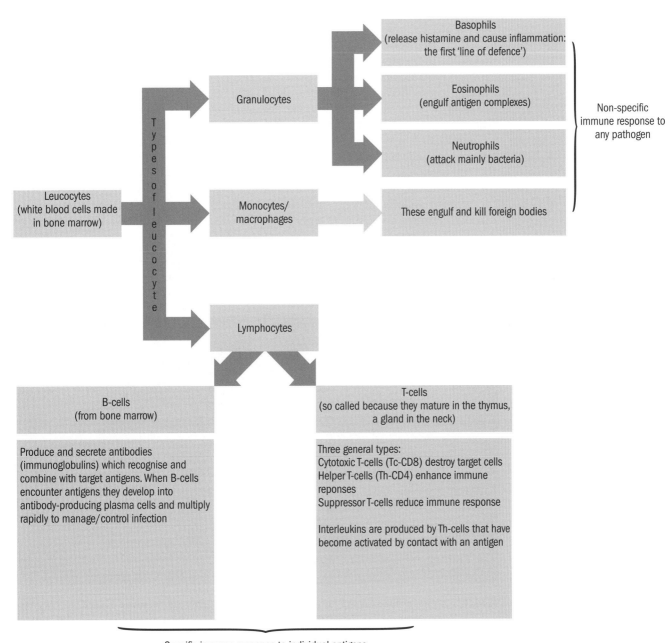

Figure 5.2 The immune system (adapted from Hayward, 1998)

People often catch a cold soon after a period of stress (such as final exams) because stress seems to reduce the immune system's ability to fight off cold viruses (we're 'run down'). Goetsch and Fuller (1995) refer to studies that show decreases in the activity of *lymphocytes* among medical students during their final exams (e.g. Kiecolt–Glaser *et al.*, 1984). Lymphocytes ('natural killer cells') are a particular type of white blood cell, which normally fight off viruses and cancer cells. Levels of immunoglobulin A (IgA) increase immediately after an oral exam (if it appeared to go well), but *not* after written exams (suggesting that the stress isn't relieved until much later – when the results come out!) (Petit–Zeman, 2000).

Of course, none of these findings means that stress actually *causes* infections. Stress makes us more susceptible to infectious agents by temporarily suppressing immune function (the *immunosuppressive effects* of stress). Stressors that seem to have this effect include exams (see above) and the death of a spouse (see Chapter 20). For example, Schliefer *et al.* (1983) found that the immune systems of men whose wives had died from breast cancer functioned less well than before their wife's death.

Interleukin-b is produced soon after tissue damage, helping to remodel connective tissue in wounds and to form collagen (scar tissue). Kiecolt–Glaser *et al.* (1995) compared the rate of wound healing in two groups: (a) a group of 13 'high-stress' women, caring for relatives with Alzheimer's disease; and (b) a 'stress-free' matched control group. All the women underwent a 3.5 mm full thickness punch biopsy on their non–dominant forearm. Healing took significantly longer in the caregivers than in the controls (48.7 versus 39.3 days).

It's a 'double whammy' situation – the prolonged GAS response makes us ill in specific ways, but the suppression of the immune stem makes us prey to any infection that comes along. Including cancer.

KEY STUDY 5.2 Using psychological techniques to boost the immune system (Norton, 2000)

- Norton reports on a study in which women with breast cancer were encouraged to visualise their white blood cells waging war against the cancer cells. This was intended to boost their immune system in a way that could help them fight the disease.

- This *guided imagery* was combined with progressive muscle relaxation, as well as standard surgery, chemotherapy and radiotherapy.

- Compared with women in a control group (given only the medical treatment), those who used the psychological techniques had higher numbers of mature T-cells, activated T-cells and cells carrying T-cell receptors (see Figure 5.2). These are important for attacking malignant cells.

- At the end of the nine-month study, these women also had higher levels of lymphokines (activated killer cells), which help prevent the disease from spreading. The women reported a better quality of life and fewer side-effects from medical treatments.

I wish we could have used this with Pat, a 68-year-old woman I met on my first community placement. She'd had a mastectomy for breast cancer followed by radiotherapy. A wound abscess developed and was excised, the wound being left to heal by 'secondary intention' (left open to heal through granulation of tissue). As this took a while and needed daily dressings, I got to know Pat well.

Moderators and mediators of stress

Moderator variables are antecedent conditions (such as personality, ethnic background and gender) that interact with exposure to stress to affect health outcome. *Mediator variables* intervene in the link between stress exposure and health outcome – for example, appraisal (Folkman and Lazarus, 1988b). If they *reduce* the impact of a stressful event, they're called 'protective' or 'buffering' variables – they soften or cushion the impact (Bartlett, 1998).

Personality

What's now referred to as the *Type A Behaviour Pattern* (TABP) was originally called 'Type A personality' – a stable personality trait (Friedman and Rosenman, 1974). TABP is now conceptualised as a stereotypical set of behavioural responses, including:
◎ *competitiveness* and *achievement orientation*
◎ *aggressiveness* and *hostility*
◎ *sense of time urgency*.

Many early studies showed that people who display TABP were at much greater risk of high BP and CHD, compared with 'Type Bs'. However, these risks are only *relative*: the vast majority of 'Type As' *don't* develop CHD and many Type Bs *do* (Davison and Neale, 1994). Also, most studies have found that TABP assessed immediately following a heart attack *doesn't* predict future attacks. This suggests that TABP *isn't* a distinct risk for CHD in those already at risk of the disorder (Penny, 1996).

However, there seem to be clear physiological differences between Type As and Bs in response to stress – even when the person isn't conscious (Fletcher, 1995). Krantz *et al.* (1982, in Fletcher, 1995) found that, compared with Type Bs, Type A patients undergoing coronary bypass surgery showed greater BP changes while anaesthetised (by as much as 30 mmHG) and were much more likely to have complications during surgery that could be attributed to enhanced sympathetic NS activity.

According to Temoshok (1987), *Type C personalities* are cancer-prone. The Type C personality has difficulty expressing emotion and tends to suppress or inhibit emotions, particularly negative ones such as anger. While there's no clear-cut evidence that these personality characteristics can actually cause cancer, it does seem likely that they influence the progression of cancer and, hence, the survival time of cancer patients (Weinman, 1995).

Greer and Morris (1975) found that women diagnosed with breast cancer showed significantly more emotional suppression than those with benign breast disease (especially among those under 50). This had been a characteristic for most of their lives. Cooper and Faragher (1993) reported that experiencing a major stressful event is a significant predictor of breast cancer. This was especially so in women who didn't express anger but used denial as a form of coping.

Pat was a 'Type C' personality. She had a tragic history, starting at eight years old when her mother died. Pat's second baby was badly deformed (Pat had taken thalidomide) and died soon after birth. The drug damaged Pat's liver – she was hospitalised and separated from her first child for six months. When she was 40 her husband died suddenly of a heart attack. She lives with a man and has other children, but never married. She'd never discussed her problems with anyone except Sally, the District Nurse.

KEY STUDY 5.3 Beating breast cancer (Greer *et al.*, 1979)

- Greer *et al.* studied women who'd had a mastectomy after being diagnosed with breast cancer.

- Those who reacted either by *denying* what had happened ('I'm being treated for a lump, but it's not serious') or by showing *fighting spirit* ('This is not going to get me') were significantly more likely to be free of cancer five years later than women who stoically accepted it ('I feel an illness is God's will …') or were described as 'giving up' ('Well, there's no hope with cancer, is there?').

- A follow-up at 15 years (Greer, 1991; Greer *et al.*, 1990) confirmed the improved prognosis. Survival was almost three times lower in the stoical or 'giving up' women. This difference obtained independently of factors such as age, menopausal status, clinical stage, type of surgery, tumour size and post-operative radiotherapy.

- According to Hegarty (2000): 'Such research … appears to give scientific support to the advice … "to think positive" in the face of a diagnosis of cancer. It suggests the value of having psychological resources which will allow individuals to adapt to, rather than succumb to, a severe threat to their well-being. It might even be possible to teach such strategies to people who neither have nor use them.'

Pat was miserable about the loss of a breast; she told Sally (the District Nurse) she felt sexually unattractive and repulsed by her own body. She found it difficult to cope with the messiness of the wound, her sore skin and the possibility of progression of her malignancy. Her attitude was 'stoical', accepting her illness as the last in a long line of misfortunes. According to Greer et al.'s (1990) study, this would adversely affect her prognosis.

Self-esteem

This is an important factor in moderating stress (Carson and Kuipers, 1998, in Burnard *et al.*, 2000). The study of CMHNs in Wales described above found that those with high self-esteem/self-worth used a wide range of coping skills to deal with work stress. However, 40 per cent of respondents reported low self-esteem and felt others had little respect for them. Low self-esteem scores were associated with higher levels of psychological distress, greater emotional exhaustion, lower use of coping skills and increased alcohol consumption.

Positive and resilient self-esteem is a crucial resource in combating the negative implications for an individual that often accompany stressful events (Turner and Roszell, 1994, in Carson *et al.*, 1997). Research has shown a significant inverse relationship between self-esteem and symptoms of depression (the lower the former, the greater the latter) (Pearlin and Lieberman, 1979, in Carson *et al.*, 1997). Although self-esteem hasn't featured much in the literature on nursing stress, Carson *et al.* believe it's reasonable to predict that nurses with high self-esteem will have lower levels of stress and burnout and better coping skills than those with low self-esteem.

The Claybury CPN (Community Psychiatric Nurse) Study (Carson *et al.*, 1997) was a survey of stress, coping and burnout in 245 MHNs and 323 ward-based nurses in five large mental hospitals and two district hospital psychiatric units. A range of standardised measures was used, including the modified Rosenberg Self-Esteem Scale (see Chapter

ASK YOURSELF …
- Can you think of ways in which sexism might adversely affect women's health?

- Do women have access to protective factors that men don't?

16), the General Health Questionnaire (a well-validated measure of psychological distress) and the Maslach Burnout Scale (Maslach and Jackson, 1986). Overall, the results confirmed the prediction that levels of stress, burnout and use of coping skills are related to levels of self-esteem in MHNs.

*Isn't it essential to know **why** they had low self-esteem? Pat's was affected by her feeling of sexual unattractiveness. Not knowing what to do lowers my self-esteem; knowing how to cope with a situation makes me feel more confident.*

COPING WITH STRESS

WHAT DO WE MEAN BY COPING?

Lazarus and Folkman (1984) define coping as 'constantly changing cognitive and behavioural efforts to manage external and/or internal demands that are appraised as taxing or exceeding the resources of the person'. (This mirrors the definition of stress as the individual's belief that his/her available biological, psychological and social resources aren't sufficient to meet the demands of the situation.)

DIFFERENT KINDS OF COPING

According to Roger and Nash (1995), the term 'coping' conjures up ideas about being able to handle any situation that comes our way. But in relation to stress, they distinguish between *maladaptive* and *adaptive* coping styles, as follows.

◎ *Maladaptive* styles involve failing to adjust appropriately to our environment and experiencing misery and unhappiness as a result. They can take the form of *emotional* and *avoidance* coping styles.
◎ *Adaptive* styles involve an appropriate adjustment to the environment and gaining from the experience. These can be either *detached* or *rational*.

In fact, the term 'maladaptive coping' is a contradiction in terms (see Table 5.2).

Pat apparently 'coped' with several major crises in her past life by suppressing her emotions and 'soldiering on'. Whether or not this, and the 'life events' themselves, contributed to her cancer can't be known. But avoidance coping might have adversely affected her recovery.

Cohen and Lazarus (1979) have classified all the coping strategies that a person might use into five general categories.

1. **Direct action response:** the individual tries to directly change or manipulate his/her relationship to the stressful situation, such as escaping from/removing it.
2. **Information seeking:** the individual tries to understand the situation better and to predict future events that are related to the stressor.
3. **Inhibition of action:** doing nothing. This may be the best course of action if the situation is seen as short term.
4. **Intrapsychic or palliative coping:** the individual reappraises the situation (for example, through the use of psychological defence mechanisms – see below and Table 6.3, page 116) or changes the 'internal environment' (through drugs, alcohol, relaxation or meditation).
5. **Turning to others** for help and emotional support.

Table 5.2 Maladaptive and adaptive coping, and their short- and long-term consequences (adapted from Roger and Nash, 1995)

Maladaptive coping

Emotional
Feeling overpowered and helpless
Becoming miserable, depressed, angry
Taking frustrations out on other people
Preparing for the worst possible outcome and seeking sympathy from others
Short-term benefits: expression of emotion
Long-term consequences: increasingly overwhelmed by problem

Avoidance
Sitting tight and hoping it all goes away
Pretending there's nothing the matter if people ask
Thinking about something else and talking about it as little as possible
Trusting in fate and believing things will sort themselves out
Short-term benefits: temporary relief as problem blocked out
Long-term consequences: blocking out cannot be sustained

Adaptive coping

Detached
Not seeing the problem or situation as a threat
Keeping a sense of humour
Taking nothing personally and seeing the problem as separate from yourself
Resolving the issue by getting things into proportion
Short-term benefits: able to stand back and take stock of problem
Long-term consequences: prevents overidentification with problem

Rational
Using past experience for working out how to deal with the situation
Taking action to change things
Taking one step at a time and approaching the problem with logic
Giving the situation full attention and treating it as a challenge to be met
Short-term benefits: logic determines resolution of problem
Long-term consequences: problems put into perspective

ASK YOURSELF ...
• Which of these coping responses best describes your typical response to stressful situations?

• How about your best friend or partner?

• Does the way you cope depend on the nature of the stressor?

These five categories of coping overlap with the distinction between *problem-focused* and *emotion-focused* coping (Lazarus and Folkman, 1984).

Pat definitely used avoidance coping at first; she wouldn't look at her scar, discuss her cancer or go out in case her wound leaked through the dressing. She'd told Sally she felt helpless, dependent on nurses and no longer in control of her own life.

98

Sally used the 'rational' approach to manage Pat's problems, concentrating first on the wound. She used effective padding, replaced painful adhesive tape with Netelast for comfort, and encouraged Pat to wear soft, loose-fitting tops to disguise the bulky dressing. She did a weekly wound measure to demonstrate healing to Pat and promote optimism.

STRESS MANAGEMENT

Much of what we've said about coping with stress refers to what people do in a largely *spontaneous* way. In this informal sense, we all 'manage our stress' more or less effectively. But, more formally, *stress management* refers to a range of psychological techniques used in a quite deliberate way, in a professional setting, to help people reduce their stress. These techniques may be used singly or in combination.

◎ In the case of *biofeedback* (discussed in Chapter 3 in relation to pain control), the focus is on treating the symptoms of stress rather than the stressor itself.

◎ The same is true of a number of procedures used to bring about a state of relaxation, in particular *progressive muscle relaxation* – such as the Alexander technique (see Maitland and Goodliffe, 1989) – meditation and hypnosis.

◎ *Cognitive restructuring* refers to a number of specific methods aimed at trying to change the way individuals think about their life situation and self, in order to change their emotional responses and behaviour. This approach is based largely on the work of Beck (*the treatment of automatic thoughts*) and Ellis (*rational emotive therapy*), two major forms of *cognitive behaviour therapy* (see Chapter 3 and Gross, 2005). This approach provides information to reduce uncertainty and to enhance people's sense of control.

Night duty and an unanticipated emergency were both new experiences for me and the theory of stress helped me understand my response to both of them. I recall clearly the physical effects of staying awake and working all night, and the 'alarm' stage of the GAS response. But the most stressful part of the night was my feeling of inadequacy when Mr Hendon vomited blood. I didn't know how to respond to that particular situation. On reflection, however, I realise I learned a great deal. Adam taught me how to aspirate the naso-gastric tube and let me do it several times. I learned about checking blood and managing the transfusion line, and the importance of keeping accurate records. I did use the experience and skills I already had to help with the routine work and to reassure Mrs Hendon. And now I'm using the 'information seeking' and 'rational' methods of coping, which Roger and Nash (1995) say are adaptive measures. I've also read up on GI bleeding and hypovolaemic shock. Overall, this incident has increased my confidence; I think understanding the theory and knowing how to cope practically will reduce my stress in a similar situation.

CHAPTER SUMMARY

◎ Stress has been defined as a **stimulus** (corresponding to the **engineering model**), a **response** (corresponding to the **physiological model**) and as **interaction** between an organism and its environment (corresponding to the **transactional model**).

◎ The physiological model is based on Selye's **General Adaptation**

Syndrome/GAS, which comprises the **alarm reaction**, **resistance** and **exhaustion**.

◎ The alarm reaction involves changes in the sympathetic branch of the ANS, which are collectively called the **fight-or-flight syndrome**. This is associated with the **ANS–adrenal–medulla system/sympatho-adrenomedullary axis**.

◎ Resistance is associated with the **anterior pituitary-adrenal cortex system/hypothalamic–pituitary–adrenal axis**.

◎ Exhaustion is related to **psychophysiological disorders** ('**diseases of adaptation**').

◎ Potential causes of stress (**stressors**) include **disruption of circadian rhythms** (as in shift work), **life changes** (as measured by the **Social Readjustment Rating Scale/SRRS**) and **occupation-linked stressors**.

◎ Nursing is a high-stress occupation, sharing many stressors with those working in the emergency services. Routinely dealing with death and people's pain and distress demands **emotional labour**, which may not be acknowledged or valued as readily as the more physical aspects of nursing.

◎ Some of the more stressful areas of nursing include coronary care units/CCUs, cancer wards/units, intensive care units/ICUs, Accident and Emergency/A&E, and mental health nursing.

◎ **Burnout** is an occupational hazard for a variety of health care professionals, especially those working with the terminally ill, as in HIV units.

◎ Chronic stress makes us ill through repeated increases in heart rate and blood pressure/BP, increased blood cholesterol and by suppressing the functioning of the **immune system** (the **immunosuppressive effects** of stress).

◎ **Personality** and **self-esteem** represent **moderators** of the effects of stress.

◎ The **Type A Behaviour Pattern/TABP** is associated with increased risk of high BP and coronary heart disease/CHD, while **Type C personalities** may be cancer-prone.

◎ So-called **coping** with stress can be both **adaptive** and **maladaptive**.

◎ All coping strategies can be classified as either **direct action response**, **information seeking**, **inhibition of action**, **intrapsychic/palliative coping** or **turning to others for emotional support**. These overlap with the distinction between **problem-focused** and **emotion-focused** coping.

◎ **Stress management** can take the form of **biofeedback**, **progressive muscle relaxation** and **cognitive restructuring**.

PERSONALITY AND HEALTH BEHAVIOUR

6

INTRODUCTION AND OVERVIEW

Wood (1988) defines personality simply as 'patterns of behaviour that distinguish us from each other'. To the extent that each of us 'has' a personality that's stable and relatively permanent, our behaviour will be consistent from one situation to another. An alternative view is that behaviour is largely determined by situational factors and that it will vary considerably across situations (see Gross, 2005).

For over 2000 years many physicians have believed that our personality type has an influence on our physical and mental health, and that personality acts as a moderator of the effects of stress (see Chapter 5). So, the 'choleric' person, who easily gets angry, runs a risk of apoplexy, the 'melancholic' type is prone to depression, and both of these differ from the 'sanguine' individual who has a more optimistic outlook on life and apparently better health prospects. This ancient classification has a modern incarnation in the form of Eysenck's personality theory.

Personality theorists differ with respect to whether they're trying to:

◎ compare individuals in terms of a specified number of traits or dimensions common to everyone (the *nomothetic approach*), or
◎ identify individuals' unique characteristics and qualities (the *idiographic approach*).

Eysenck's and Cattell's theories are nomothetic, while the *humanistic* theories of Maslow and Rogers are idiographic (see Chapters 2 and 16). Humanistic theories share a concern for the characteristics that make us distinctively human, including our experience of ourselves as people. Arguably the most famous theory of all, namely Freud's *psychoanalytic theory*, also has elements of both (again see Chapter 2).

Gosling (1995) maintains that:

> ... an understanding of personality can provide the nurse with important guidelines regarding how best to understand an individual patient's illness and how best to care for each patient as an individual. Furthermore, the study of personality can provide insight into how each individual nurse approaches his or her role in caring for the patient.

From my diary (11): *Year 2/Medical Ward*

I've been on the ward a week and today Adam, a Staff Nurse and my mentor, suggested I help him with the medicine round. I gave Phyllis (a 70-year-old woman admitted for investigations of anaemia) her tablets. She had great difficulty in swallowing them and became more and more agitated and apologetic. Adam reassured her, telling her to take her time and that I'd stay with her. I noticed that each time she tried to swallow a tablet she rubbed her leg in an agitated way.

As I knew her quite well (she'd been in several days) I tried to calm her by sitting down and chatting to her. She has severe arthritis, so I asked her if her leg was hurting. She shook her head and explained that when she was in the children's home – she'd told me before she'd been orphaned at the age of four – she was made to sit at the table until she'd eaten everything. As she always had a poor appetite she was often left alone to finish her meal and used to rub her leg 'to help the food down'. She smiled as if it was a joke.

THE PSYCHOMETRIC APPROACH (EYSENCK AND CATTELL)

Psychometric means 'mental measurement' and a major tool used to measure personality is *factor analysis* (FA). FA is a statistical technique, based on correlation, which attempts to reduce large amounts of data (such as scores on personality questionnaires) to much smaller amounts. Essentially, the aim is to discover which test items correlate with one another and which don't, and then to identify the resulting correlation clusters (or factors).

EYSENCK'S TYPE THEORY

What are 'types'?

The term 'type' was formerly used to describe people who belonged either to one group or category or another, so that it was impossible for a particular individual to be considered a member of both. For example, according to the Ancient Greek theory of the 'four temperaments' or 'four humours' (Galen, second century AD), a person was either:

◎ *choleric* (due to an excess of yellow bile)
◎ *sanguine* (due to an excess of blood)
◎ *melancholic* (due to an excess of black bile), or
◎ *phlegmatic* (due to an excess of phlegm – see the 'Introduction and Overview').

These four humours are included in the inner circle of Eysenck's diagram (see Figure 6.1). But unlike Galen's four humours, Eysenck's types are *personality dimensions*, which represent continua along which everyone can be placed.

I suppose Phyllis, being thin, pale and worried-looking, would have been typed as melancholic!

EXTROVERSION (E), NEUROTICISM (N) AND PSYCHOTICISM (P)

Eysenck (1947) factor-analysed 39 items of personal data (including personality ratings) for each of 700 neurotic soldiers, screening them for brain damage and physical illness.

Two uncorrelated factors emerged: *introversion–extroversion* (E) and *neuroticism (emotionality)–stability* (N). These two dimensions are assumed to be normally distributed: most people will score somewhere in the middle of the scale, and very few at either extreme. 'Typical' introverts and extroverts are 'idealised extremes' (or *ideal types*).

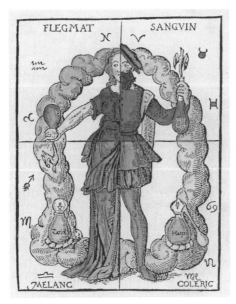 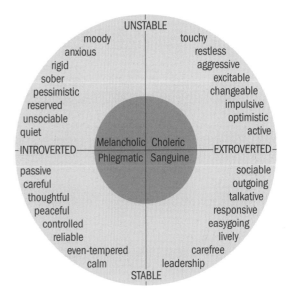

Figure 6.1 Personality has been dissected into component parts for thousands of years; what is interesting is how these ideas relate to the modern concept of personality traits, as shown by Eysenck's dimensions of personality (from Eysenck, 1965)

Box 6.1 Typical introverts and extroverts (Eysenck, 1965)

- The *typical introvert* is a quiet, retiring sort of person, introspective, fond of books rather than people; he's reserved and distant except to intimate friends. He tends to plan ahead, 'looks before he leaps' and distrusts the impulse of the moment. He doesn't like excitement, takes matters of everyday life with proper seriousness, and likes a well-ordered mode of life. He keeps his feelings under close control, seldom behaves in an aggressive manner, and doesn't lose his temper easily. He's reliable, somewhat pessimistic and places great importance on ethical standards.

- The *typical extrovert* is sociable, likes parties, has many friends, needs to have people to talk to, and doesn't like reading or studying by himself. He craves excitement, takes chances, often sticks his neck out, acts on the spur of the moment and is generally an impulsive individual. He likes practical jokes, always has a ready answer, and generally likes change; he's carefree, easy-going, optimistic and likes to 'laugh and be merry'. He prefers to keep moving and doing things, tends to be aggressive and lose his temper quickly; altogether his feelings aren't kept under tight control and he's not always a reliable person.

As regards neuroticism, the typical high N scorer could be described as:

> … an anxious, worrying individual, moody and frequently depressed; he is likely to sleep badly and to suffer from various psychosomatic disorders. He is overly emotional, reacting too strongly to all sorts of stimuli and finds it difficult to get back on an even keel after each emotionally arousing experience. (Eysenck, 1965)

By contrast, the typical low N scorer (stable) individual:

... tends to respond emotionally only slowly and generally weakly and to return to baseline quickly after emotional arousal; he is usually calm, even-tempered, controlled and unworried. (Eysenck, 1965)

A third dimension, *psychoticism* (P) (Eysenck and Eysenck, 1985), has also been identified. This was originally uncovered in a 1952 study of psychiatric patients, but is less well established than the other two dimensions. Just as E and N are unrelated to each other, so they are both unrelated to P. According to Eysenck and Eysenck (1975):

A high [P] scorer ... may be described as being solitary, not caring for people; he is often troublesome, not fitting in anywhere. He may be cruel and inhumane, lacking in feelings and empathy, and altogether insensitive. He is hostile to others, even his own kith and kin, and aggressive, even to loved ones. He has a liking for odd and unusual things, and a disregard for danger; he likes to make fools of other people, and to upset them.

Unlike E and N, P isn't normally distributed – both normals and neurotics score low on P. Eysenck also believes that P overlaps with other psychiatric labels, in particular 'schizoid', 'psychopathic' and 'behaviour disorders'. The difference between normals and psychotics, as well as that between normals and neurotics, is one of *degree* only (see Gross, 2005).

From what I know of her, I'd guess Phyllis is more introvert than extrovert. She spends most of her time reading, apart from when she's doing things for other patients. And I think she'd score higher than normal on the N scale, she's easily agitated, and 'jumpy' if you catch her unawares. To be honest, for a few seconds I was impatient with her anxiety; I'd anticipated being able to complete the medicine round with Adam (who is a good teacher) and I was enjoying the learning experience. But I'm pleased I quickly dismissed the feeling as uncaring.

The biological basis of personality

Eysenck attempts to explain personality differences in terms of the kinds of nervous system individuals inherit.

◎ The main function of the *ascending reticular activating system* (ARAS) is to maintain an optimum level of alertness or 'arousal'. It does this by enhancing the incoming sensory data to the cortex through the excitation of neural impulses, or by 'dampening them down' through inhibition. Extroverts have a 'strong nervous system'. Their ARAS is biased towards the *inhibition* of impulses, with the effect of reducing the intensity of any sensory stimulation reaching the cortex (they're *chronically underaroused*). For introverts, the bias is in the opposite direction: the intensity of any sensory stimulation reaching the cortex is *increased* (they're *chronically overaroused*).

◎ As far as N is concerned, it's the *reactivity* (or *lability*) of the sympathetic branch of the autonomic nervous system that's crucial – in particular, differences in the *limbic system*, which controls the ANS. The person who scores high on N has an ANS that reacts particularly strongly and quickly to stressful situations compared with less emotional or more stable individuals (see Chapter 5).

◎ The biological basis of P is much more uncertain, but Eysenck (1980) has suggested that it may be related to levels of the male hormone, *androgen*, and/or other hormones.

This helps explain why Phyllis sleeps badly – as an introvert, she's chronically over-aroused.

> **Box 6.2 Evidence relating to biological differences between introverts and extroverts**
>
> • According to Eysenck (1970), introverts have lower pain thresholds and extroverts are more susceptible to the adverse effects of sensory deprivation. For example, one demonstration of the 'stimulus hunger' of extroverts is their willingness to go to great lengths to obtain a 'reward' of loud music or bright lights, which introverts work hard to avoid.
>
> • According to Hampson (1995), evidence for the role of the ARAS and arousal mechanisms in E is inconclusive, but great advances have been made since the mid-1980s in understanding the genetics of personality. As a result of large-scale twin, adoption and family resemblance studies, it's now widely concluded that about 50 per cent of the variation in self-report personality measures may be due to heredity (Loehlin *et al*., 1988). (But see Gross, 2005, for a discussion of the limitations of family resemblance, twin and adoption studies.)

We're taught pain is an intensely individual experience. Eysenck's ARAS theory is a convincing explanation of different pain thresholds. It means Phyllis could be more likely to need analgesics than someone with an extrovert personality.

Drugs and personality

According to Wilson (1976), we'd expect introverts to be more difficult to sedate using a drug such as sodium amytal, because they're supposed to be more aroused. A particularly powerful technique involves *sedation/sleep threshold*, in which a barbiturate (which depresses the CNS) is injected by continuous infusion until the participants either go to sleep or reach some specified level of drowsiness (defined behaviourally or physiologically). The amount of drug needed is a measure of tolerance of sedation (Claridge and Davis, 2003).

Using this method, it's repeatedly been shown that anxiety (clinically diagnosed) neurotics, and their 'normal' (non-clinical) counterparts (introverted neurotics or *dysthymics*) show extremely high drug tolerance (resistance to sedation) (Claridge and Herrington, 1960, 1962). Both groups were much more difficult to sedate than extroverted neurotics (*hysterics*), who are more easily sedated than normal participants (who score in the middle ranges on E and N).

Although nearly 50 years old, these studies still represent a valid observation about biology and the pharmacology of personality and psychological disorders (Claridge and Davis, 2003).

This is further evidence that could explain why Phyllis sleeps badly. It seems a 'normal' amount of night sedation is inadequate for her particular needs.

For the same reasons, regardless of an individual's normal position on the scale, *stimulant* drugs should shift behaviour in the direction of introversion, while depressant drugs (such as alcohol) should have the opposite effect.

ASK YOURSELF ...

• In terms of introverted and extroverted behaviour, what should be the effect of (a) stimulant and (b) depressant drugs (see Chapter 7)?

• Who should be easier to sedate – introverts or extroverts?

Anxiolytic (*anti-anxiety*) drugs should increase emotional stability, *adrenergic* drugs (those that mimic the effects of adrenaline) should decrease it, *hallucinogens* should increase psychotic behaviour and *anti-psychotic* drugs (*narcoleptics*) should decrease it. According to Eysenck (1995), empirical studies have, on the whole, supported these causal hypotheses.

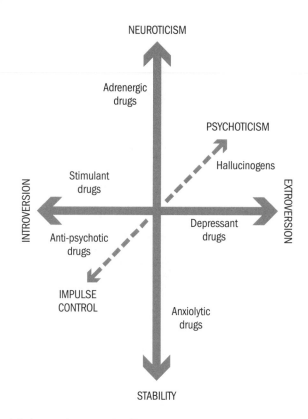

Figure 6.2 Drug addiction and personality (Eysenck, 1983). Source Eysenck, H.J. (1995) 'Trait theories of personality'. In S.E. Hampson & A.M. Coleman (Eds) *Individual Differences and Personality*. London, Pearson Education

Eysenck's theory and health

◎ According to Claridge and Davis (2003), Eysenck can take most of the credit for the *dimensional* approach to understanding psychological disorders. In using FA to identify the basic dimensions of *normal* personality, he always had in mind the need to describe and explain the *abnormal*. He believed that the various psychological disorders recognised in psychiatry actually define the *extremes* of his personality dimensions.

◎ Eysenck's view was that disorders *aren't* diseases in the medical sense. Rather, they're *behavioural* disturbances, an exaggerated form of response patterns that characterise the personality dimensions. For example, anxiety neurotics are the clinical counterparts of individuals high on N and I. While he was quite successful in mapping N onto *neurosis*, he was less successful in mapping P onto *psychosis*. The question is still open as to whether P has anything to do with psychosis at all. It seems

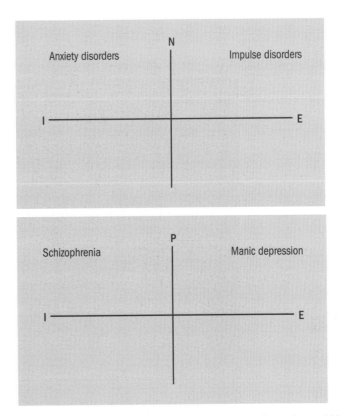

Figure 6.3 Eysenck's location of non-psychotic disorders in two dimensions of N/I-E (top) and psychotic disorders in two dimensions of P/I-E (bottom) (from Claridge & Davis, 2003)

to be more relevant to psychopathic and other anti-social behaviours than to psychotic disorders such as schizophrenia (Claridge and Davis, 2003).

◎ According to Wood (1988), the one basic mistake that researchers have made is to look for links between *specific* personality patterns (say, aggression or emotional suppression) and *particular* diseases: 'Perhaps personality is more like diet. If it is not good then you may be more susceptible to a whole range of different complaints, not just, say, breast cancer or coronary thrombosis.'

◎ Friedman and Booth-Kewley (1987, in Wood, 1988) examined hundreds of studies of personality and disease. They concluded that people who are anxious, depressed and hostile may be prone to problems such as asthma and arthritis, and not just to heart disease. Instead of simply being 'coronary prone' or 'cancer prone', there may be a 'disease prone' personality that arises when a series of negative emotions occurs in the same person at the same time. And what may underlie this 'disease-prone personality' is the most deep-seated personality factor of all – namely, emotional stability (Eysenck's N).

◎ At one extreme are people who remain calm even in the face of near disaster; at the other are those who react to even mild stresses with fear, anxiety, nervousness or anger. These emotions cause mental paralysis, preventing the person from doing what's necessary to deal with the situation. But this lack of emotional balance or resilience also has consequences for physical health. For example, emotionally unstable people report more symptoms, such as neurotic men with clean coronary arteries feeling more chest pain than more stable men whose arteries really are blocked (Bass and Wade, 1984, in Wood, 1988).

CRITICAL DISCUSSION 6.1 Personality and smoking

- According to Cohen (1979, in Furnham and Heaven, 1999), personality may either represent a specific and direct causal factor in disease or it mediates/buffers the effect of causal factors. A third possibility is that personality factors influence certain types of health-related behaviours, which are either health-promoting or detrimental to health (see Chapter 4). An example of the latter is smoking.

- Smoking is an important lifestyle factor associated with CHD, as well as lung and throat cancers. Because smoking is (to some degree) a voluntary behaviour (see Chapter 7), its role in heart disease assumes an additional interest for personality psychologists: how do smokers and non-smokers differ (Furnham and Heaven, 1999)?

- Furnham and Heaven cite evidence that smokers have higher E scores than non-smokers and, as E scores rise, so does cigarette consumption. One study found that smoking was associated with E, impulsiveness and sensation-seeking. Another reported that both E and N correlated with smoking, with deep inhalers forming the most neurotic group. Male smokers had higher average E scores than female smokers.

- One Canadian study (Patton et al., 1993, in Furnham and Heaven, 1999) also found that current smokers (as opposed to those who'd never smoked and quitters) scored high on P. But female smokers were significantly higher on P than any of the other groups.

- However, personality variables such as E, N and P may be only three of a much longer list of factors that predict smoking (particularly among young people), such as peer pressure and conformity to group norms (see Chapter 12), having parents who smoke, school performance, self-esteem and the 'status' afforded by smoking (Furnham and Heaven, 1999).

Phyllis smokes. 'Only two or three a day,' she said when assessed: 'I'm a worrier and I can't give it up.' The N element?

CATTELL'S TRAIT THEORY

Cattell's factors are source *traits*, which he believed to be the fundamental dimensions of personality, the underlying roots or causes of clusters of behaviour (surface traits). Whereas surface traits may correspond to common-sense ways of describing behaviour and may sometimes be measured by simple observation, they're actually the result of interactions among the source traits. Valid explanations of behaviour must concentrate on source traits as the structural factors that determine personality.

Cattell identified three sources of data relevant to personality.

1. *L-data* (L for 'life') refer to ratings by observers. Cattell regarded these as the best source, but he also recognised that they're notoriously difficult to obtain; great skill and time are needed to make accurate ratings.

2. *Q-data* (Q for 'questionnaire') refer to scores on personality questionnaires. His 16 factors (source traits) are measured by the widely used *Cattell 16 PF* (personality factor)

questionnaire, which is intended for use with adults (see Table 6.1). This isn't exclusively of the 'yes/no' variety (there may be three choices – yes/occasionally/no).

3. *T-data* (T for 'tests') refer to objective tests specially devised to measure personality, such as galvanic skin response/GSR (a measure of anxiety) and reaction time. T-data are objective, primarily in the sense that the purpose of the test is concealed from the participant.

Table 6.1 The 16 source traits measured by Cattell's 16 PF questionnaire (based on Cattell, 1965)

Description	Name of trait	Description
Warm-hearted, outgoing, easy-going, sociable	**A** Affectia vs Sizia	Reserved, cool, detached, aloof
Abstract thinker, intellectual interests [high score]	**B** Intelligence	Concrete thinker, practically minded [low score]
Emotionally stable, calm, mature	**C** Ego strength vs Dissatisfied emotionality	Emotionally unstable, easily upset, immature
Assertive, aggressive, dominant, competitive	**E** Dominance vs Submissiveness	Submissive, modest, mild, accommodating
Happy-go-lucky, enthusiastic	**F** Surgency vs Desurgency	Pessimistic, subdued, sober, cautious, serious
Persevering, conscientious, moralistic [high score]	**G** Superego strength	Expedient, disregard for rules, law unto oneself [low score]
Adventurous, gregarious, uninhibited	**H** Parmia vs Threctia	Shy, timid, diffident, inhibited
Tender-minded, sensitive, gentle, clinging	**I** Premsia vs Harria	Tough-minded, self-reliant, realistic, no-nonsense
Suspicious, jealous, self-opinionated	**L** Protension vs Alexia	Trusting, adaptable, easy to get along with
Unconventional, imaginative, bohemian	**M** Autia vs Praxernia	Conformist, conventional, influenced by external realities
Shrewd, calculating, worldly	**N** Shrewdness vs Naivety	Simple, unpretentious, lacking insight

Table 6.1 *continued*

Description	Name of trait	Description
Insecure, worrying, self-reproaching [high score]	**O** Guilt proneness	Self-assured, confident, complacent, spirited [low score]
Liberal, free-thinking	**Q1** Radicalism vs Conservatism	Conservative, traditional
Preference for own decisions	**Q2** Self-sufficiency vs Group dependence	Group dependent, a follower
Controlled, socially precise [high score]	**Q3** Self-sentiment Strength	Undisciplined, careless of social rules [low score]
Relaxed, composed [high score]	**Q4** Ergic tension	Overwrought, tense, frustrated [low score]

DIFFERENCES BETWEEN CATTELL AND EYSENCK

◎ Cattell believes there's a fundamental *discontinuity* between normals and, say, schizophrenics – that is, there's a *qualitative* difference between them (and not merely a quantitative one, as Eysenck maintains).

◎ Cattell, much more than Eysenck, acknowledges how behaviour can fluctuate in response to situational factors. His definition of personality as that which 'determines behaviour in a defined situation and a defined mood' (Cattell, 1965) implies that behaviour is never totally determined by source traits. Although personality factors remain fairly stable over time, they constitute only one kind of variable influencing overt behaviour. Others include (a) *mood and state factors* (e.g. depression, arousal, anxiety, fatigue and intoxication), and (b) *motivational factors* (innate, biological drives and culturally acquired drives).

Phyllis probably was made more anxious by thinking she was delaying me. This is consistent with Cattell's recognition that mood, motivation and situational factors can influence behaviour.

Personality and the nurse

Gosling (1995) cites a study by Lewis (1983) of almost 1000 British student nurses. They differed from a comparison group of undergraduates in the following ways:

◎ female nurses scored higher on Factor F and lower on Q1 – they were more spontaneous and quick to act, but less inventive and creative

◎ male nurses scored higher on G (they were more conscientious) and lower on N (less socially analytical and shrewd)

◎ those who completed their training were more socially confident, self-confident and more group-orientated (Factors H, O and Q1) compared with those who didn't.

ASK YOURSELF ...
- Which of Cattell's source traits do you think are of particular importance in nursing?

- Are these different for female and male nurses?

Perhaps it's not surprising that these characteristics may be necessary to successfully complete the initial years of training; nursing isn't only about the application of procedures, but is also about caring for people and being able to relate effectively as a professional to other professionals in a caring environment (Gosling, 1995). UK nursing tutors rated interpersonal qualities ('good communication skills', 'being a good listener', 'ability to get on with people') as more important than intellectual ones when considering the suitability of applicants for both traditional and Project 2000 courses (Cater, 1993, in Gosling, 1995).

Would psychometric testing help in nurse selection? It's used in many other professions. However, I know I've learned caring skills, like quickly recognising distress such as Phyllis showed, and how to respond to patients' anxiety; it's made me calmer and more confident.

MULTI-TRAIT THEORIES AND THE 'BIG FIVE'

Eysenck's and Cattell's theories are examples of *multi-trait theories*. Multi-trait theories try to include all aspects of personality and assume that individual differences can be described in terms of a particular profile on the same set of traits. Since the 1980s, there's been a vast amount of research to discover a small but comprehensive number of basic trait dimensions that can account for the structure of personality and individual differences.

There's a growing consensus that personality can adequately be described by five broad constructs or factors, commonly referred to as the 'big five' (see Table 6.2) (Costa and McCrae, 1992; Digman, 1990; Goldberg, 1993; McCrae and Costa, 1989).

Table 6.2 The 'big five' personality factors

	Desirable traits	**Undesirable traits**
(I) Extroversion (corresponds to Eysenck's construct)	Outgoing, sociable, assertive	Introverted, reserved, passive
(II) Agreeableness	Kind, trusting, warm	Hostile, selfish, cold
(III) Conscientiousness	Organised, thorough, tidy	Careless, unreliable, sloppy
(IV) Emotional stability (or **neuroticism**) (corresponds to Eysenck's construct)	Calm, even-tempered, imperturbable	Moody, temperamental, narrow
(V) Intellect/openness to experience	Imaginative, intelligent, creative	Shallow, unsophisticated, imperceptive

Eysenck's types are still two of the big five!

HUMANISTIC THEORIES (ROGERS AND MASLOW)

Humanistic theories have their philosophical roots in *phenomenology* and *existentialism*, and some would say they're more 'philosophical' than 'psychological'. They're concerned with characteristics that are distinctively and uniquely human, in particular experience, uniqueness, meaning, freedom and choice. We have first-hand experience of ourselves as people, and Rogers' theory in particular is centred around the self-concept (see Chapter 16 and Gross, 2005).

What Rogers and Maslow have in common is their positive evaluation of human nature, a belief in the individual's potential for personal growth (*self-actualisation*). But while Maslow's theory is commonly referred to as a 'psychology of being' (self-actualisation is an end in itself and lies at the peak of his *hierarchy of needs*), Rogers' is a 'psychology of becoming' (it focuses on the *process* of becoming a 'fully functioning person').

I needed to remind myself (see Chapter 1) that phenomenology means how we individually (subjectively) experience what happens, and existentialism is the belief that individuals are free and responsible for their own development. These are the basic principles of individualistic care and patient autonomy!

MASLOW'S HIERARCHY OF NEEDS (HoN)

Although Maslow's focus on needs makes it relevant to motivation, his theory is commonly discussed in relation to personality. (The book in which he first proposed his hierarchy of needs (HoN) was *Motivation and Personality*, 1954). He believes that human beings are subject to quite different sets of motivational states or forces:

◎ those that ensure survival by satisfying basic physical and psychological needs (physiological, safety, love and belongingness, and esteem – *deficiency* or *D-motives*), and

◎ those that promote the person's self-actualisation – realising one's full potential, 'becoming everything that one is capable of becoming' (Maslow, 1970), especially in the intellectual and creative domains (*growth*, *being* or *B-motives*).

As Maslow states: 'We share the need for food with all living things, the need for love with (perhaps) the higher apes, [and] the need for Self-Actualisation with [no other species].'

Behaviours that relate to survival or deficiency needs are engaged in because they satisfy those needs (a *means to an end*). But those that relate to self-actualisation are engaged in for their own sake, because they're intrinsically satisfying. The latter include the fulfilment of ambitions, the acquisition of admired skills, the steady increase of understanding about people, the universe or oneself, the development of creativeness in a particular field or, most important, simply the ambition to be a good human being. It's simply inaccurate to speak in such instances of tension reduction, which implies the overcoming of an annoying state, for these states aren't annoying (Maslow, 1968).

The hierarchical nature of Maslow's theory is intended to highlight the following points:

◎ Needs lower down must be satisfied before we can attend to needs higher up. For example, if you're reading this while you're hungry, tired or in pain, you probably won't absorb much about Maslow. You can probably think of exceptions, such as the mountain climber who risks his/her life for the sake of adventure (what Maslow would call a 'peak' experience – if you'll forgive the pun!).

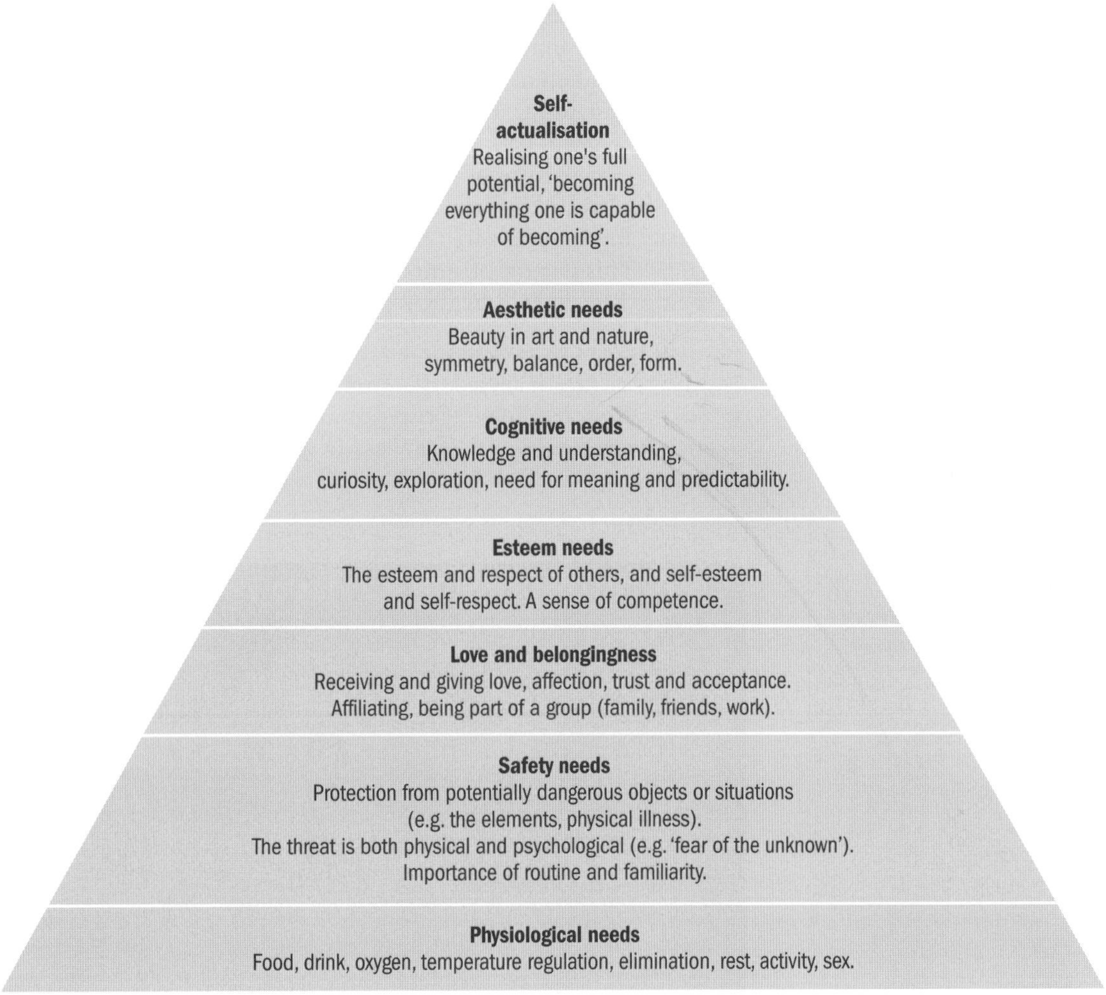

Figure 6.4 Maslow's hierarchy of needs (based on Maslow, 1954)

> **ASK YOURSELF ...**
> - Do you believe Maslow's hierarchy is a useful way of thinking about human motivation and individual differences?
>
> - Has he omitted any important needs?
>
> - To what extent might the hierarchy reflect the culture and historical period in which Maslow lived and wrote?
>
> - How relevant/useful is it when applied to nursing theory and practice?

◎ Higher-level needs are a later evolutionary development: in the development of the human species (*phylogenesis*), self-actualisation is a fairly recent need. This applies equally to the development of the individual (*ontogenesis*): babies are much more concerned with their bellies than with their brains. But it's always a case of one need *predominating* at any one time, *not* excluding all other needs.

◎ The higher up the hierarchy we go, the more the need becomes linked to life experience and the less 'biological' it is. Individuals will achieve self-actualisation through different activities and by different routes: 'A musician must make music, an artist must paint, a poet must write, if he is to be ultimately at peace with himself. What a man can be, he must be' (Maslow, 1968). This captures nicely the idiographic nature of Maslow's theory (see above).

◎ The higher up the hierarchy we go, the more difficult it becomes to achieve the need. Many human goals are remote and long-term, and can be achieved only in a series of steps. This pursuit of aims/goals that lie very much in the future is unique to human beings, although individuals differ in their ability to set and realise such goals.

Phyllis, like most patients in acute care, is probably more concerned with D-motives now. But her poor health obviously affects her B-motives, the quality of her life. Her arthritic knees and general lack of energy prevent her being so actively involved in the church charity work she enjoys. She likes to go to the chapel each day and looks forward to her visit from the hospital chaplain.

ASK YOURSELF ...

• Do you agree with Torrance and Jordan's view of nursing theory and practice?

• Give your reasons. (It might be useful to look back over Chapters 3 and 5, where a variety of evidence is given suggesting that even lower-level (deficit) needs – and how nurses might help patients satisfy them – should be understood in a broader context than the 'skin' of the individual patient.)

CRITICAL DISCUSSION 6.2 Maslow's hierarchy of needs and nursing

• According to Torrance and Jordan (1995), Maslow's account of human needs emphasises the central role for the biological sciences in nursing theory and practice.

• Nurses encounter individuals with ill health and disease on a daily basis and therefore clinical nursing practice is moulded around the individual's physiological and psychological responses to these health problems.

• Although nursing practice clearly has a role beyond illness (e.g. health education and promotion), its main focus remains with people who are ill.

• Torrance and Jordan argue that, in the broader view, nursing aims to help with both deficit and growth needs, but it has to ensure that immediate physiological and safety needs are met. If the nurse/patient relationship is effective in meeting these basic needs, it can then offer assistance in meeting higher-level needs.

• However, it does appear that people become patients because illness interferes with their ability to meet the lower-level needs from their own resources.

Models of nursing (such as Roper-Logan-Tierney) ensure we meet Phyllis's biological and safety needs by assessing her basic activities of living and her degree of dependency. But they also address higher levels of the hierarchy, i.e., to consider Phyllis as an individual, her psychological and social needs, and her developmental progress. I recognise her high anxiety levels are a significant element in her care.

PSYCHOANALYTIC THEORY (FREUD)

As we saw in Chapter 2, *psychodynamic* implies the active forces within the personality that motivate behaviour, in particular the unconscious conflict between the id, ego and superego. Freud's was the first of this kind of theory and all psychodynamic theories stem, more or less directly, from Freud's *psychoanalytic theory*.

THE PSYCHIC APPARATUS

Freud believed that the personality (or *psychic apparatus*) comprises three parts: the id, ego and superego (see Figure 6.5).

◎ The *id* 'contains everything that is inherited, that is present at birth, that is laid down in the constitution – above all, therefore, the instincts' (Freud, 1923/1984). The wishes and impulses arising from the body's needs build up a pressure or tension (*excitation*), which demands immediate release or satisfaction. Since the id's sole aim is to reduce excitation to a minimum, it is said to be governed by the *pleasure principle*. It is – and remains – the infantile, presocialised part of the personality. The two major id instincts are sexuality and aggression (see Gross, 2005).

◎ The *ego* is 'that part of the id which has been modified by the direct influence of the external world' (Freud, 1923/1984). It can be thought of as the 'executive' of the personality, the planning, decision-making, rational and logical part of us. It enables us to distinguish between a wish and reality (which the id cannot do), and is governed by the *reality principle*. While the id demands immediate gratification of our needs and impulses, the ego will postpone satisfaction until the appropriate time and place (*deferred gratification*). The 'ego represents ... reason and common sense, in contrast to the id, which contains the passions' (Freud, 1923/1984).

◎ Not until the *superego* has developed can we be described as moral beings. It represents the *internalisation* of parental and social moral values: 'It observes the ego, gives it orders, judges it and threatens it with punishment, exactly like the parents whose place it has taken' (Freud, 1933). It is in fact the *conscience* that threatens the ego with punishment (in the form of guilt) for bad behaviour, while the *ego-ideal* promises the ego rewards (in the form of pride and high self-esteem) for good behaviour. These correspond to punishing and rewarding parents, respectively.

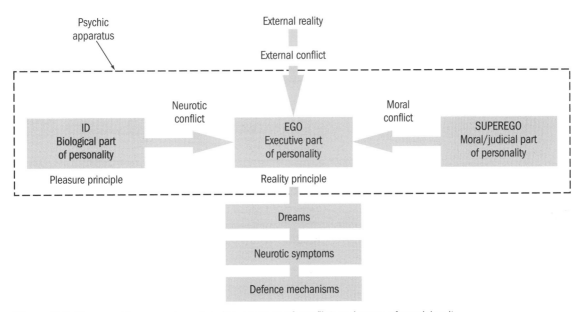

Figure 6.5 The psychic apparatus, showing sources of conflict and ways of resolving it

Most of the time I'm compromising between what I want to do and what I should do! Phyllis's anxiety frustrated my self-seeking wish (id) to complete the medicine round with Adam. But my conscience told me I was being selfish and should put Phyllis's needs first (superego). After a few minutes I (ego) fetched two spoons and crushed the remaining tablets, and she took them with some mashed banana. She was so pleased, it made me feel guilty I'd resented her! (Superego again.)

Freud believed that conflict within the personality is unavoidable, because the ego is being 'pulled' in two opposing directions by the id and the superego. The ego's solution comes in the shape of three forms of compromise, namely *dreams* and *neurotic symptoms* (see Gross, 2005), and *defence mechanisms*.

DEFENCE MECHANISMS

The *ego defence mechanisms* are, by definition, unconscious, and this is partly what makes them effective. They involve some degree of self-deception, which, in turn, is related to their distortion of 'reality' (both internal and external). This prevents us from being overwhelmed by temporary threats or traumas, and can provide 'breathing space' in which to come to terms with conflict or find alternative ways of coping. As short-term measures, defence mechanisms are advantageous, necessary and 'normal', but as long-term solutions to life's problems they're usually regarded as unhealthy and undesirable (see Chapter 5, page 97).

Table 6.3 Some major ego defence mechanisms

Name of defence mechanism	Description	Example(s)
Repression	Forcing a threatening or distressing memory/feeling/ wish out of consciousness and making it unconscious	A five-year-old child repressing its incestuous desire for the opposite-sex parent
Displacement	Transferring our feelings from their true target onto a harmless, substitute target (e.g. 'kicking the cat')	Frustration caused by problems at work expressed as domestic violence; phobias
Denial	Failing/refusing to acknowledge/perceive some aspect of reality	Refusing to accept that you have a serious illness, or that your partner is going off you
Rationalisation	Finding an acceptable excuse (a 'cover story') for some really quite unacceptable behaviour/ situation	'Being cruel to be kind'; 'I only did it because I love you'

Table 6.3 *continued*

Name of defence mechanism	Description	Example(s)
Reaction-formation	Consciously feeling/thinking the opposite of your true (unconscious) feelings/thoughts	Being considerate/polite to someone you strongly dislike – even going out of your way to be nice to them
Sublimation	A form of displacement in which a (socially positive) substitute activity is found for expressing some unacceptable impulse	Playing sport to redirect aggressive urges
Identification	Incorporating/introjecting another person into one's own personality – making them part of oneself	Identification with the aggressor (boys)/anaclitic identification (girls) (see Gross, 2005)
Projection	Displacing your own unacceptable feelings/characteristics onto someone else	'I hate you' becomes (through reversal of subject/object) 'you hate me'
Regression	Reverting to behaviour characteristic of an earlier stage of development	Losing your temper, comfort eating, sleeping more when depressed
Isolation	Separating contradictory thoughts/feelings into 'logic-tight' compartments	Talking about some traumatic experience without any display of emotion – or even giggling about it

Some of these are very familiar tactics that I recognise I – and others – use! Phyllis hadn't repressed the memory of those mealtimes, but she seems to have repressed her emotion about what must have been a traumatic experience, repeated many times. She didn't appear distressed – in fact, she joked about it. This is an example of a defence mechanism: isolating an emotion to stop it hurting. She also says she isn't worried about the cause of her anaemia, which is probably denial. I first observed this when caring for Gail, a young terminally ill patient (see my diary entry in Chapter 20, page 372 and comments pages 374–375).

LEVELS OF CONSCIOUSNESS

According to Freud, thoughts, memories and other psychic material could operate at one of three levels: *conscious*, *pre-conscious* and *unconscious*. What we're consciously aware of at any one time represents the mere tip of an iceberg – most of our thoughts and ideas are either not accessible at that moment (pre-conscious) or are totally inaccessible (unconscious), unless special techniques such as free association and dream interpretation are used (see Gross, 2005).

The ego represents the conscious part of the mind, together with some aspects of the superego (namely, those moral rules and values we are able to express in words). The unconscious comprises: (a) id impulses; (b) all repressed material; (c) the unconscious part of the ego (the part involved in dream work, neurotic symptoms and defence mechanisms); and (d) part of the superego (for example, the vague feelings of guilt or shame that are difficult to account for). Freud depicted the unconscious as a *dynamic force* and not a mere 'dustbin' for all those thoughts and feelings that are too weak to force themselves into awareness. This is best illustrated by the process of repression (Thomas, 1985).

According to Freud, in the absence of a physical cause, Phyllis's poor appetite and insomnia might be the product of unconscious (repressed) feelings from her traumatic childhood. However, no one would presume that. The stroking of her leg is a neurotic symptom.

Psychic determinism

Much of our behaviour (and our thoughts and feelings) has *multiple* causes, some conscious, some unconscious. Freud called this *overdetermination*. By definition, we know only about the conscious causes, which we normally take to be the reasons for our actions. But if some of the causes are also unconscious, then the reasons we give for our behaviour can never tell the whole story (and the unconscious causes may be the more important). This means that we don't know ourselves as well as we'd like, or as well as we think we do ('irrational man').

Overdetermination is one aspect of *psychic determinism* – the view that all behaviour is purposive or goal-directed and that everything we do, think and feel has a cause. It follows that so-called 'accidents' (things that 'just happen') do have a cause after all – and the cause may actually turn out to be the 'victim'. For instance, the 'accident-prone' person isn't an unfortunate victim of circumstances, but is unconsciously bringing the accidents about – perhaps in an attempt to punish him/herself in some way. While not denying the existence of events that lie beyond people's control, Freud believed that it's more common for an 'accident' to be the consequence of our own, unconscious wishes and motives.

Freud's ideas make me suspect that the experiences of Phyllis's childhood have something to do with why she can't swallow her tablets.

AN EVALUATION OF FREUD'S THEORY

Is the theory scientific?

Popper's criticism that Freud's theory is *unfalsifiable* and, therefore, unscientific, is discussed in Chapter 2. However, it would be a serious mistake to regard *reaction formation* (the example used by Popper) as typifying Freudian theory, and the sheer volume of research suggests that Freudian theory cannot be dismissed as lightly as Popper and Eysenck would like on the grounds of it being 'unscientific'. According to

Kline (1989), the view adopted by almost all experimental psychologists involved in the study of Freud's theory is that it should be seen as a collection of hypotheses. As Fisher and Greenberg (1977) argue, some of these hypotheses will turn out to be true, others false, when put to Popper's test of falsifiability.

Some hypotheses are undoubtedly more critical to the overall theory than others. For example, if no evidence could be found for repression, this would alter considerably the nature of psychoanalysis (Kline, 1989).

Freud obtained his 'data' from his work as a psychoanalyst with emotionally disturbed patients. The case study relies on the reconstruction of childhood events and, as used by Freud, is generally considered to be the least scientific of all empirical methods used by psychologists (see Chapter 1). It's open to many types of distortion and uncontrolled influences (see Gross, 2005).

How representative were Freud's patients?

One of the standard criticisms made of Freud's database is that his patients were mainly wealthy, middle-class Jewish females, living in Vienna at the turn of the twentieth century. This makes them highly unrepresentative of the population to whom his theories were generalised. If these people were also neurotic, how can we be sure that what Freud discovered about them is true of 'normal' individuals? However, Freud regarded neurosis as continuous with normal behaviour – that is, neurotics are suffering only from *more extreme* versions of problems experienced by all of us (see Eysenck's theory, above).

More serious, perhaps, is the criticism that Freud studied only adults (with the very dubious exception of 'Little Hans' – see Gross, 2005) and yet he put forward a theory of personality development. How many steps removed were his data from his theory? According to Thomas (1985), the analyst interprets, through his or her theoretical 'lens', ostensibly symbolic material derived from the reported dreams, memories, and so on, of neurotics about apparent experiences stemming from their childhood one or more decades earlier. However, this in itself doesn't invalidate the theory – it merely makes the study of children all the more necessary.

 So Freud's work was based on retrospective case histories of non-representative samples, and he put forward a theory of childhood based on studies of adults. He broke all the 'scientific' rules!

The nature of Freudian theory

Freud's theory has great hermeneutic strength – that is, it provides methods and concepts that enable us to interpret and 'unpack' underlying meanings (Stevens, 1995; see also Chapter 2). Stevens claims that: 'Although Freud wanted to create a nomothetic theory … in effect he finished up with a set of "hermeneutic tools" – concepts and techniques that help us to interpret underlying meanings …'

There's no doubting the tremendous impact that Freud has had, both within psychology and outside it. The fertility of psychoanalytic theory, in terms of the debate, research and theorising it has generated, makes it one of the richest in the whole of psychology. According to Kline (1989): '… Freudian theory is still a powerful intellectual force. To claim that it is dead, as do many experimental psychologists – at least by implication for it rarely influences their thinking – must be either ignorance or wishful thinking.'

Kline argues that Freudian theory is still useful; is it because he helps us answer the 'why' questions? It doesn't please the behaviourists, who prefer more scientific methods – but then neither do the idiographic, qualitative approaches used frequently in nursing research. Maslow and Freud's theories show us how an understanding of the motivations and life experience of patients contributes to their better care.

I noted Phyllis's difficulty (and the solution) on her care plan; I also discussed it with Adam, and he's requested that her medications be written up as liquids. By staying with Phyllis today, I learned something valuable about taking, as well as giving, medications – and Adam's promised I can do the round again with him tomorrow!

CHAPTER SUMMARY

◎ The **psychometric** theories of Eysenck and Cattell are **nomothetic**, while the **humanistic** theories of Maslow and Rogers are **idiographic**. Freud's **psychoanalytic theory** has elements of both.

◎ Eysenck uses the term 'type' for sets of correlated traits or **personality dimensions**, specifically **introversion–extroversion** (E) and **neuroticism–stability** (N), which are both normally distributed, and **psychoticism** (P), which isn't.

◎ E and N are widely accepted as being reliable and valid, but there's much more doubt about P.

◎ Extroverts are chronically **underaroused**, while introverts are chronically **overaroused**. Compared with low N scorers, the sympathetic branch of the ANS reacts particularly strongly to stressful situations in high N scorers. The biological basis of P is much more uncertain, but male hormones may be involved.

◎ Compared with Eysenck, Cattell acknowledges the influence of situational factors on behaviour, as well as mood and state factors, and motivational factors.

◎ There's a growing consensus that personality can adequately be described by five broad constructs/factors (the '**big five**'), namely **extroversion**, **agreeableness**, **conscientiousness**, **neuroticism/emotional stability** and **intelligence/openness to experience**.

◎ **Humanistic theories** are rooted in **phenomenology** and **existentialism**, and are concerned with uniquely human characteristics, including **self-actualisation**.

◎ Maslow's **hierarchy of needs** distinguishes survival, deficiency or **D-motives** and growth, being or **B-motives**.

◎ Freud's **psychoanalytic theory** was the original **psychodynamic** theory, in which unconscious motivating forces play a central role. **Dreams**, **neurotic symptoms** and **defence mechanisms** represent three types of **compromise** through which the ego tries to meet the conflicting demands of the id and superego.

◎ **Defence mechanisms** involve some degree of **self-deception** and **distortion of reality** that, in the short term, prevent us from being overwhelmed by anxiety. But, as long-term solutions, they're unhealthy and undesirable.

◎ Our behaviour is **overdetermined** (one aspect of **psychic determinism**).

◎ Although Freud intended to produce a nomothetic theory, his work can be thought of as a set of **hermeneutic tools** that help to interpret underlying **meanings**. Although this kind of theory is difficult to test empirically, it has influenced our everyday understanding of ourselves.

SUBSTANCE USE AND ABUSE

7

INTRODUCTION AND OVERVIEW

In the context of hospitals and doctors' surgeries, a drug is normally understood to mean a medicine ('pills'/'tablets') and is assumed to be beneficial. According to the World Health Organization (WHO, in Sykes, 1995), a drug is 'any substance or product that is used or intended to be used to modify or explore physiological systems or pathological states for the benefit of the recipient'.

However, for thousands of years, people have taken substances to alter their perception of reality and societies have restricted the substances their members are allowed to take. These substances, which we usually call drugs, are *psychoactive*, denoting a chemical substance that alters conscious awareness through its effect on the brain. Most drugs fit this definition. Some – for example, aspirin – are *indirectly* psychoactive: their primary purpose is to remove pain, but being headache-free lifts our mood. Others, however, are *designed* to change mood and behaviour. These are collectively referred to as *psychotherapeutic* drugs, such as those used in the treatment of anxiety, depression and schizophrenia (see Gross, 2005).

This chapter is concerned with psychoactive drugs used to produce a temporarily altered state of consciousness for the purpose of *pleasure*. These include *recreational drugs*, which have no legal restrictions (such as alcohol, nicotine and caffeine) and *drugs of abuse*, which are illegal. However, just as recreational drugs can be abused (such as alcohol), so illegal drugs are taken recreationally (such as ecstasy). 'Substance abuse', therefore, doesn't imply particular types of drug, but refers to the extent to which the drug is used and the effects – emotional, behavioural and medical – on the abuser.

What counts as a recreational drug or a drug of abuse changes over time within a particular society, as well as between societies. For example, cocaine had been freely available over the counter in a huge variety of tonics and pick-me-ups before the 1930s, and was an ingredient of the original blend of Coca-Cola in the 1890s. At that time, it was seen as a harmless stimulant (Plant, 1999); now it's a Class A drug. Conversely, in the UK cannabis was reclassified in 2004 from a Class B to a Class C drug (still illegal but seen as less dangerous and carrying a more lenient, if any, punishment).

According to Veitia and McGahee (1995):

> Cigarette smoking and alcohol abuse permeate our culture and are widespread enough to be considered ordinary addictions ... The degree to which these drugs permeate our culture and the extent to which they are accepted by our society distinguish them from other addictive but illegal substances such as heroin.

From my diary (13): Year 2/Medical Ward

Mr Bates (Brian) is a 50-year-old man who is alcohol dependent and has a cirrhotic liver and ascites. Adam, my mentor, knows Brian well as he appears at about six-monthly intervals with haematemesis and/or malaena. When I helped admit him, Brian looked thin, pale, sweaty, dyspnoeic and was in obvious discomfort; an abdominal paracentesis was planned for an hour later. He was given oxygen; a blood transfusion and IV fluids were started. Adam inserted a naso-gastric tube. As we needed to monitor Brian's fluid balance and he was unable to pass urine into a urinal, the HO told Brian he must have an indwelling catheter. Brian became agitated and then very aggressive, shouting that he 'couldn't stand any more tubes' when the doctor tried to persuade him. Adam asked the doctor to leave the problem with him and gradually talked Brian into a calmer mood. We then helped him out of bed (with some difficulty) and on to a commode to pass urine.

> **ASK YOURSELF ...**
> • What do you understand by the term 'addiction'?

DEFINING ABUSE

THE CONCEPT OF ADDICTION

Until recently, the study and treatment of drug problems were organised around the concept of *addiction*: people with drug problems have problems because they're addicted to the drug (Hammersley, 1999). Addicts are compelled by a physiological need to continue taking the drug, experience horrible physical and psychological symptoms when trying to stop, and will continue taking it despite these symptoms because of their addictive need. Their addiction will also change them psychologically for the worse, they will commit crimes to pay for the drug, neglect their social roles and responsibilities, and even harm the people around them. In addition, some drugs are considered inherently much more addictive than others (see below), and substance users can be divided into addicts and non-addicts.

Criticisms of the concept

◎ It's an oversimplification. Most professionals who deal with people with any kind of problem – medical, criminal, educational, social – will have seen many clients who aren't exactly addicts, but whose drug use seems to have contributed to, or worsened, their other problems (Hammersley, 1999).

◎ It's based on the *addiction-as-disease model*. While medical models such as this are generally persuasive, because they offer a diagnosis, a definition and a pathology, they also appear to relieve the 'addict' of responsibility for his/her behaviour (Baker, 2000). This is discussed further below, in relation to alcohol dependence (see pages 128–130).

It seems to be accepted by Brian and the nurses that his primary diagnosis is 'alcoholism' (i.e. he's addicted to the recreational, and legal, drug of alcohol).

According to Hammersley (1999), the more modern view is to see drug problems as two-fold: *substance abuse* and *substance dependence* (hence the title of this chapter). This view is adopted in the American Psychiatric Association's (2000) *Diagnostic and Statistical Manual of Mental Disorders* (DSM-IV-TR – see Boxes 7.1 and 7.2). 'Addiction' is now usually used to refer to a field of study covering substance use, abuse and dependence, rather than to a theory of why people become dependent.

ASK YOURSELF ...
- What do terms such as 'workaholic', 'shopaholic' and 'chocaholic' tell you about the nature of addictive behaviour?

- Can you define addiction in a way that can cover such non-drug behaviours?

- What might they all have in common?

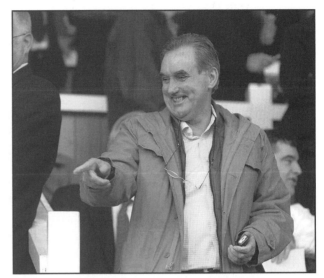

George Best, gifted footballer and famous alcoholic

Is there more to addiction than drugs?

Rather than rejecting the concept of addiction, some researchers argue that the concept should be *broadened*, in order to cover certain recent forms of 'addictive' behaviour that don't involve chemical substances at all. The addiction can be to a substance or an activity: shopping, gambling, eating (or abstaining from eating – see Gross, 2005), television, computer games, the Internet, sex and exercise could equally fit this definition (Griffiths, 1995). Drawing on current definitions of substance dependence, pathological gambling and eating disorders, Walters (1999) suggests that addiction may be defined as 'the persistent and repetitious enactment of a behaviour pattern', which includes:

◎ *progression* (increase in severity)
◎ *preoccupation* with the activity
◎ *perceived loss of control*
◎ *persistence* despite negative long–term consequences.

Brian's history shows that, according to Walters' (1999) definition, he's addicted to alcohol. He's well aware his 'diseases' are caused by alcohol but persists in his drinking pattern.

SUBSTANCE USE AND ABUSE

According to Hammersley (1999), abuse is the use of a substance in a harmful or risky manner, without medical sanction. The concept is something of a compromise, because it's debatable whether *any* use of a substance can be entirely risk-free. It also suggests that some risks are negligible, while others are substantial. Hammersley claims: 'The health risks of tobacco smoking now seem so substantial that all smoking is probably abuse – there is no negligible-risk use of tobacco ...' But he believes that most other drugs *can* be used in ways that make risks negligible.

Box 7.1 The DSM-IV-TR criteria for substance abuse

- A maladaptive pattern of substance use leading to clinically significant impairment or distress, as manifested by one (or more) of the following, occurring within a 12-month period:

  1. recurrent substance use resulting in a failure to fulfil major role obligations at work, school or home (e.g. repeated absences or poor work performance related to substance use, substance-related absences, suspensions, or expulsions from school; neglect of children or household)

  2. recurrent substance use in situations where it is physically hazardous (e.g. driving an automobile or operating a machine when impaired by substance use)

  3. recurrent substance-related legal problems (e.g. arrests for substance-related disorderly conduct)

  4. continued substance use despite having persistent or recurrent social or interpersonal problems caused or exacerbated by the effects of the substance (e.g. arguments with spouse about consequences of intoxication, physical fights).

- The symptoms have never met the criteria for substance dependence for this class of substance.

Brian obviously abuses alcohol. He is chronically ill, hasn't been employed for years, and has lost his driving licence due to convictions for 'drunk driving'.

DEPENDENCE

How does dependence differ from abuse?

Box 7.2 DSM-IV-TR criteria for substance dependence

- A maladaptive pattern of substance use leading to clinically significant impairment or distress, as manifested by three (or more) of the following, occurring at any time in the same 12-month period:

  1. Tolerance, as defined by either of the following:

     (a) a need for markedly increased amounts of the substance to achieve intoxication or desired effect

     (b) markedly diminished effect with continued use of the same amount of the substance.

  2. Withdrawal, as manifested by either of the following:

     (a) the characteristic withdrawal syndrome for the substance (varies from substance to substance)

     (b) the same (or a closely related) substance is taken to relieve or avoid withdrawal symptoms.

  3. The substance is often taken in larger amounts and over a longer period than was intended.

4. There is a persistent desire or unsuccessful efforts to cut down or control substance use.

5. A great deal of time is spent in activities necessary to obtain the substance (e.g. visiting multiple doctors or driving long distances), use the substance (e.g. chain-smoking) or recover from its effects.

6. Important social, occupational or recreational activities are given up or reduced because of substance use.

7. The substance use is continued despite knowledge of having a persistent physical or psychological problem that is likely to have been caused or exacerbated by the substance (e.g. current cocaine use despite recognition of cocaine-induced depression, or continued drinking despite recognition that an ulcer was made worse by alcohol consumption).

Specify if:

- *With physiological dependence*: evidence of tolerance or withdrawal (i.e. either item 1 or 2 is present).

- *With psychological dependence*: no evidence of tolerance or withdrawal (i.e. neither item 1 nor 2 is present).

Brian's medical notes record if he doesn't drink he gets the 'shakes', which indicates physical dependency, and becomes 'stressed' (aggressive) under any kind of pressure (e.g. having a catheter inserted), which indicates psychological dependency.

The concept of dependence is based around a constellation of symptoms and problems, not just on the idea of physiological need for a drug. Only items 1 and 2 in Box 7.2 refer to physiological dependence. Anyone who fits three or more of these criteria would be diagnosed as substance-dependent. Dependence, therefore, is quite varied, and few people fit all seven criteria (Hammersley, 1999).

Even restricting dependence to physiological dependence, the picture is more complex than it might at first appear. Different drugs may involve specific effects, such as opiates raising pain thresholds. As Sykes (1995) points out, the search for analgesics that don't have addictive potential continues, but it's possible that the effectiveness of opiates and similar drugs in reducing severe pain is partly due to the pleasurable mood they induce – so the search may fail (see Chapter 3).

Most substance-dependent people have tried to give up several times, always returning to use after weeks, months or even years. They often report strong craving or desire for the substance, and are at particular risk of resuming use when stressed, anxious, depressed, angry or happy. They also often feel they have difficulty controlling the amount they take, once they start. When they relapse, they often return very quickly to their old, often destructive, habits.

Brian said he's given up 'giving up'.

Physiological vs psychological dependence

As Box 7.2 shows, *physiological dependence* is related to *withdrawal* and/or *tolerance* (which relates to the traditional concept of *addiction*), while *psychological dependence* isn't. However, being deprived of a substance that's highly pleasurable can induce anxiety. Since the symptoms of anxiety (rapid pulse, profuse sweating, shaking, and so on) overlap with withdrawal symptoms, people may mistakenly believe that they're physiologically dependent. Psychological dependence is, though, part of the overall *dependence syndrome* (see Figure 7.1).

Does this mean Brian's 'shakes' may be the result of psychological, not physiological, dependence?

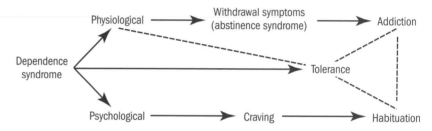

Figure 7.1 Summary of major components of dependence syndrome

A good example of the difference between the two types of dependence is imipramine, used to treat depression (see Gross, 2005). When it's stopped after prolonged use, there may be nausea, muscle aches, anxiety and difficulty in sleeping, but there's *never* a compulsion to resume taking it (Lowe, 1995). However, Lowe claims that 'psychological' dependence has little scientific meaning beyond the notion that drug taking becomes part of one's habitual behaviour. Giving it up is very difficult, because the person has become *habituated* to it:

> Habituation is the repeated use of a drug because the user finds that use increases pleasurable feelings or reduces feelings of anxiety, fear, or stress. Habituation becomes problematic when the person becomes so consumed by the need for the drug-altered state of consciousness that all his or her energies are directed to compulsive drug-seeking behaviour … (Lowe, 1995)

Physiologically addictive drugs, such as heroin and alcohol, typically cause habituation *as well*. Most widely used recreational drugs, including cannabis, cocaine, LSD, PCP (see Table 7.1) and *methylenedioxymethamphetamine* (*MDMA*, otherwise known as '*ecstacy*'), *don't* cause physiological dependence – but people *do* become habituated.

Some dependent people can stay dependent for long periods *without* suffering any other problems. This applies particularly to people who otherwise fit well into society and who haven't experienced financial, legal or health problems as a result of their substance use – such as many smokers. Some very heavy drinkers 'only' damage their livers, and even some heroin or cocaine users fit this pattern. Nevertheless, '… one of the most striking things about the counselling of substance dependent people is that they will continue to use the substance even when they have suffered very severe problems as a result …' (Hammersley, 1999). Some of these severe problems are discussed in the section below on the effects of drugs.

When a stimulus (and the response to it) becomes so familiar, it's perceived as normal and perhaps necessary. Brian obviously sees alcohol as necessary in his life. To help nurses understand habituation, David Cooper (in Alexander et al., 2006) suggests stopping a favourite substance for a week and noting the effects. I tried giving up coffee. The physical symptoms (headache and tiredness) of caffeine withdrawal were mild, but I resented being deprived of the pleasure of drinking it and after two days became very bad tempered!

CLASSIFYING DRUGS

Psychoactive drugs have been classified in several different ways. For example, Hamilton and Timmons (1995) identify three broad groups:

1. **stimulants** temporarily excite neural activity, arouse bodily functions, enhance positive feelings and heighten alertness; in high doses, they cause overt seizures
2. **depressants** (or sedatives) depress neural activity, slow down bodily functions, induce calmness and produce sleep; in high doses, they cause unconsciousness
3. **hallucinogens** produce distortion of normal perception and thought processes; in high doses, they can cause episodes of psychotic behaviour.

A fourth category is *opiates*. These also depress activity in the CNS, but have an *analgesic* property – that is, they reduce sensitivity to pain without loss of consciousness. The Royal College of Psychiatrists (1987) identified *minor tranquillisers* as a separate category, but in Table 7.1 they've been included under the general category of depressants. *Cannabis* doesn't fall easily into any of these other categories.

I feel uncomfortable to think that I, and most of my friends, are addicted to a stimulant drug: caffeine. Alcohol in large quantities is a depressant – that is, it dampens down stimuli.

THE EFFECTS OF DRUGS

ALCOHOL

Despite the difficulties in assessing the relationship between level of intake and harmful effects, certain 'safe levels' are widely accepted (Gelder *et al.*, 1999). These are expressed in terms of *units* of alcohol; one unit is equal to eight grammes of ethanol (the equivalent of half a pint of beer, a small glass of wine, a glass of sherry, or a standard (pub) measure of spirits).

For *men*, up to *28 units* per week, and for *women*, up to *21 units* is considered safe (Ogden, 2004), provided the whole amount isn't taken all at once and that there are occasional drink-free days. Anything over 50 and 35 units, respectively, is considered 'dangerous'. The British legal driving blood alcohol limit is 80 mg per 100 ml (equivalent to two or three drinks).

How does alcohol affect us?

According to Motluk (1999), it's possible to identify a number of stages, based on the amount of alcohol consumed.

◎ With our first drink, and with blood alcohol levels remaining fairly low, *stimulation* is the first effect. At these low levels, alcohol sensitises one of the brain's major excitatory message pathways, the *N*-methyl-*D*-aspartate (NMDA) system (not to be

ASK YOURSELF ...
• Either from your own experience, or from observing others, how would you describe the effects of alcohol?

Table 7.1 Some examples of the major categories of psychoactive drugs

Major category	Examples/slang name(s)
Depressants (sedatives)	*alcohol* *barbiturates*: 'downers', 'barbs', various other names derived from names or colour of pill/capsule (e.g. 'blueys') *tranquillisers*: 'tranx' *solvents*
Stimulants	*caffeine* *nicotine* *amphetamines*: 'uppers', 'speed', 'sulphate', 'sulph', 'whizz' *MDMA:* 'ecstasy', 'E', plus many names derived from shape and colour of drugs *cocaine:* 'coke', 'snow', 'crack', 'freebase', 'base', 'wash', 'rock'
Opiates	*morphine*: 'junk', 'skag', 'H', 'smack' *heroin* *codeine* *methadone*: 'amps' (injectable), 'linctus' (oral)
Hallucinogens	*lysergic acid diethylamide (LSD)*: 'acid' *mescaline* *psilocybin*: 'magic mushrooms', 'mushies' *phencycladine (PCP)*: 'angel dust'
Cannabis	*cannabis sativa*: 'pot', 'dope', 'blow', 'draw', 'smoke' *herbal cannabis*: 'grass', 'marijuana', 'ganja' *cannabis resin*: 'weed', 'the herb', 'skunk' *cannabis oil*: 'hash', 'hashish'

(Based on Cooper, 1995)

confused with ecstasy!). This makes certain NMDA receptors more readily activated by the brain's main neurotransmitter, glutamate. Some of the most sensitised brain regions are the cortex (thinking), hippocampus (remembering) and nucleus accumbens (NA) (pleasure-seeking), and our inhibitions begin to decrease.

◎ After two or three drinks, alpha rhythms (a brain wave indicating a relaxed state in awake adults) increase, extra blood flows to the prefrontal cortex and to the right temporal cortex. Mood is heightened and we may even feel euphoric.

◎ After three or four drinks, a turning point is reached, reflecting the complex 'biphasic' relationship with alcohol. With our blood now awash with alcohol, the very NMDA receptors that helped to perk us up after just one drink are refusing to respond. Also, the brain's *gamma-aminobutyric acid (GABA) system* becomes activated. GABA is an *inhibitory* neurotransmitter, which dulls activity (it's the system activated by benzodiazepines, such as Valium). From this point, alcohol begins to act more like a *depressant/sedative*. The hippocampus and thalamus are both slowed down.

◎ Any more drinks and our speech and other motor functions begin to fail us. The cerebellum seems to be most affected by this stage. A common experience is that the room is spinning. This is called *positional alcohol nystagmus*: a booze-induced version of an eye reflex normally triggered by the inner ear's balance organs when they detect head rotation (Motluk, 1999).

◎ A blood alcohol concentration of 500 mg per 100 ml is considered lethal. At that concentration, the brain centres that keep us breathing shut down.

Brian's blood must be permanently 'awash with alcohol', as his liver function is grossly impaired and his tolerance levels are high. Presumably, for him alcohol acts as a sedative, which relieves his 'stress'.

Box 7.3 Some physiological effects of alcohol

- Ethanol is a *diuretic*, so you end up *expelling* more water than you drink. It acts on the pituitary gland, blocking production of the hormone *vasopressin*, which directs the kidneys to reabsorb water that would otherwise end up in the bladder. So, the body borrows water from other places, including the brain, which shrinks temporarily. Though the brain itself cannot experience pain, it's thought that dehydration shrivels the *dura* (a membrane covering the brain). As this happens, it tugs at pain-sensitive filaments connecting it to the skull. Water loss might also account for pains elsewhere in the body (see Chapter 3).

- Frequent trips to the toilet also result in loss of essential sodium and potassium ions, which are central to how nerves and muscles work. Subtle chemical imbalances caused by ion depletion could account for a cluster of symptoms, including headaches, nausea and fatigue.

- Alcohol also depletes our reserves of sugar, leading to hypoglycaemia. The body's store of energy-rich glycogen in the liver is broken down into glucose; this quickly becomes another constituent of urine. This can account for feelings of weakness and unsteadiness the morning after.

(Based on New Scientist, 1999)

Heavy drinkers suffer malnutrition. Since alcohol is high in calories, appetite is suppressed. It also causes vitamin deficiency, by interfering with absorption of vitamin B from the intestines; long term, this causes brain damage. Other physical effects include liver damage, heart disease, increased risk of a stroke and susceptibility to infections due to a suppressed immune system (see Chapter 5). Women who drink while pregnant can produce babies with *foetal alcohol syndrome* (see Gross, 2005).

Brian looked undernourished and on admission was dehydrated. His immune system is being weakened by internal stress and his health is deteriorating – his last admission was only three months ago with acute bronchitis.

Alcohol and memory

Alcohol interferes with normal sleep patterns. Although it causes sedation, alcohol also suppresses rapid eye movement (REM) sleep (where dreaming takes place) by as much as 20 per cent (see Gross, 2005). There also appears to be a link between alcohol-induced sleepiness and memory loss. People who get drunk and then forget what happened have memory impairments similar to those suffered by people with sleep disorders, such as daytime sleepiness (Motluk, 1999). In both cases, the person cannot recall how they got home, or what happened while at work or at the pub. It's the *transfer* of information into long-term memory that seems to be disrupted. The GABA signals that induce the sleepiness can interfere with both the early and late stages of memory formation (*stimulus registration* and *consolidation*, respectively). Chemicals that mimic GABA can do this, and there are many GABA receptors in the hippocampus. Another memory disorder associated with chronic alcohol consumption is *Korsakoff's syndrome* (see Gross, 2005).

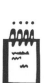

Eddie is 61 and has Korsakoff's syndrome. Gross (2005) describes this as a memory disorder associated with prolonged and heavy use of alcohol; there is an inability to process new information into long-term memory (anterograde amnesia) and to remember past events (retrograde amnesia). Eddie has been on the ward for seven weeks waiting for a bed in a care home. Each time he needs the toilet we have to take him, as he can't remember where it is. One night he was found passing urine in the day room. The night nurse admitted she felt very cross with him, it took effort to remind herself Eddie is unable to help his behaviour.

Who drinks, and why?

The heaviest drinkers are young men in their late teens/early twenties, but there have been recent increases among 15–16 year olds. Fewer women drink dangerous amounts, but the rates among women are rising faster than in men, especially those in professional and managerial jobs (Gelder *et al.*, 1999).

A recent Mori poll (in Waterhouse *et al.*, 2000) showed that 17 per cent of those under 25 say they drink in order to get 'trolleyed'. A European School Survey Project on Alcohol and Other Drugs indicated that more than half of 15–16-year-old British teenagers admitted 'binge drinking' in the previous month. Under-16s are drinking twice as much as they were ten years ago (Ahmed, 2004). The UK survey by the Alcohol and Health Research Centre in Edinburgh of more than 2600 school students (2001), revealed that 57 per cent of boys and 54.8 per cent of girls had drunk five or more drinks in a row in the previous 30 days. Among 16–24 year olds, 38 per cent of men and 21 per cent of women regularly drink twice the recommended daily limit (Waterhouse *et al.*, 2000; see above).

The increased **abuse** of alcohol by young people indicates changing psychosocial/environmental causes rather than biological ones. Brian's medical history showed he started drinking heavily as a teenager, with a gang of friends.

Brian's past unsuccessful attempts to cut down/give up his drinking would have affected his belief he could give up drinking (perceived behavioural control). This is similar to Diana, an obese patient who kept failing to lose weight (see diary entry on page 62). This is an example of the 'normative' social and environmental elements of the Theory of Planned Behaviour Model (see Chapter 4).

STIMULANTS

Cocaine

Cocaine hydrochloride is a powerful CNS stimulant extracted from the leaves of the coca shrub, native to the Andes mountains in South America. The Peruvian Indians originally discovered that chewing the leaves could increase stamina and relieve fatigue and hunger. While they still chew the leaves, elsewhere in the world it's inhaled in powder form, injected into the veins in liquid form, or smoked. When smoked, the drug reaches the brain in 5–10 seconds, much faster than the other methods. It can also be swallowed, rubbed on the gums or blown into the throat.

Typically, the user experiences a state of euphoria, deadening of pain, increased self-confidence, energy and attention. There's also a 'crash' when the drug wears off.

Even in small amounts, the stimulating effects can cause cardiac arrest and death. Recent research suggests that young people who use cocaine (and amphetamines) may be increasing their risks of having a stroke (brain haemorrhage) (Laurance, 2000). The growing pandemic of cocaine use in western society is overshadowing the traditional risk factors for stroke, such as high blood pressure. This is much more common in older people, as are strokes, but it's becoming increasingly common for people under 30 to suffer strokes after taking drugs.

Cocaine (and amphetamines) produces a surge in blood pressure. People with abnormal blood vessels in their brain, such as a cerebral aneurysm, are at greatest risk. But, it's also possible that the drug taking caused the deformed blood vessels (Laurance, 2000). Repeated inhalation constricts the blood vessels in the nose. The nasal septum may become perforated, necessitating cosmetic surgery.

Formication refers to the sensation that 'insects' ('coke bugs') are crawling beneath the skin. Although this is merely random neural activity, users sometimes try to remove the imaginary insects by cutting deep into their skin. Cocaine definitely produces *psychological dependence*, but there's much more doubt regarding *physiological dependence*, *tolerance* and *withdrawal*.

Increased levels of the neurotransmitter dopamine probably account for the euphoric effect, while raised levels of noradrenaline explain the increased energy. Cocaine stimulates neural circuits that are normally triggered by reinforcing events such as eating or sex. The 'crash' is caused by the fairly sudden depletion of dopamine and noradrenaline.

Box 7.4 Crack

- *Crack* is a form of cocaine, which first appeared in the 1980s.

- It's made using cocaine hydrochloride, ammonia or baking soda, and water. When heated, the ammonia or baking soda produces a 'cracking' sound. The result is a crystal, which has had the hydrochloride base removed (hence 'free basing' to describe its production).

- Its effects are more rapid and intense than cocaine's, but the 'crash' is also more intense.

Unlike heroin-dependent people, most cocaine users will get over their drug problem *without* professional help (Hammersley, 1999).

Amphetamines can induce psychological, if not necessarily physiological, dependency. This is why amphetamines should not be prescribed for obesity or depression (British National Formulary, 2005).

OPIATES

These are derived from the unripe seed pods of the opium poppy ('plant of joy'). One constituent of opium is *morphine*, from which *codeine* and *heroin* can be extracted.

Morphine and heroin

In general, the opiates depress neural functioning and suppress physical sensations and responses to stimulation. In Europe, *morphine* was first used as an analgesic during the Franco-Prussian War (1870–1871). However, it quickly became apparent that it produced physiological dependence (the 'soldier's disease'). The German Bayer Company developed *heroin* (the 'hero' that would cure the 'soldier's disease') in order to prevent this dependence, but, unfortunately, it also causes physiological dependence and has many unpleasant side-effects.

Heroin can be smoked, inhaled or injected intravenously. Puffing the heated white powder ('chasing the dragon') is now the preferred method, because syringes are seen as dirty and dangerous (Khan, 2003). The immediate effects (the 'rush') are described as an overwhelming sensation of pleasure, similar to sexual orgasm but affecting the whole body. Such effects are so pleasurable that they override any thoughts of food or sex. Heroin rapidly decomposes into morphine, producing feelings of euphoria, well-being, relaxation and drowsiness.

Long-term users become more aggressive and socially isolated, as well as less physically active. Opiates in general may damage the body's immune system, leading to increased susceptibility to infection. The impurity of the heroin used, users' lack of adequate diet, and the risks from contaminated needles, all increase health risks. Overdoses are common.

Heroin produces both *physiological* and *psychological dependence*. *Tolerance* develops quickly. *Withdrawal symptoms* initially involve flu-like symptoms, progressing to tremors, stomach cramps, and alternating chills and sweats. Rapid pulse, high blood pressure, insomnia and diarrhoea also occur. The skin often breaks out into goose bumps resembling a plucked turkey (hence '*cold turkey*' to describe attempts to abstain). The legs jerk uncontrollably (hence '*kicking the habit*'). These symptoms last about one week, reaching a peak after about 48 hours.

Some patients fear pain-relieving drugs will cause addiction (Walker et al., 2004). However, McCaffery and Beebe (1994, in Alexander et al., 2006) argue that this dependence rarely appears in a clinical setting, since analgesic opioids are usually titrated and gradually reduced as pain diminishes. However, I remember that last week Clare, a young woman of 19 with Crohn's disease who comes in frequently with acute abdominal pain, was written up for IV morphine. She had a cannula in situ so IV drugs would have been more comfortable in the short term but Sister referred to the possibility of inducing dependency and asked the House Officer to change the prescription to IM.

Box 7.5 Heroin and endorphins

- The brain produces its own opiates (*opioid peptides* or *endorphins* – see Chapter 3).

- When we engage in important survival behaviours, endorphins are released into the fluid that bathes the neurons. Endorphin molecules stimulate *opiate receptors* on some neurons, producing an intensely pleasurable effect just like that reported by heroin users.

- Regular use of opiates overloads endorphin sites in the brain and the brain stops producing its own endorphins (Snyder, 1977). When the user abstains, neither the naturally occurring endorphins nor the opiates are available. Consequently, the internal mechanism for regulating pain is severely disrupted, producing some of the withdrawal symptoms described earlier.

Methadone

This is a synthetic opiate (or opioid) created to treat the *physiological dependence* on heroin and other opiates. Methadone acts more slowly than heroin and doesn't produce the heroin 'rush'. While heroin users may be less likely to take heroin if they're on methadone, they're likely to become at least *psychologically dependent* on it. By the early 1980s, long-term prescribing of methadone (methadone maintenance) began to be questioned, both in terms of effectiveness and the message it conveyed to users.

However, the HIV/AIDS epidemic has made harm minimisation a priority. The dispensing of injecting equipment and condoms in 'needle exchange' schemes has been combined with attempts to persuade users to substitute oral methadone for intravenous heroin. This reduces the risk of transmitting both HIV and other blood-borne viruses, such as hepatitis B (Lipsedge, 1997). Hepatitis B rates among all injecting drug users are over 20 per cent, and hepatitis C rates have reached almost 40 per cent in new injectors (Drugscope, in Crouch, 2003).

CANNABIS

This is second only to alcohol in popularity. The *cannabis sativa* plant's psychoactive ingredient is *delta-9-tetrahydrocannabinil (THC)*. THC is found in the branches and leaves of the male and female plants (*marijuana*), but is highly concentrated in the resin of the female plant. *Hashish* is derived from the sticky resin and is more potent than marijuana (see Table 7.1). 'Skunk' is herbal cannabis grown from selected seeds by intensive indoor methods and is twice as potent as hash or weed.

Cannabis is usually smoked with tobacco, or eaten. When smoked, THC reaches the brain within seven seconds. Small amounts produce a mild, pleasurable 'high', involving relaxation, a loss of social inhibition, intoxication and a humorous mood. Speech becomes slurred and coordination is impaired. Increased heart rate, reduced concentration, enhanced appetite and impaired short-term memory are also quite common effects. Some users report fear, anxiety and confusion.

Large amounts produce hallucinogenic reactions, but these aren't full blown as with LSD. THC remains in the body for up to a month, and both male sex hormones and the female menstrual cycle can be disrupted. If used during pregnancy, the foetus may fail to grow properly, and cannabis is more dangerous to the throat and lungs than cigarettes. While tolerance is usually a sign of physiological dependence, with cannabis *reverse tolerance* has been reported: regular use leads to a *lowering* of the amount needed to produce the initial effects. This could be due to a build-up of THC, which takes a long time to be metabolised. Alternatively, users may become more efficient inhalers and so perceive the drug's effects more quickly. *Withdrawal* effects (restlessness, irritability and insomnia) have been reported, but they seem to be associated only with continuous use of very large amounts. *Psychological dependence* almost certainly occurs in at least some people.

ASK YOURSELF ...
- Do you agree with the reclassification of cannabis?
- Do you think it should be legalised (decriminalised)?
- Why/why not?

CRITICAL DISCUSSION 7.1 Cannabis and the drugs debate

- Greenfield (in Ahuja, 2000) considers cannabis to be pretty potent. It takes 0.3 mg to induce the same kind of effects as 7000 mg of alcohol, primarily feelings of well-being and relaxation. This potency suggests that specific cannabis receptors exist in the brain.

- 3.3 million Britons (one in ten 16–59-year-olds) are estimated to have used the drug in 2004. A quarter of 15–24-year-olds used it in 2002 (Burke and Asthana, 2004). In 2005, 1 per cent of 11-year-olds, 17 per cent of 14-year-olds and 26 per cent of 15-year-olds used cannabis (Roberts, 2006).

- The brain continues to develop in adolescence (see Chapter 17) and cannabis may interfere with the frontal cortex's ability to control response inhibition and emotional regulation, and to analyse problems and plan. Sustained use over several years may result in cognitive impairment, affecting memory and the organisation and integration of complex information (Roberts, 2006).

- In 2004 and 2005, 1420 patients were admitted to hospital as a result of excessive use of cannabis. This compares with 490 admissions in 2001 (Roberts, 2006).

- Several recent studies have demonstrated the links between cannabis and schizophrenia. Murray, consultant psychiatrist at the Maudsley Hospital in London, estimates that 25,000 of the 250,000 people with schizophrenia in the UK could have avoided the illness if they had not used cannabis. He also believes that most psychiatrists would now say that cannabis causes (non-schizophrenic) psychosis (in Roberts, 2006).

- While these studies don't prove that cannabis is harmful for everyone, nor is it 'harmless'. Some experts have compared the risks to the link between smoking and lung cancer/heart disease: it's safer to abstain but vulnerable people are at greater risk. The number of people who are vulnerable to the effects of cannabis is probably tiny (Burke and Asthana, 2004).

THEORIES OF DEPENDENCE

According to Lowe (1995), '… It is now generally agreed that addictive behaviours are multiply determined phenomena, and should be considered as biopsychosocial entities'. Similarly, Hammersley (1999) maintains that dependence is a complex behaviour that takes several years to develop. So, it's unlikely that one theory or factor could account for all of it. Most researchers believe that social, personal, family and lifestyle factors are important, as well as the action of the drug itself. However, it's not yet understood fully how these work and interact. According to Hammersley, theories of dependence have two dimensions. These are concerned with the extent to which dependence is:

1. supposedly caused by *biological*, as opposed to *social*, factors
2. the result of *abnormal/pathological* processes, as opposed to the *extreme end* of *normal* processes.

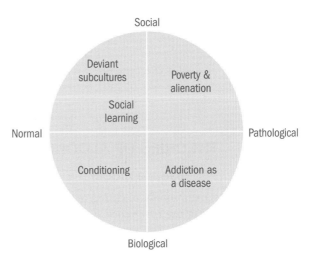

Figure 7.2 Five main theories of addiction (from Hammersley, 1999)

STAGES OF SUBSTANCE USE

The traditional approach to 'breaking the habit' (whether this involved alcohol or tobacco) was total abstinence, and this is still the philosophy of Alcoholics Anonymous (AA). However, this relatively unsuccessful approach has now largely been replaced by a research emphasis on cessation *as a process*, as demonstrated in Prochaska and DiClemente's (1984) Stages of Change (SoC) model.

> **Box 7.6 The Stages of Change (SoC) model (Prochaska and DiClemente, 1984) and the nurse's role (based on Crouch, 2003)**
>
> 1. **Precontemplation:** the person is basically unaware of having a problem/fails to acknowledge it (denial – see Chapter 6). Most nurses (especially those in A&E) see people in this stage. In A&E in particular, the person returns week after week, month after month, always in crisis. Not surprisingly, the nurse ends up regarding substance misusers as a waste of time: they're not health-seeking, and the nurse's main role is harm reduction. Opportunities for harm reduction often arise in A&E, such as information leaflets regarding needle exchanges. This is an essential first step towards change. However, following the establishment of 2000 exchanges during the 1980s (distributing 27 million needles annually), the health promotion message is getting lost and drug users are once again sharing equipment.
> 2. **Contemplation:** the person begins to recognise that they have a problem and becomes prepared to do something about it.
> 3. **Preparation:** the person is now seriously considering taking some action to change their behaviour.
> 4. **Action:** some initial behaviour change takes place.
> 5. **Maintenance:** the behaviour change is sustained for a period of time.
> 6. **Relapse:** eventually, most of those who relapse will return to the action stage.

The SoC model helps explain how a person can remain ambivalent about change over many years (Crouch, 2003). Individuals don't progress through the stages in a straightforward, linear fashion, but may switch back and forth (the 'revolving door'); this illustrates the *dynamic* nature of cessation (Ogden, 2004).

In the rest of this section, we shall consider one major theory (*addiction as a disease*) of one particular case of substance dependence (*alcohol dependence*).

THEORIES OF ALCOHOL DEPENDENCE

The disease model

Rush, widely regarded as the father of American psychiatry, is commonly credited with being the first major figure to conceptualise alcoholism as a 'disease', in the early 1800s. At about the same time, the British doctor, Trotter, likened alcoholism to a mental disorder. Both men saw it as a product of a distinct biological defect or dysfunction, much like cancer, diabetes or TB (Lilienfeld, 1995).

In 1935, a doctor and former alcoholic, Smith, and Wilson (a stockbroker) founded Alcoholics Anonymous (AA) in the USA. AA assumes that certain individuals possess a physiological susceptibility to alcohol analogous to an allergy: a single drink is sufficient to trigger an unquenchable desire for more, resulting in an inevitable loss of control.

Perhaps the most influential champion of the disease model was Jellinek, a physiologist. Based on questionnaire data with AA members, Jellinek (1946, 1952) proposed that alcoholism was a biological illness with a highly characteristic and predictable course (see Gross, 2005).

Evaluating the disease model

According to Lilienfeld (1995), the course of alcoholism appears to be far more variable than Jellinek proposed (there aren't clear-cut stages that alcoholics go through), and many drinkers don't fit into any of Jellinek's 'species'. For example, Cloninger (1987) proposed that *Group 1* alcoholics are at risk for 'Type 1' alcoholism:

◎ they drink primarily to reduce tension, are predominantly female, are prone to anxiety and depression, and tend to have relatively late onset of problem drinking.
By contrast, *Group 2* alcoholics are at risk for 'Type 2' alcoholism:

◎ they drink primarily to relieve boredom, give free rein to their tendency towards risk-taking and sensation-seeking, are predominantly male, prone to anti-social and criminal behaviour, and tend to have relatively early onset of drinking behaviour (see Chapter 6).

Although the evidence for Cloninger's model is tentative and indirect, it challenges the disease model in a quite fundamental way. If he's correct, alcoholism may represent the culmination of two very different (and, in fact, essentially opposite) pathways (Lilienfeld, 1995).

Nevertheless, the disease model was the single most influential theory for much of the twentieth century. It's still the dominant view underlying psychiatric and other medically orientated treatment programmes, but has been much less influential among psychologically-based programmes since the 1980s.

Alcohol dependence syndrome (ADS – Edwards, 1986) is a later version of the disease model. It grew out of dissatisfaction with 'alcoholism' and with the traditional conception of alcoholism as disease. 'Syndrome' adds flexibility, suggesting a group of concurrent behaviours that accompany alcohol dependence. They needn't always be observed in the same individual, nor are they observable to the same degree in everyone. For example, instead of loss of control or inability to abstain, ADS describes 'impaired control'. This implies that people drink heavily because, at certain times and for a variety of psychological and physiological reasons, they choose not to exercise control (Lowe, 1995). Lowe maintains: 'Simple disease models have now been largely replaced by a more complex set of working hypotheses based, not on irreversible physiological processes, but on learning and conditioning, motivation and self-regulation, expectations and attributions.'

Lowe's approach is more compatible with the biopsychosocial model of health and illness, and is concerned with time and process elements (like the Health Action Process Approach model – see Chapter 4). This is too late to help Eddie, and perhaps also for Brian, but I can see it might be effective in the early treatment of alcohol dependence.

TREATING ALCOHOL DEPENDENCE

The AA approach

According to Powell (2000), the more general concept of addiction as a 'disease of the will' has become popular. It has been broadly applied to other forms of addiction and is adopted by the AA's 'sister' organisations, Narcotics Anonymous (NA), Gamblers Anonymous (GA), Workaholics Anonymous (WA), Sex Addicts Anonymous (SAA) and even Survivors of Incest Anonymous (SIA).

Strictly, what AA offers isn't 'treatment' at all. Instead, it adopts a spiritual framework, requiring alcoholics to surrender their will to a 'higher power' (or God), confess their wrongs and try to rectify them. This requires an acceptance of abstinence as a goal, and usually works better for those who are heavily dependent (Hammersley, 1999; see Gross, 2005).

This may be effective but isn't it just substituting one dependency for another?

Aversion therapy

In *aversion therapy* (a form of behaviour therapy based on classical conditioning – see Chapter 2), some undesirable response to a particular stimulus is removed by associating the stimulus with another, aversive (literally, 'painful') stimulus. For example, alcohol is paired with an emetic drug (which induces severe nausea and vomiting), so that nausea and vomiting become a conditioned response (CR) to alcohol.

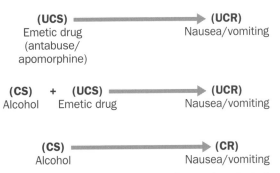

Figure 7.3 Diagrammatic illustration of aversion therapy for treating alcoholism.

ASK YOURSELF ...

- Look back at Chapter 3 (page 50) and the account of the treatment of anticipatory nausea and vomiting (ANV) in cancer patients undergoing chemotherapy.

- Apply these same principles of classical conditioning to describe how nausea and vomiting would be made a CR to alcohol.

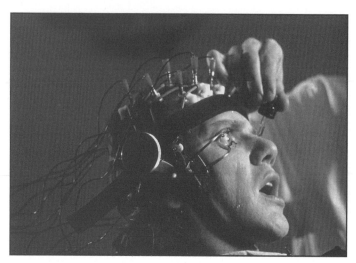

Malcolm McDowell in a scene from *Clockwork Orange*. His eyes are clamped open, forcing him to watch a film portraying acts of violence and sadism, as part of aversion therapy. He'd earlier been given an emetic drug, so that extreme nausea and violence will become associated

Patients would, typically, be given warm saline solution containing the emetic drug. Immediately before the vomiting begins, they're given a 4 oz glass of whisky, which they're required to smell, taste and swill around their mouth before swallowing. (If vomiting hasn't occurred, another straight whisky is given and, to prolong nausea, a glass of beer containing emetic.) Subsequent treatments involve larger doses of injected emetic, or increases in the length of treatment time, or a widening range of hard liquors (Kleinmuntz, 1980). Between trials, the patient sips soft drinks to prevent generalisation to all drinking behaviour and to promote the use of alcohol substitutes.

Meyer and Chesser (1970) found that about half their alcoholic patients abstained for at least one year following treatment, and that aversion therapy is better than no treatment at all. Lang and Marlatt (1982, in Ogden, 2004) concluded that use of antabuse was more effective than electric shock, but it requires the patient to take the drug and also ignores the multiplicity of reasons behind their drink problem. According to Tucker *et al.* (1992, in Davison *et al.*, 2004), aversion therapy, if used at all, seems best applied in the context of broadly based programmes that address the patient's particular life circumstances, such as marital conflict, social fears and other factors often associated with problem drinking.

Antabuse works for some, but not others. It breaks down alcohol into acetaldehyde, which accumulates in the body. This produces various aversive symptoms, including flushing and nausea, and can sometimes prove fatal (Starr and Chandler, 1995).

And it has nothing to say about why people **become** dependent – which is surely the first step in helping to avoid/treat the condition?

Reflecting on this experience shows that, however it's caused and however it's defined, we treat many patients for diseases caused by dependency on alcohol and other substances. Learning about the physiological elements of the condition has made me more sympathetic to patients who are dependent; initially I felt more concern for Clare's potential addiction than for Brian and Eddie's. However, Lowe's (1995) biopsychosocial approach to alcohol dependency makes me realise that many individual experiences (stress, keeping up with fashion) may start a reactive process that becomes self-reinforcing and, for some (the reason is still unknown), out of control. By the time they get to Brian's stage, it seems too late. I plan to find out if health education plays a part in the care we give patients in the early stages of alcohol-related illness.

CHAPTER SUMMARY

◎ Drugs are **psychoactive** substances. They may be used **therapeutically** or for **pleasure**, the latter being subdivided into **recreational** and **drugs of abuse**.

◎ Which drugs are legal or illegal changes over time within the same society, and between societies. Cigarette smoking and alcohol abuse are so widespread that they may be considered 'ordinary addictions'.

◎ The concept of **addiction** has been criticised for being oversimplified and for reflecting the **disease model**. The more modern view is to see drug problems as involving **substance abuse** and **dependence**. This view is adopted by DSM-IV-TR.

◎ Some researchers argue that the concept of addiction should be **broadened**, so as to cover forms of addictive behaviour that don't involve chemical substances at all. Addictive behaviours may display the same components, regardless of the particular substance or activity involved.

◎ DSM-IV-TR defines abuse and dependence in terms of several criteria. **Dependence** can be either **psychological** or **physiological**, the latter indicated either by **tolerance** or **withdrawal**. Both types of dependence are part of the **dependence syndrome**.

◎ Physiologically addictive drugs, such as alcohol and heroin, typically also cause **habituation**. Most widely used recreational drugs, including cannabis, cocaine and ecstasy, produce habituation without causing physiological dependence.

◎ Major categories of drugs include **depressants (sedatives)**, **stimulants**, **opiates**, **hallucinogens (psychedelics)** and **cannabis**.

◎ **Alcohol** is a depressant, although its initial effect is to stimulate the brain. With increasing amounts of alcohol, the brain generally slows down, and the breathing centres may eventually shut down.

◎ Alcohol can produce several life-threatening physical diseases in the drinker, as well as causing **foetal alcohol syndrome**. It also impairs **memory** function, an extreme form being **Korsakoff's syndrome**.

◎ Stimulants include **cocaine**, which causes only psychological dependence, and **MDMA** (or **ecstasy**).

◎ **Morphine** and **heroin** are opiates. Heroin produces both psychological and physiological dependence, and withdrawal symptoms are severe and extremely unpleasant. It is thought that regular use of opiates causes the brain to stop producing its own **endorphins**.

◎ **Methadone** is an orally taken synthetic opiate created to treat physiological dependence on heroin and other opiates. Users may well become psychologically dependent.

◎ **Cannabis** doesn't fit neatly into the other categories. It comes in different forms and can be taken in a variety of ways. There is some evidence of **reverse tolerance**, and psychological dependence is likely for some people.

◎ **Theories of dependence** differ according to whether the causes are seen as **biological** or **social**, and whether dependence is seen as **pathological** or the **extreme end** of **normal processes**.

◎ The single most influential theory of alcohol dependence is the **disease model**. Supporting evidence is also very limited. **Alcohol dependence syndrome (ADS)** is a more flexible version of the disease model.

◎ **Aversion therapy**, based on **classical conditioning**, aims to make alcohol an aversive CS, by associating it with an aversive UCS (such as antabuse). Its effectiveness is limited and its side-effects may prove fatal.

SOCIAL PERCEPTION

8

INTRODUCTION AND OVERVIEW

Social (or person) perception refers to the perception of people (as opposed to physical objects – see Figure 8.1). The focus of this chapter is on *interpersonal perception* or *ordinary personology*, the process by which 'ordinary people come to know about each other's temporary states (such as emotions, intentions and desires) and enduring dispositions (such as beliefs, traits and abilities) from their actions (Gilbert, 1998). This is included in what Fiske and Taylor (1991) call *social cognition*, '… the process by which people think about and make sense of other people, themselves, and social situations'. According to Fiske (2004), social cognition builds on *attribution theory*, which is discussed in Chapter 9.

Traditionally, person perception has been concerned with *impression formation*, and the research was carried out largely from the perspective of *the perceiver*.

◎ Is certain information about a person more influential than others (*central vs peripheral traits*)?

◎ Is the order in which we learn things about someone important (the *primacy–recency effect*)?

◎ Do we have ready-made beliefs about how individuals' characteristics 'belong together' (*implicit personality theory*)?

◎ Do we have ready-made beliefs about groups, which we then apply to individuals (*stereotyping*)?

We'll also discuss impression formation from the *actor's* point of view (that is, the person being perceived), by considering some of the ways in which we try to influence others' impressions of us (*impression management/self-presentation*).

Since the 1980s, these traditional perspectives of person perception have largely been replaced by that of *social cognition*. The study of impression formation was very 'cognitive', in that it was concerned with the content of our thoughts about others. But social cognition reflected the *information-processing approach*, which has become psychology's dominant paradigm since the 1950s (see Chapter 1). This is concerned less with the content and more with the often unconscious, automatic processes that underlie our (usually) conscious impressions of others.

From my diary (7): Year 1/Orthopaedic Ward

I had – eventually – a very satisfying experience today! I noticed a new patient as soon as I came onto the ward and did a double-take: she looked about 60, with grey, matted hair and was huddled in her bed with a wary expression. When she saw me looking at her she shrank back into her pillows and looked away.

At handover, Staff Nurse told us Vera was 55 years old and was, as I'd assumed, 'in a terrible state', generally unkempt with very long, uncared-for nails. She lived alone in a neglected flat where she'd fallen and fractured her wrist.

After handover, Maggie (my mentor) asked me if I'd like to try to persuade Vera to have a shower. She refused point blank. I didn't know what to do, but then noticed she was wearing a beautiful silver bracelet, which seemed incongruous on her grubby arm. I admired it and she said she never took it off. I asked her why and she told me it was the last thing her husband had given her before he was killed in an accident (five years ago). I sat down by the bed and spent a long time chatting to her. In the end, I did manage to get her into the shower and wash her hair. Afterwards, after a great deal more persuasion, she let the podiatrist attend to her nails. It was very rewarding to see her looking so different – and behaving differently too.

PERCEIVING OBJECTS AND PERCEIVING PEOPLE

According to Fiske (2004), when we form impressions of other people it seems to happen *immediately* ('automatically'). But in fact we:

> … search the social horizon unaware that [we] are using mental binoculars and that things are much farther away than they appear. All our experience … is actually *mediated* or filtered through a psychological lens, our perceiving apparatus. Although we experience the world as if we take in a literal, unfiltered copy, each person passes reality through a different lens …

We're aware only of the *end product* of this process, which is our experience of the person. Part of Heider's (1958) common-sense psychology (equivalent to ordinary personology) is this direct experience of the world, which he contrasts with the *scientific* analysis of how people perceive it (see Chapter 9).

This applies equally to perception of objects (see Gross, 2005). As Figure 8.1 shows, both social (or person) and object perception involve *selection*, *organisation* and *inference*. Applied to perceiving people, this might mean:

◎ focusing on people's physical appearance or on just one particular aspect of their behaviour (*selection*)

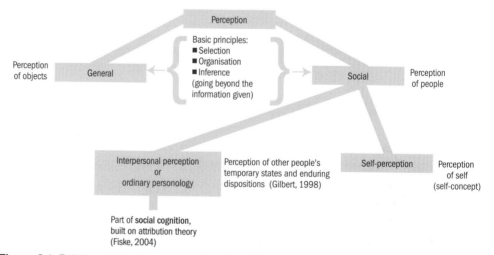

Figure 8.1 Relationship between general and social perception

ASK YOURSELF ...
• In what ways does perceiving people differ from perceiving objects?

◎ trying to form a complete, coherent impression of a person (*organisation*)

◎ attributing characteristics to someone for which there's no direct or immediate evidence, as in stereotyping (*inference*).

◎ People *behave* (but objects don't). It's often behaviour that provides the data for making inferences about what people are like.

◎ People are *causal agents* – that is, they intend to act on their environment (Fiske and Taylor, 1991).

◎ People *interact* with other people (but they don't interact with objects or objects with each other). One person's behaviour can influence another's, so that behaviour is *mutually influential*.

◎ People anticipate being observed, and this is related to *self-presentation* (Fiske and Taylor, 1991; see below).

◎ People are generally more *changeable* than objects, and it's harder to verify the *accuracy* of observations about people (what they're 'really' like) (Fiske and Taylor, 1991; see also Chapter 6).

◎ People *perceive* and *experience* (but objects cannot). One person's perception can influence the other's (especially his/her non-verbal behaviour), so that each person's perception of the other is at least partly a product of the other's perception of him/her. As Fiske and Taylor (1991) put it, social perception is *mutual perception*.

My first impression of Vera was, like everyone's, I think, very negative. When I heard about her home circumstances I felt even more disapproving. I think she probably perceived my attitude from the way I looked at her as I went past.

ASK YOURSELF ...
• In what ways can we all be considered psychologists?

ARE WE ALL PSYCHOLOGISTS?

Everyone tries to 'figure people out', explain, predict and, very often, control others' behaviour, as part of their everyday living in a social world. These also happen to be the three traditionally accepted aims of science, including psychology (see Chapter 2). Gahagan (1984) defines interpersonal perception as 'the study of how the layperson uses theory and data in understanding people'. One component of this definition is the study of the *lay person as a psychologist*. According to Nisbett and Ross (1980):

> We are all psychologists. In attempting to understand other people and ourselves, we are informal scientists who construct our own intuitive theories of human behaviour. In doing so, we face the same basic tasks as the formal scientist ...

'Intuitive theories' is another way of referring to 'implicit personality theories' (see below, page 148).

THE PERSON AS THINKER

We've already noted that social psychology has always been strongly cognitive. People are thinking organisms, who 'reside' between stimulus and response (an S–O–R model as opposed to an S–R model – see Chapter 2 and Gross, 2005). According to Fiske and Taylor (1991), the person as thinker has been presented in four ways:

1. *Consistency seeker.* Several theories of attitude change are built on the assumption that people try to be consistent in their ideas and opinions, as well as between these and their behaviour. The most influential is Festinger's (1957) *cognitive dissonance theory* (see Chapter 10).

2. *Naïve scientist.* According to attribution theories, we try to infer unobservable causes from observable behaviour; this makes us all amateur scientists (see above). This view was first proposed by Heider (1958), the 'father of attribution theory'.

3. *Cognitive miser.* People are limited in their capacity to process information. They take shortcuts whenever they can, adopting strategies that simplify complex problems. This might lead them to draw biased and hence inaccurate conclusions (Nisbett and Ross, 1980; see also Chapter 9).

4. *Motivated tactician.* This refers to a development of the cognitive miser view, 'putting back' the motivational and emotional variables. The motivated tactician is a 'fully engaged thinker who has multiple cognitive strategies available and chooses among them based on goals, motives, and needs' (Fiske and Taylor, 1991).

I confess I thought that Vera might have been drinking and had fallen over; I suppose I was trying to work out cause and effect. That certainly turned out to be biased and inaccurate.

FORMING GLOBAL IMPRESSIONS OF PEOPLE

CENTRAL VERSUS PERIPHERAL TRAITS

Certain information we have about a person (certain traits we believe they possess) may be more important in determining our overall impression of that person than other information. This was demonstrated in Asch's (1946) classic study.

KEY STUDY 8.1 Building our impressions around something warm or cold (Asch, 1946)

- Asch presented participants with a stimulus list of adjectives describing a fictitious person. For one group, the adjectives were: intelligent, skilful, industrious, warm, determined, practical and cautious. A second group had the same list, except that the word 'cold' replaced the word 'warm'.

- Both groups were then presented with a response list of 18 different adjectives and were asked to underline those that described the target person.

- The two groups chose significantly and consistently different words from the response list. For example, the 'warm' group saw the character as generous, humorous, sociable and popular, while the 'cold' group saw him as having the opposite traits. There were also certain qualities attributed to him equally by both groups (reliable, good-looking, persistent, serious, restrained, strong and honest).

- When 'polite' and 'blunt' were used instead of 'warm' and 'cold', participants underlined almost identical words in the response list.

- Asch concluded that 'warm–cold' represented a *central trait* or *dimension*, while 'polite–blunt' represented a *peripheral trait* or *dimension*.

- The central traits that seem to influence our global perception in this way are implicitly *evaluative* – that is, they're to do with whether the person is likeable or unlikeable, popular or unpopular, friendly or unfriendly, kind or cruel, and so on.

Kelley (1950) replicated Asch's findings using a *real* (as opposed to hypothetical) person (see Gross, 2005).

THE PRIMACY–RECENCY EFFECT

The other major explanation of global perception concentrates on the *order* in which we learn things about a person:

◎ the *primacy effect* refers to the greater impact of what we learn first about someone ('first impressions count')

◎ the *recency effect* refers to the greater impact of what we learn later on.

Initial support for a primacy effect came in another study by Asch (1946). He used two lists of adjectives describing a hypothetical person: one in the order intelligent, industrious, impulsive, critical, stubborn and envious; the other in the reverse order. Participants given the first list formed a favourable overall impression, while those given the second list formed an unfavourable overall impression.

My first impression of Vera was, I admit, unfavourable. I remember now that at handover Vera's physical self-neglect and lack of hygiene were the first things staff mentioned, even before the diagnosis.

A *negative* first impression may be more resistant to change than a positive one. One explanation for this is that negative information carries more weight, because it's likely to reflect socially undesirable traits or behaviour and, therefore, the observer can be more confident in attributing the trait or behaviour to the person's 'real' nature. (This is relevant to Jones and Davis's attribution theory – see Chapter 9, pages 161–165.) It may be more adaptive for us to be aware of negative traits than positive ones, since the former are potentially harmful or dangerous.

Luchins (1957) found that, although the primacy effect may be important in relation to strangers, as far as friends and other people whom we know well are concerned, the recency effect seems to be stronger. For example, we may discover something about a friend's childhood or something that happened to them before we knew them, which might change our whole perception of them. How well do we (or can we) know anybody?

Patients are often not with us long enough to find out much, but sometimes just one piece of information, like Vera telling me about her husband, can lead to better understanding.

According to Ward (1990), the way a patient is first greeted by a nurse may influence their perception both of the nurse and of the forthcoming treatment, and may serve to heighten or reduce their anxiety (see Chapter 3). Ward reports a study designed to examine the interaction between nurses and patients when they first meet in the A&E department at a large general hospital. The method used was non-participant observation.

> **KEY STUDY 8.2 Nurse–patient interaction in A&E (Ward, 1990)**
>
> - A video camera recorded 26 patients called in, 11 by trained nurses, 12 by student nurses in the second week of their allocation to the department, and 3 by doctors.
>
> - Typically, the staff member called out the patient's name to the waiting room in general, then turned to the patient when they started to rise from their seat. Very few of the nurses went to the patient, even where the patient had crutches or obvious difficulty in walking, was carrying luggage or had children with them.
>
> - Student nurses were more likely to go up to the patient than were the trained staff, who waited until the patient was with them. Some of the trained nurses and the doctors called the patient's name and then immediately disappeared back into the treatment area. The students were also more likely to remain facing the patient, while the trained staff often turned their back on the patient. Doctors seemed even more reluctant to venture into the waiting room.
>
> - There appeared to be an invisible line that staff, especially trained nurses and doctors, were reluctant to cross. This may be a form of *territorial* behaviour.
>
> - *All* staff went back into the treatment area ahead of the patients, who would often stand back to allow the staff to go first.

ASK YOURSELF ...
- How could you explain the difference in behaviour between the trained and the student nurses?

The territorial suggestion rings true: nurses and doctors do perceive themselves as being on 'home ground'. I always feel intrusive when I start a new placement, so Vera must have felt extremely anxious and 'out of place' when first admitted.

The students were in only their second week in A&E and may not yet have become fully socialised into the norms of behaviour for the departmental staff. It's possible that their training has made them more prepared to break down barriers between the perceived roles of patient and nurse. The trained staff are likely to have become used to a ritualised way of greeting patients and, as a result, may have lost sight of the seriousness with which most patients view their injury or illness and their attendance at the department. If this is true, the ritual may help protect staff from the stress involved in this situation (Ward, 1990; see also Chapter 5).

The importance of personal space

Inevitably, nurses engage in close proximity and bodily contact – often of a very intimate nature – with patients. This 'invasion' of *personal space* may help determine the patient's impression of the nurse.

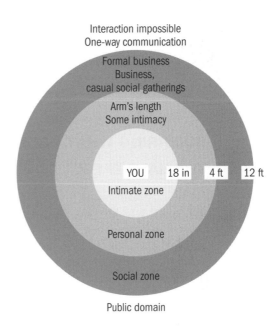

Interaction impossible
One-way communication
Formal business
Business,
casual social gatherings
Arm's length
Some intimacy

YOU | 18 in | 4 ft | 12 ft

Intimate zone

Personal zone

Social zone

Public domain

Figure 8.2 Hall's four zones of personal space (from Nicholson, 1977)

Personal space is a sort of invisible bubble that surrounds us. Hall (1959, 1966) identified four main regions or zones of personal space (as shown in Figure 8.2).

There are important *cultural differences* regarding the rules governing personal space (*proxemic rules*), and our feelings towards others may depend on whether these rules are followed. The rules themselves are influenced by the nature of the relationship. In general, relatives and friends are allowed much closer proximity – and bodily contact – than mere acquaintances or strangers. But some strangers, such as nurses and doctors, are 'allowed in' to our intimate zone by virtue of the role relationship. Nevertheless, this needs to be treated sensitively.

Related to personal space is the concept of *privacy*. According to Barron (1990), privacy is a human need and right, which allows people to maintain individuality. It's important for the psychological well-being of hospital patients that private domains be provided that aren't open to public view or use. It's also important that nursing staff respect the right to privacy and don't invade patients' privacy without permission. Brown's study of elderly wards in both the UK and Sweden led her to conclude that, despite the development of purpose-built units and the move away from open wards (in the UK), there remains a lack of privacy for elderly people as a result of staff attitudes.

Davidson (1990) points out that 'privacy' is derived from the Latin word meaning 'peculiar to oneself'. This has obvious physical implications and another, psychological, meaning related to the choice we exercise over the thoughts and feelings we share with others: 'In the UK health-care system, privacy is often seen as a privilege for which the patient pays dearly. The provision of a room of one's own is an important part of "going private" and the health insurers place great emphasis on it in their literature' (Davidson, 1990).

Barron's (1990) comments are significant in relation to Vera. She had been isolated for so long, the notion of anyone getting close to her, let alone doing something as intimate as washing her, must have been threatening. Of course, I did pull the curtains around the bed before I attempted to attend to her but I know now I needed to do much more than that to make Vera feel secure; I was invading her psychological as well as her physical space.

INFERRING WHAT PEOPLE ARE LIKE

THE HALO EFFECT

Asch's original finding that the inclusion of 'warm' produces a more positive impression compared with the same list including 'cold' demonstrates the *halo effect*. If we're told a person is warm, then we tend to attribute to them other favourable characteristics (a *positive* halo). The reverse is true if we're told the person is 'cold' – we attribute them with a *negative* halo. The halo effect seems to illustrate very well two basic principles of perception (see Figure 8.1):

1. We like to see people in as *consistent* (or organised) a way as possible. It's easier to regard someone as having either all good or all bad qualities than a mixture of good and bad. Two quite extreme examples of this are when lovers regard each other as perfect and faultless ('love is blind') and the '*mirror-image phenomenon*', where enemies see each other as all bad (see Chapter 11).
2. The halo effect is a very general form of *implicit personality theory*. Such theories enable us to infer what people are like when we have only very limited information about them.

Does the halo effect explain why I wasn't surprised at Vera's initial response to me? Did I assume an unkempt person would also be irresponsible, anti-social, inconsiderate and unpleasant?

IMPLICIT PERSONALITY THEORIES (IPTs)

As we saw earlier, we all have 'implicit' theories about what makes people 'tick'. One kind of implicit theory is to do with how personality is structured and what traits tend to go together or cluster. Zebrowitz (1990) refers to these as 'person type' IPTs.

The importance of names

Our names are part of the central core of our self-image (see Chapter 16) and they can sometimes form the basis for others' expectations. Harari and McDavid (1973) pointed out that first names, like surnames, are often associated with particular characteristics, partly determined by the media.

KEY STUDY 8.3 Names and psychiatric diagnosis (Birmingham, in Adler, 2000)

- Birmingham, a forensic psychiatrist at Southampton University, asked 464 British psychiatrists to provide a diagnosis based on a one-page description of a 24 year old who'd assaulted a train conductor.

- When they were asked to assess 'Matthew', over 75 per cent gave him a sympathetic hearing, proposing that he was suffering from schizophrenia and in need of medical help.
- But when renamed 'Wayne', psychiatrists gave him a more sinister character: he was twice as likely as Matthew to be diagnosed as a malingerer, a drug abuser or suffering from a personality disorder (see Gross, 2005).

If Vera had been called Penelope, would I have made different assumptions about her?

The importance of physical appearance

Another kind of IPT involves inferring what somebody is like psychologically from certain aspects of their physical appearance. Allport (1954) gave examples of widely held, but totally unfounded, beliefs that fat people are jolly, high foreheads are a sign of superior intelligence, eyes too close together are a sign of untrustworthiness, and redheads have fiery tempers.

According to the *attractiveness stereotype*, we tend to perceive attractive-looking people as also having more attractive personalities. Dion *et al.* (1972) found that photographs of attractive people, compared with unattractive people, were consistently credited with more desirable qualities, including sexually warm and responsive, kind, strong, outgoing, nurturing and sensitive. So, 'what is beautiful is socially good' (Fiske, 2004). Dion and Dion (1995) observe that stereotyping based on facial attractiveness appears at least as early as six years old (see Chapter 16). They also suggest that this might be linked to the *just world hypothesis*, such that there's a positive bias towards 'winners', equivalent to 'blaming the victim' (see Chapter 9).

According to Kelly and May (1982, in Darbyshire, 1986b), there is evidence that patients are 'treated differentially according to their illnesses, putative social class, occupation, appearance, age, attitudes and behaviour'. Bordieri *et al.* (1984, in Darbyshire, 1986b) found that nurses held a highly attractive child less personally responsible for a disturbance, 'blamed' the behaviour on emotional causes, and judged the attending nurses as more responsible, compared with an unattractive child.

Darbyshire cites several other studies, which all demonstrate the 'beautiful is good' stereotype within health care. For example, Bordieri *et al.* (1983) found that attractive victims of paralysis were rated as having better prospects for recovery than less attractive victims, and Corter *et al.* (1978) reported that experienced nurses tended to attribute a better prognosis of intellectual development to attractive premature babies.

According to Richardson *et al.* (1985), mentally retarded individuals are more likely to have an atypical appearance, which can be a barrier to social intercourse, causing isolation and maladaptive behaviour. Darbyshire notes a trend towards performing facial surgery on Down's syndrome children in order to improve their looks. The social benefits of such surgery must be weighed against the ethical issues involved.

ASK YOURSELF ...

- Does this research ring true for you in your professional experience?
- Does the 'beautiful is good' stereotype relate to how nurses and doctors perceive each other?
- Could it extend to how student nurses are perceived and assessed by senior staff?

After her shower and shampoo, Vera remarked how soft her hair felt; when I'd plaited it and showed her she became quite coy about her improved appearance. And her new image had a radical effect on everyone; all the nurses began smiling at her and remarking how nice she looked. We all forgot how disapproving we'd been before.

STEREOTYPES AND STEREOTYPING

Stereotypes can be thought of as a special kind of IPT that relates to an entire social group. The term was introduced into social science by Lippmann (1922), who defined stereotypes as 'pictures in our heads'. Other definitions include:

◎ '… the process of ascribing characteristics to people on the basis of their group memberships …' (Oakes *et al.*, 1994)

◎ '… widely shared assumptions about the personalities, attitudes and behaviour of people based on group membership, for example ethnicity, nationality, sex, race and class …' (Hogg and Vaughan, 1995).

Nurses constitute another 'group membership' (see below).

Ethnic/racial stereotypes

One of the earliest studies of stereotyping was Katz and Braly's (1933) study of undergraduates at Princeton University in the USA. They were presented with a list of ethnic groups (Americans, Jews, Negroes, Turks, Germans, Chinese, Irish, English, Italians and Japanese) and 84 words describing personality. They were asked to list, for each ethnic group, the five or six traits that were 'typical' of that group.

The Princeton students showed considerable agreement, especially about negative traits. Rather disturbingly, most of the students had had no personal contact with any members of most of the ethnic groups they had to rate. Presumably, they'd absorbed the images of those groups prevalent in the media.

Gilbert (1951) studied another sample of Princeton students and this time found less uniformity of agreement (especially about unfavourable traits) than in the 1933 study. But, in a further repeat, Karlins *et al.* (1969) found a re-emergence of social stereotyping, but towards more favourable stereotypical images.

Most patients don't seem to notice my Asian origin, but last week an elderly patient with one arm in plaster declined my help with washing himself. He didn't look at me when he spoke and later I saw the HCA helping him. As usual, I felt a flash of anger but I realise now that stereotyping isn't just about racism: it's categorising people – and patients – rather than treating them as individuals. And I did it, with Vera.

ASK YOURSELF …
• Do you think that stereotypes/ stereotyping are inherently bad/wrong?

• Give reasons for your answer.

The traditional view of stereotypes: are they inherently bad?

For most of the time that psychologists have been studying stereotypes and stereotyping, they've condemned them for being both false and illogical, and dangerous, and people who use them have been seen as prejudiced and even pathological (see Chapter 11).

The research started by Katz and Braly (1933) was intended to trace the link between stereotypes and prejudice: stereotypes are public fictions arising from prejudicial influences 'with scarcely any factual basis'. So, should they be dismissed as completely unacceptable?

According to Allport (1954), most stereotypes do contain a 'kernel of truth', and Lippmann had recognised the categorisation processes involved in stereotyping as an important aspect of general cognitive functioning. Allport built on these ideas, arguing that 'The human mind must think with the aid of categories …'. However, he also believed that prejudiced people tend to make extremely simple *dichotomous* (either/or) judgements compared with tolerant, non-prejudiced people.

Sherif (1967) also argued that stereotypes aren't in themselves deficient, but serve to reflect the reality of intergroup relations. Instead of asking if they are objectively true or accurate, stereotypes need to be understood in this *intergroup* context. To this extent, they are highly flexible, since changes in the relationship with other groups will result in changes to the stereotyped images of those groups (see Chapter 11). However, according to Operario and Fiske (2004), it's precisely this broader context of stereotypes, reflected in social hierarchy and history, that defines their truly insidious nature (see Gross, 2005).

Stereotyping as a normal cognitive process

ASK YOURSELF ...
• How does this view of stereotyping relate to the view of the person as thinker (Fiske and Taylor, 1991; see above, page 143)?

If stereotypes are 'categories about people' (Allport, 1954; Brislin, 1981), and categories in general – and stereotypes in particular – are shortcuts to thinking, then from a purely cognitive point of view, there's nothing unique about stereotypes. According to Brislin (1993), stereotypes 'reflect people's need to organise, remember, and retrieve information that might be useful to them as they attempt to achieve their goals and to meet life's demands ...'.

Lippmann (1922) also argued that stereotypes serve a crucial *practical* function:

> ... the real environment is altogether too big, too complex, and too fleeting for direct acquaintance. We are not equipped to deal with so much subtlety, so much variety, so many permutations and combinations. And although we have to act in that environment, we have to reconstruct it on a simpler model before we can manage it.

'Big, complex and fleeting' describes many caring situations, so it's enlightening to consider stereotyping as a time-saving cognitive process. But, as health professionals, we should be careful about falling into that trap!

According to the *cognitive miser* perspective, stereotypes are resource-saving devices. They simplify the processing of information about other people. As Fiske (2004) says, '... under the busy conditions of ordinary interaction, people can save cognitive resources by using stereotype-consistent information ...'. This is a good example of the *selective* nature of person perception.

The accuracy of stereotypes

Definitions claim that stereotypes are *exceptionless generalisations*. But, clearly, the degree of generalisation involved is too great to make a stereotype factually true: no group is completely homogeneous and individual differences are the norm. Yet in Katz and Braly's study, the instruction to list the traits typical of each ethnic/national group was taken to mean 'true of all members of each group' (Brown, 1986). However, the early studies never actually found out what participants understood by 'typical'.

McCauley and Stitt (1978) attempted to rectify this. They concluded that what 'typical' seems to mean is *characteristic* – that is, true of a higher percentage of the group in question than of people in general (Brown, 1986). Stereotypes, then, seem to be *schemas* about what particular groups are like relative to 'people in general'. They *aren't* exceptionless generalisations. Perhaps this is how we should understand Allport's claim that stereotypes do contain a 'kernel of truth'.

Stereotypes, expectations and behaviour

Our expectations of people's personalities or capabilities may influence the way we actually treat them, which in turn may influence their behaviour in such a way that confirms our expectation (the *self-fulfilling prophecy*). This illustrates how stereotypes can (unwittingly) influence our behaviour towards others, and not just our perception and memory of them.

My approach to Vera was an example of this. Although I didn't mean it to, my disapproval must have shown in my expression or my body language. I expected resistance, and I got it!

Stereotypes and nurses' behaviour

In a small, ethnographic study of midwives' stereotypes of Asian women, Bowler (1993, in Knight, 1995) suggested that these relate to four main themes: communication problems, failure to comply with care, making a fuss about nothing, and a lack of normal (western) maternal instinct. Bowler points to several instances where care was less than optimal, because the midwives relied on their stereotypes. After observing the deliveries of six Asian women, she noted that only one was offered pain relief. The midwives may have found it too difficult to explain pain relief options to women who spoke little English, or perhaps they thought that the women did not need (or deserve) pain control because of their known 'low pain thresholds' (Bowler, in Knight; see also Chapter 3).

An American study by McDonald (1994) aimed to discover whether nurses provide greater amounts of narcotic analgesics (a) to men than to women, and (b) to white patients than to those from minority ethnic communities. The sample consisted of 180 patients (79 women, 101 men), aged 18–64, all with non-perforated appendicitis with subsequent uncomplicated appendectomy. None had a criminal or drug addiction history. The ethnic composition was: 2 per cent Asian; 12 per cent African-American; 8 per cent Hispanic; 78 per cent white.

Males received significantly more analgesics than females for the initial post-operative dose. This suggests that, if stereotyping occurs, it may not be extensive or prolonged. However, members of ethnic majorities received significantly more than members of minority groups for the total post-operative dose. McDonald finds this latter finding more difficult to explain. In addition to nurses' stereotypes, minority patients may have been less likely to express their pain, more reluctant to receive analgesics, or their complaints may have been given less credibility.

So, it would seem that it's not stereotypes themselves that are dangerous or objectionable, but how they affect behaviour. According to Operario and Fiske (2004): '… stereotypes are both (a) basic human tendencies inherent within our mental architecture; and (b) potentially damaging belief systems, depending on the power of the situation …'

This is shocking, but I'm learning how such things happen. And apart from showing how dangerous stereotypical assumptions are, it shows how complicated the accurate assessment of patients' needs can be.

> #### *ASK YOURSELF …*
> - What images of 'the nurse' do you think are held by members of the general public (as portrayed in the media, for example)?
> - What effect are these stereotypes likely to have on patients' impressions of nurses?
> - How might they be challenged/overcome?

For most, nurses are female (see below), self-sacrificing angels, handmaidens ('the good woman serving the doctor'), battleaxes or sex kittens (O'Dowd, 1998).

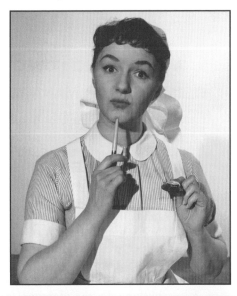

CRITICAL DISCUSSION 8.1 Nursing: a suitable profession for a man?

- According to Mason (1991), despite the circuitous route by which men become nurses, it's surprisingly easy to come up with a stereotype. A typical candidate is in his early twenties and no one in his immediate family has a medical background. He won't have thought about becoming a nurse in school and will probably have been in a totally unrelated job since 16 or 18. He will have stumbled on nursing after a couple of unfulfilling years career-wise. Despite the misgivings of friends and family, he then decides it's the career for him.

- While wanting to care for people is the prime reason given by men for entering nursing (as it is for females), in psychiatric nursing the need for physical strength to restrain patients has led to male/female ratios closer to 50:50 (Mason, 1991).

- The perceived link between male nursing and homosexuality rests on the belief that gay men are more caring than straight men. But this assumption commands little support, even among gays. And although most acknowledge that a male nurse has to be able to work well with women, there's no evidence that gay men are any better in this respect than other men (Mason, 1991).

- The subject of young female mental health patients falling in love with male nurses has always been a sensitive, but often unacknowledged, issue (Holyoake, 1998). Holyoake argues that: 'For many male nurses, popular stereotypes militate against their ability to interact with female patients without being charged with seduction or entrapment.'

ASK YOURSELF ...
- How do you feel about men becoming midwives?

- Is this an 'inappropriate' area of nursing for men?

- Are there any other 'inappropriate' areas?

- Should patients have the right to choose the gender of the nurses who care for them?

One of these stereotypes is of the male psychiatric nurse as potential abuser of women mental health care users (Stanley, 1998). While cases of such male nurses using their social power against vulnerable women do occur (and are dealt with stringently by the UKCC), there are also cases of women patients making overt moves towards male nurses, who may feel embarrassed or compromised (Gulland, 1998, in Stanley, 1998).

Two of the elderly women (with fractured femurs) have said to me that they don't want the male HCA ('that man') coming anywhere near them. Yet they're quite happy for male doctors to attend them! And most male patients seem quite happy to be cared for by female nurses.

INFLUENCING HOW OTHERS SEE US

IMPRESSION MANAGEMENT

It's difficult to think of a social situation in which we're not trying (consciously or otherwise) to manipulate how others perceive us. This fundamental aspect of social interaction is referred to as *impression management* (or *self-presentation*) (Baumeister, 1982; Leary and Kowalski, 1990), which Turner (1991) defines as 'the process of presenting a public image of the self to others'. Sometimes we may be trying to influence particular people on a particular occasion, such as in a job interview, or we may be trying to maintain an image of ourselves (as a caring or competent person, for example).

According to Leary and Kowalski (1990), impression management can increase our subjective well-being by meeting three primary motivations:

1. maximising the reward of social relationships (*belonging* – its major function)
2. enhancing self-esteem (*self-enhancement*)
3. establishing desired identities (*self-understanding*).

It's widely agreed that we usually try to influence others in a positive way – that is, we want them to have a favourable impression of us (Schlenker, 1980; Turner, 1991).

In books such as *The Presentation of Self in Everyday Life* (1971), Goffman, the Canadian sociologist, offers a 'dramaturgical' analysis of social interaction. To create a successful impression requires the right setting, props (e.g. the way you are dressed), skills and a shared understanding of what counts as 'backstage'. For example, the person who takes *self-disclosure* too far (see below) may be regarded as bringing onto stage what should be kept 'backstage', and so creates an unfavourable impression.

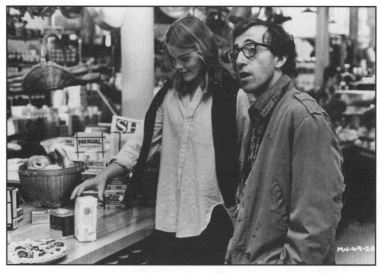

Woody Allen (in *Manhattan*) typically plays a character who's unlucky in love. This is partly due to his inappropriate self-disclosure

How is impression management carried out?

Impression management requires us to 'take the role of the other'. We must be able, psychologically, to step into someone else's shoes to see how we look from their viewpoint, and to adjust our behaviour accordingly. Fiske and Taylor (1991) and Fiske (2004) identify several components of impression management, ways of adjusting our behaviour to take into account other people's viewpoints.

This underpins the whole concept of individualised care – talking to Vera and learning about her background did help change the way I behaved towards her.

Table 8.1 Major components involved in impression management (based on Fiske, 2004; Fiske and Taylor, 1991)

In **behaviour matching**, we try to match the target person's behaviour. For example, if the other person is self-disclosing, we'll tend to do so to a comparable degree.

When we **conform to situational norms**, we use our knowledge of what's appropriate behaviour in a particular situation to adopt that behaviour ourselves. For every social setting, there's a pattern of social interaction that conveys the best identity for that setting (the 'situated identity'). **High self-monitors** (see text below) are more likely to make a favourable impression.

Appreciating or flattering others (**ingratiation**) can sometimes produce a favourable response from the target person, especially if it's done sincerely. But if seen for what it is, flattery (or laughing at their jokes, etc.) can backfire on the flatterer, who'll be seen as deliberately trying to achieve his/her own ends (a hypocrite or sycophant – an 'arse-licker' in popular terminology).

If we show **consistency** among our beliefs, or between our beliefs and behaviour, we're more likely to impress other people favourably. Inconsistency is usually seen as a sign of weakness.

Our **verbal and non-verbal behaviours** should match, which they usually do if we're sincere. But if we're flattering, or in some other way being dishonest, the non-verbal channel will often 'leak', giving away our true feelings. When people perceive an inconsistency between what someone says and what they're trying to convey with their body, the latter is usually taken as revealing the 'true' message (Argyle *et al.*, 1972; Mehrabian, 1972).

Self-promotion is an attempt to be seen as *competent*, but this can conflict with the wish to be *liked*. Also, there's the danger of being seen as conceited, and, at worst, a fraud.

Intimidation is meant to convey the impression of being *dangerous* ('don't mess with me'). But empty threats can produce a loss of credibility (as with parents and children).

In **exemplification**, the person wants to be seen as *worthy*, *moral* and *saintly*. The downside is being seen as sanctimonious, 'holier than thou' ('a pain').

Supplication is the strategy of last resort. The aim is to be seen as *helpless* ('strategic incompetence'), but the downside is being perceived as lazy, calculating and manipulative.

Most of these make us seem insincere and manipulative! But as self-monitoring is a skill we're expected to develop through reflection on practical and psychological aspects of care, it provides useful insights. I think when I first approached Vera, my verbal and non-verbal language probably didn't match.

Are some positive impressions more positive than others?

One exception to the rule that we always try to create favourable impressions in others is *behavioural self-handicapping*. You might protect yourself from anticipated failure by engaging in behaviours that will produce insurmountable obstacles to success. So, when the inevitable failure happens, you've a ready-made excuse.

Alternatively, you may blame, in advance, things about yourself that could explain the failure (apart from your lack of competence). For example, lecturers at exam time get quite used to students telling them how badly they're going to do because of lack of sleep, not having been well, having been unable to revise, always getting anxious about exams, and so on (*self-reported handicaps*).

One way of thinking about self-handicapping is to see it as an attempt to influence the kind of *attribution* other people make about our behaviour. We want them to see our failures as caused by factors 'beyond our control' and that don't, therefore, threaten the positive impression they have of us (and that we have of ourselves). Making excuses for, as well as confessing, our socially undesirable behaviour after it has occurred can also be explained in attributional terms (Weiner, 1992; see also Chapter 9).

Like defence mechanisms, some of these strategies are uncomfortably familiar!

SELF-MONITORING

While people in general are concerned with the impressions they make on others, people differ in the extent to which they can and do exercise intentional control over their self-presentation. *Self-monitoring* refers to how much people attend to the social situation as a guide for their behaviour, as opposed to their own internal states (Snyder, 1974, 1987). *High self-monitors* are particularly talented in this way compared with *low self-monitors* (Snyder, 1995).

◉ *High self-monitors* are concerned with behaving in a socially appropriate manner and so are more likely to monitor the situation (rather than themselves), looking for subtle cues as to 'how to behave'. They're more skilled in using facial expressions and their voices to convey particular emotions, and can interpret others' non-verbal communication more accurately compared with low self-monitors (Ickes and Barnes, 1977; Snyder, 1979). But, carried to an extreme, their perceptiveness and social sensitivity can make them look like self-interested opportunists who change themselves and their opinions to suit the situation (Snyder, 1987). Their behaviour shows greater *cross-situational inconsistency* – they behave differently in different situations.

◉ *Low self-monitors* remain 'themselves' regardless of the situation, rarely adapting to the norms of the social setting. They monitor their behaviour in relation to their own enduring needs and values. Carried to an extreme, they can be seen as insensitive, inflexible and uncompromising (Snyder, 1987). They show greater *cross-situational consistency*.

According to Fiske (2004):

Both levels of self-monitoring can be useful in the social world. Groups need people who are sensitive to norms and flexible about adjusting to them, and groups also need people who stand up for enduring principles, so a mix of high and low self-monitors is arguably good for group survival.

As nurses we are expected to be good 'team players' and also assertive in challenging traditional norms. I think it's difficult to be both.

SELF-DISCLOSURE

How accurately others perceive us is determined partly by how much we reveal to them about ourselves (*self-disclosure*). Wiemann and Giles (1988) define this as 'the voluntary making available of information about one's self that would not ordinarily be accessible to the other at that moment'.

According to Jourard (1971), we disclose ourselves through what we say and do (as well as what we omit to say and do). This means that we have greater control over some aspects of self-disclosure than others since, generally, we have greater control over verbal than non-verbal behaviour. However, Jourard believes that the decision to self-disclose (or to become 'transparent') is one taken freely, and the aim in disclosing ourselves is to 'be known, to be perceived by the other as the one I know myself to be'. Jourard believes that we can learn a great deal about ourselves through mutual self-disclosure, and our intimacy with others can be enhanced. It's a way of both achieving and maintaining a healthy personality, but only if the self-disclosure meets the criterion of *authenticity* (or honesty).

Factors influencing disclosure include:

◎ *reciprocity* – the more personal the information we disclose to someone, the more personal the information they're likely to disclose to us
◎ *norms* – the situation we're in often determines how much (or what kind of) disclosure is appropriate
◎ *trust* – generally, the more we trust someone, the more prepared we are to self-disclose to them
◎ *quality of relationships* – Altman and Taylor's (1973) *social penetration theory* maintains that the more intimate we are with somebody, the greater the range of topics we disclose to them and the more deeply we discuss any particular topic
◎ *gender* – women generally disclose more than men, and Jourard (1971) argues that men's limited self-disclosure prevents healthy self-expression and adds stress to their lives.

ASK YOURSELF …
• Think of your various relationships. What determines the nature and extent of what you disclose to other people?

• To what extent is self-disclosure expected/permitted in your nurse role?

My experience with Vera showed me how easily assumptions can be made – and changed – by appearance or minimal information, and I felt guilty (again) at making a hasty judgement about her. I feel much more aware of the dangers of misperceptions now. In future, I'll try not to jump to 'shortcut' conclusions, especially those based on Derbyshire's (1986) 'beautiful is good' stereotype!

Trying to appear 'professional' (i.e. confident and capable) to patients can make it difficult to be too open with them, to know how far to go. This is one benefit of group tutorials. It's a relief to be able to express misgivings and worries about our experiences honestly; we do feel closer as a result. And I'm sure that without chatting to Vera and gaining her trust, I wouldn't have obtained her cooperation.

CHAPTER SUMMARY

◎ **Interpersonal perception** refers to how we all attempt to explain, predict and, to some degree, control the behaviour of other people. In these ways, we can all be thought of as psychologists.

◎ Both object and person perception involve **selection**, **organisation** and **inference**. But only people behave, interact with each other, perceive and experience.

◎ Four views of people as thinking organisms have been identified, seeing us as **consistency seekers**, **naïve scientists**, **cognitive misers** and **motivated tacticians**.

◎ **Central traits** exert a major organising influence on our overall impression of a person, while **peripheral traits** have little or no influence. An alternative, but not contradictory, explanation is that overall impressions and inferences about additional traits reflect our **implicit personality theories** (IPTs).

◎ While most of the evidence supports a **primacy effect** with regard to strangers, a **recency effect** may be more powerful with regard to people we know well.

◎ The **halo effect** is one kind of IPT, which enables us to infer what people are like when we have only limited information about them. IPTs may be based on people's names and their physical attractiveness.

◎ **Stereotypes** represent a special kind of IPT, and they characterise entire **groups**. Traditionally, researchers studied stereotypes in relation to prejudice and regarded them as false, illogical **overgeneralisations**.

◎ **Stereotyping** affects our **expectations** of others and may also influence people's **behaviour** towards members of outgroups.

◎ We try actively to influence the impression that others form of us through **impression management/self-presentation**. Strategies used to create favourable impressions include **behaviour matching**, **appreciating/flattering others**, **showing consistency among our beliefs**, and **matching our verbal and non-verbal behaviours**.

◎ **High self-monitors** try to match their behaviour to the situation, while **low self-monitors** are more likely to 'be themselves'.

◎ Important factors that influence **self-disclosure** include **reciprocity**, **norms**, **trust**, **quality of relationship** and **gender**.

ATTRIBUTION

9

INTRODUCTION AND OVERVIEW

Attribution theory deals with the general principles governing how we select and use information to arrive at causal explanations for behaviour. As we noted at the beginning of Chapter 8, attribution is an important aspect of social perception, theories of which flourished from the 1950s to the 1970s. Most of our impressions of others are based on their overt behaviour and the setting in which it occurs. How we judge the causes of someone's behaviour (the 'actor') will have a major influence on the impression we form about them. Was their behaviour something to do with them 'as a person', such as their motives, intentions or personality (an *internal* cause)? Or was it something to do with the situation, including some other person or some physical feature of the environment (an *external* cause)?

Unless we can make this sort of judgement, we cannot really use the person's behaviour as a basis for forming an impression of them. Although we might mistakenly attribute the cause to the person instead of the situation, an attribution still has to be made. This applies as much to nurses and doctors trying to explain the causes of patients' illnesses as it does to social interaction in general.

Rather than being a single body of ideas and research, attribution theory is a collection of diverse theoretical and empirical contributions sharing several common concerns. Six different traditions form the 'backbone' of attribution theory (Fiske and Taylor, 1991). Three are discussed in this chapter:

◎ Heider's (1958) *'common-sense' psychology*
◎ Jones and Davis's (1965) *correspondent inference theory*
◎ Kelley's (1967, 1972, 1983) *covariation* and *configuration models*.
The other three are not:
◎ Shachter's (1964) *cognitive labelling theory* (of emotion – see Gross, 2005)
◎ Bem's (1967, 1972) *self-perception theory* (of attitude change – see Chapter 10)
◎ Weiner's (1986) *attributional theory of motivation* (see Gross, 2005).

The models and theories of Heider, Jones and Davis, and Kelley see people as being logical and systematic in their explanations of behaviour. In practice, however:

> … Using an intuitive and relatively automatic process, people do not think about making attributions; they just do it. People are experts at understanding other people – at least we all think we are – but we do not actually understand how we do it until we reflect on it. And attribution theory is one way of systematically reflecting on it. (Fiske, 2004)

One of the most important aspects of the nurse's role is assessment. To make an accurate assessment, we use our perceptual abilities to make judgements about people's character and personality, and use this information to help us predict their future behaviour and how they're likely to respond to us. Most of us pride ourselves on our effective assessment skills, but psychological research suggests that we may not always be as accurate as we'd like to think (Sayer, 1992).

From my diary (8): Year 1/Orthopaedic Ward

There was a bit of a panic on the ward this morning. Everyone was busy getting ready to admit elective surgery patients when Charge Nurse (CN) asked where Mr Inman was; he'd been in overnight following a reduction of a left Colles fracture under general anaesthetic. I couldn't find him. When I told the CN, he said he had to be found and to look again. He sounded bad-tempered so I hurried off to do as he asked. When I still couldn't find him, I told Maggie (the Staff Nurse and my mentor). She looked concerned, explaining that Mr Inman had Von Willebrand's disease, a type of haemophilia. He was supposed to have another blood test to check if he needed a further injection of DDAVP (Desmopressin) before being discharged. Everyone was very worried and eventually Maggie phoned his house. I heard her tell CN that Mr Inman was at home and then I had to go to help admit patients.

ATTRIBUTION AND THE NAÏVE SCIENTIST

The process by which we make judgements about internal/external causes is called the *attribution process*. It was first investigated by Heider (1958). According to Antaki (1984), attribution theory promises to 'uncover the way in which we, as ordinary men and women, act as scientists in tracking down the causes of behaviour; it promises to treat ordinary people, in fact, as if they were psychologists …'.

HEIDER'S 'COMMON-SENSE' PSYCHOLOGY

Heider argued that the starting point for studying how we understand the social world is the 'ordinary' person. He asked, 'How do people usually think about and infer meaning from what goes on around them?' and 'How do they make sense of their own and other people's behaviours?' These questions relate to what he called 'common-sense' psychology: the 'ordinary' person is a naïve scientist who links observable behaviour to unobservable causes, and these *causes* (rather than the behaviour itself) provide the meaning of what people do.

What interested Heider was the fact that members of a culture share certain basic assumptions about behaviour. These assumptions belong to the belief system that forms part of the culture as a whole and distinguishes one culture from another. We explain people's behaviour in terms of:
◎ *dispositional* (or personal/internal) factors, such as ability or effort, and
◎ *situational* (or environmental/external) factors, such as circumstances or luck.
When we observe somebody's behaviour, we're inclined to attribute its cause to one or other of these two general sources. This represents one of the culturally shared beliefs about behaviour that forms part of common-sense psychology.

Although Heider didn't formulate his own theory of attribution, he inspired other psychologists to pursue his original ideas. As well as his insight relating to personal and situational factors as causes of behaviour, three other ideas have been particularly influential (Ross and Fletcher, 1985):

1. when we observe others, we tend to search for enduring, unchanging and dispositional characteristics
2. we distinguish between intentional and unintentional behaviours
3. if some event takes place when the effect occurs, we're likely to regard that event as the cause.

JONES AND DAVIS'S CORRESPONDENT INFERENCE THEORY (CIT)

CORRESPONDENT INFERENCES AND INTENTIONALITY

ASK YOURSELF ...
- Can you think of an equivalent example involving a nurse, his/her display of caring behaviour, and a patient's correspondent inference about the nurse's caring disposition?

Jones and Davis (1965) were very much influenced by Heider. They argued that the goal of the attribution process is to be able to make *correspondent inferences*. We need to be able to infer that both the behaviour and the intention that produced it correspond to some underlying, stable feature of the person (a *disposition*). An inference is 'correspondent' when the disposition attributed to an actor 'corresponds' to the behaviour from which the disposition is inferred. For instance, if someone gives up his seat on the bus to allow a pregnant woman to sit down, we'd probably infer that he's 'kind and unselfish'. This is a correspondent inference, because both the behaviour and the disposition can be labelled in a similar way ('kind and unselfish'). But if we attribute the behaviour to compliance with someone else's demands ('he' is a husband whose wife has told him to give up his seat), then we wouldn't be making a correspondent inference.

We assume people behave in a way that matches the kind of person they are. I inferred that Mr Inman was, at best, a thoughtless man to leave the ward without telling anyone and cause such worry.

According to Jones and Davis, a precondition for a correspondent inference is the attribution of *intentionality*. They specify two criteria or conditions for this. We have to be confident that the actor:

1. is capable of having produced the observed effects, and
2. knew the effects the behaviour would produce.

I was irritated by Mr Inman for wasting our time when we were so busy. I can see that underlying my irritation was the assumption that he knew he should have a blood test before he left, and knew the concern his not having one would cause.

ASK YOURSELF ...
- How might these two criteria (especially the second one) influence a nurse's perception of, say, a patient with vascular disease who has always been a heavy smoker?

The nurse might assume that smokers know their behaviour could lead to vascular disease. So, their smoking means they intend to inflict long-term damage to their health in exchange for short-term satisfaction (see Chapter 4). The nurse interprets this as an undesirable internal quality (disposition) of the person and makes a negative judgement. This logic can be applied to a whole range of behaviours, from substance abuse to unprotected casual sex, and from eating an unhealthy diet to taking an overdose (Walsh, 1995).

This reminds me, uncomfortably, of my initial attitude to Diana's smoking and weight gain (see my comments on pages 63 and 67). I'm supposed to have learned from that!

THE ANALYSIS OF UNCOMMON EFFECTS

Having made these preliminary decisions, how do we then proceed to infer that the intended behaviour is related to some underlying disposition? One answer is the *analysis of uncommon effects*. When more than one course of action is open to a person, a way of understanding why s/he chose one course rather than another is to compare the consequences of the chosen option with the consequences of those that weren't. In other words, what's *distinctive* (or *uncommon*) about the effects of the choice that's made?

For example, you've a strong preference for one particular university, even though there are several that are similar with regard to size, reputation, type of course, and so on. The fact that all the others require you to be in residence during your first year suggests that you've a strong preference for being independent and looking after yourself.

Generally, the fewer differences between the chosen and the unchosen alternatives, the more confidently we can infer dispositions. Also, the more negative elements involved in the chosen alternative, the more confident still we can be of the importance of the distinctive consequence. (If living out of residence means a lot of extra travelling or is more expensive, then the desire to be self-sufficient assumes even greater significance.)

OTHER FACTORS AFFECTING DISPOSITIONAL ATTRIBUTIONS

Because the analysis of uncommon effects can lead to ambiguous conclusions, other cues must also be used.
◎ *Choice* is self-explanatory: is the actor's behaviour influenced by situational factors or a result of free will?
◎ *Social desirability* relates to the norms associated with different situations. Because most of us conform most of the time, the need to explain other people's behaviour doesn't often arise. We base our impressions of others more on behaviour that is in some way unusual, novel, bizarre or anti-social than on behaviour that's expected or conventional.

Most patients wait until they're told they can go (social desirability). I don't know why Mr Inman decided to act differently.

ASK YOURSELF …
- Do you agree with this account of social desirability?

- Give your reasons.

- Can you think of an example from your own experience that is consistent with this account?

- Can it help explain why patients might be 'blamed' for their illness?

'Deviant' behaviour seems to provide more information about what the person is like, largely because when we behave unconventionally we're more likely to be ostracised, shunned or disapproved of (which, presumably, people don't want). Cases of professionals behaving in unprofessional ways, especially when they breach fundamental ethical codes and actually commit crimes, illustrate this point very clearly.

But it can also apply to nurses' perception of patients. For example, nurses expect people to behave in health-promoting ways (this is the 'norm' – see Chapter 4). So, when they do the opposite, such as smoking or eating a poor diet, this is 'conspicuous' and we use it as the basis of making an internal attribution. In this instance, a correspondent inference may be made regarding an *undesirable* disposition and behaviour (unlike the example above of the caring nurse). This is another way in which we may *blame* the patient.

Without his DDAVP injection Mr Inman could have been in danger from internal bleeding. And he didn't have instructions about his follow-up care either. I think I assumed he was careless of his welfare, or just too impatient to wait. Both were internal attributions.

Social desirability can also be explained in terms of the *positivity bias*.

Box 9.1 The positivity bias, vigilance and the 'Pollyanna principle'

- We usually see people as 'good', trustworthy, and so on (the *positivity bias*) (Fiske, 2004).

- According to the 'Pollyanna principle' (Matlin and Stang, 1978), people seek the pleasant and avoid the unpleasant, communicate good news more often than bad, judge pleasant events as more likely than unpleasant events, recall pleasant life experiences more accurately than unpleasant experiences, rate themselves better than the average and as more happy than not, and evaluate each other positively.

- Positivity is offset by *vigilance*: unexpected bad behaviour grabs people's attention. Why is this?

- According to Fiske (2004): (a) if negative events are perceived as rare, they should provide more information about the individual – they set the person apart from the norm; (b) negative events might also be more diagnostic – that is, allow more confident categorisation of the person as a particular kind or other, regardless of the norm.

Roles refer to another kind of conformity. When people in well-defined roles behave as they're expected to, this tells us relatively little about their underlying dispositions (they're 'just doing their job'). But when they display out-of-role behaviour, we can use their actions to infer 'what they're really like'. This is similar to the effects of social desirability, except that the norms are associated with particular social positions within an overall social context rather than with the context or situation itself.

I knew Mr Inman had been a teacher, so I suppose I expected him to behave in a 'professional' way. I also expected him to be a 'good patient'. His acting out of role made it more likely I would assume he was impatient or inconsiderate.

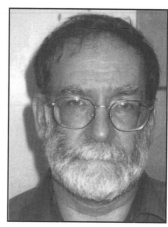

Harold Shipman, General Practitioner convicted of the murder of more than 250 of his patients

Prior expectations are based on past experiences with the same actor. The better we know someone, the better placed we are to decide whether his/her behaviour on a particular occasion is 'typical'. If it's 'atypical', we're more likely to dismiss it, or play down its significance, or explain it in terms of situational factors.

If, like Mr Inman, they do something unusual, we regard it as an important clue to their real character (uncommon effect). However, if we know them, we assume it was something in the situation that made them act 'out of character'.

We couldn't judge whether Mr Inman's behaviour was 'normal'; with short-stay patients information is usually focused on the medical/nursing procedure.

An evaluation of Jones and Davis's correspondent inference theory

While there are data consistent with Jones and Davis's theory, several weaknesses have been identified.

◎ Eiser (1983) has argued that intentions aren't a precondition for correspondent inferences. When someone is called 'clumsy', that dispositional attribution doesn't imply that the behaviour was intentional. In Eiser's view, behaviours that are unintended or accidental are beyond the scope of Jones and Davis's theory.

Health professionals are dealing all the time with people who have no control over what they do, and observing behaviour that isn't intentional.

◎ Also, it isn't just undesirable or unexpected behaviour that's informative. 'Conforming' behaviour can also be informative, as when behaviour confirms a stereotype (Hewstone and Fincham, 1996; see also Chapter 8).

◎ Although CIT continues to attract interest, most of the studies supporting it didn't measure causal attributions (Gilbert, 1995). Indeed, the model focuses on the covariation (correlation) of actions and their *consequences* as the key to attribution (Fiske, 2004). Inferring a disposition isn't the same as inferring a cause, and each appears to reflect different underlying processes (Hewstone and Fincham, 1996).

◎ Both of Kelley's models discussed next are concerned with the processes that determine whether an internal or external attribution is made for a behaviour's cause. Focusing on the covariation of actions and their potential causes is *complementary* to CIT (Fiske, 2004).

Hewstone and Fincham (1996) seem to be saying that, even if Mr Inman was normally 'difficult', it didn't mean the cause of this particular incident was, as I thought, internal. My attribution, affected by the negative consequences of his action, was wrong; Maggie found out what happened.

After breakfast someone had told Mr Inman that he could go home, so he went to the bathroom to dress. When he got back a few minutes later, two nurses were hurriedly making up his bed with clean linen; his possessions dumped (he said) on a chair outside the curtains. Everyone seemed frantically busy, so he quickly phoned for a taxi. He went to the office to say goodbye and 'thank you', but saw the CN deep in conversation with two doctors. He thought they saw him but ignored him so Mr Inman decided it must be too important to interrupt. Back in the ward, it was even busier than before, with several people waiting for admission. Mr Inman said he felt like an intruder – his one thought was to get out of the way. So he left.

ASK YOURSELF ...

• One of your fellow students (let's call her Sally) is late for psychology class one morning.

• How might you explain her late arrival?

• What kinds of information would you need in order to make a causal attribution?

KELLEY'S COVARIATION AND CONFIGURATION MODELS

THE COVARIATION MODEL

Kelley's *covariation model* (1967) tries to explain how we make causal attributions where we have some knowledge of how the actor usually behaves in a variety of situations and how others usually behave in those situations. The *principle of covariation* states that, 'An effect is attributed to one of its possible causes with which, over time, it covaries.'

In other words, if two events repeatedly occur together, we're more likely to infer that they're causally related than if they very rarely occur together. If the behaviour to be explained is thought of as an *effect*, the *cause* can be one of three kinds, and the extent to which the behaviour covaries with each of these three kinds of possible cause is what we base our attribution on. To illustrate the three kinds of causal information, let's take the hypothetical example of Sally, who's late for her psychology class.

◎ *Consensus* refers to the extent to which other people behave in the same way. In this example, are other students late for psychology? If all (or most) other students are late, then consensus is *high* (she's in good company), but if only Sally is late, consensus is *low*.

◎ *Distinctiveness* refers to the extent to which Sally behaves in a similar way towards other, similar 'stimuli' or 'entities'. Is she late for other subjects? If she is, then distinctiveness is *low* (there's nothing special or distinctive about psychology), but if she's late only for psychology, then distinctiveness is *high*.

◎ *Consistency* refers to how stable Sally's behaviour is over time. Is she regularly late for psychology? If she is, consistency is *high*, but if she's not (this is a 'one-off'), then consistency is *low*.

Kelley believes that a combination of *low consensus* (Sally is the only one late), *low distinctiveness* (she's late for all her subjects) and *high consistency* (she's regularly late) will lead us to make a *person* (*internal* or *dispositional*) attribution. In other words, the cause of Sally's behaviour is something to do with Sally, such as being a poor timekeeper.

However, any other combination would normally result in an external or situational attribution. For example, if Sally is generally punctual (*low consistency*), or if most students are late for psychology (*high consensus*), then the cause of Sally's lateness might be 'extenuating circumstances' in the first case or the subject and/or the lecturer in the second.

ASK YOURSELF ...

• Can you relate consensus, distinctiveness and consistency information to components of Jones and Davis's correspondent inference theory?

Table 9.1 Causal attributions based on three different combinations of causal information (based on Kelley, 1967)

Consensus	Distinctiveness	Consistency	Causal attribution
Low	Low	High	Person (actor/internal)
Low	High	Low	Circumstances (external)
High	High	High	Stimulus/target (external)

We can't use the idea of consistency and distinctiveness on short-term patients like Mr Inman; we don't know them for long enough to establish what is 'normal' for them. But it might apply to longer-term patients (e.g. those in traction on the orthopaedic ward).

Evaluation of Kelley's covariation model

◎ According to Gilbert (1998), the similarities between Kelley's covariation model and CIT are often overlooked:

   (a) *consensus* is similar to Jones and Davis's *social desirability* (if consensus is high, then the behaviour is socially desirable)

   (b) *distinctiveness* is similar to Jones and Davis's concern with *uncommon/unique effects* (the more distinctive the choice, the more it has to do with the unique effects of the choice)

   (c) *consistency* reflects an enduring *disposition* (as opposed to temporary circumstances).

◎ Despite a number of empirical studies supporting Kelley's model, not all three types of causal information are used to the same extent. For example, Major (1980) found that participants show a marked preference for consistency over the other two, with consensus being the least preferred.

In this case, I used high consensus (most patients wait until told to go) as salient information to judge Mr Inman's action. I now understand his behaviour also displayed low consistency (he is usually considerate) and high distinctiveness (he felt out of control in a strange situation).

◎ However, consensus information can have more of an impact if it's made more salient (for example, if it's contrary to what we might expect most people to do – Wells and Harvey, 1977). Consistent with Wells and Harvey's proposal is Hilton and Slugoski's (1986) *abnormal conditions focus model*. This can help explain why the three types of causal information aren't used to the same extent.

> **Box 9.2 The abnormal conditions focus model (Hilton and Slugoski, 1986)**
>
> - According to Hilton and Slugoski, Kelley's three types of information are useful to the extent that the behaviour requiring explanation contrasts with the information given. So, with *low consensus* information, the *person* is abnormal, whereas with *low consistency* information, the *circumstances* are abnormal. With *high distinctiveness* information, the *stimulus/target* is abnormal.
> - Just because people make attributions as if they're using covariation 'rules' doesn't necessarily mean they are (Hewstone and Fincham, 1996). Kelley seems to have overestimated people's ability to assess covariation. He originally compared the social perceiver to a naïve scientist (as did Heider), trying to draw inferences in much the same way as the formal scientist draws conclusions from data. More significantly, it's a *normative* model that states how, ideally, people should come to draw inferences about others' behaviour. However, the actual procedures that people use aren't as logical, rational and systematic as the model suggests. (This criticism also applies to Jones and Davis's CIT – see the section on error and bias below.)

My conclusions weren't based on reason, partly because I didn't have all the necessary information, and I was cross!

THE CONFIGURATION MODEL

Kelley recognised that in many situations (most notably when we don't know the actor), we might not have access to any or all of the covariation model's three types of information. Indeed, often the only information we have is a single occurrence of the behaviour of a particular individual. Yet we still feel able to explain the behaviour. The configuration model was Kelley's attempt to account for attributions about such single occurrence behaviours.

Yes! It would be the same in a significant number of caring situations – GP's surgery, Outpatients, X-ray, AE, Day surgery and Operating departments.

Causal schemata

When we make 'single event attributions' we do so using *causal schemata* (Kelley, 1972, 1983). These are general ideas – or ready-made beliefs, preconceptions and even theories (Hewstone and Fincham, 1996) – about 'how certain kinds of causes interact to produce a specific kind of effect' (Kelley, 1972). According to Fiske and Taylor (1991), causal schemata provide the social perceiver with a 'causal shorthand' for making complex inferences quickly and easily. They're based on our experience of cause–effect relationships and what we've been taught by others about such relationships. They come into play when causal information is otherwise ambiguous and incomplete.

Is this like stereotyping in social perception?

The two major kinds of causal schemata are *multiple necessary schemata* and *multiple sufficient schemata*.

> **Box 9.3 Multiple necessary and multiple sufficient schemata**
>
> - **Multiple necessary causes:** experience tells us that to be able to insert a naso-gastric tube you need theoretical knowledge, skill, confidence and the ability to obtain the cooperation of the patient, all of which indicate a commitment to learning/caring. Lack of any of these could lead to failure. So, in this sense, success is more informative than failure. Thus, there are many causes needed to produce certain behaviours – typically, those that are unusual or difficult.
> - **Multiple sufficient causes:** with some behaviours, any number of causes are sufficient to explain their occurrence. For example, a person might work in a hospital shop because of a desire to help, loneliness or boredom – any of these is a sufficient cause. If the helper is also disabled, or perhaps a very busy person, it requires extra effort, so it is likely to increase (augment) our opinion that the motive is altruistic.

According to the *discounting principle* (Kelley, 1983), 'Given that different causes can produce the same effect, the role of a given cause is discounted if other plausible causes are present.' Multiple sufficient schemata are also associated with the *augmenting principle*. This states that, 'The role of a given cause is augmented or increased if the effect occurs in the presence of an inhibitory factor.' So, we're more likely to make an internal attribution (to effort and ability) when a student passes an exam after, say, suffering the death of a relative than would be the case for a student who'd passed without having suffered such a loss.

If a person had to learn English before training as a health professional, we could assume greater dedication?

ERROR AND BIAS IN THE ATTRIBUTION PROCESS

As we've already seen, people are far less logical and systematic (less 'scientific') than required by Kelley's covariation model. We also noted that both this and Jones and Davis's CIT are *normative* models: they describe people's *ideal* attribution processes. 'Normative' here means a model of people thinking according to the highest standards, an idealised view of how people would think if provided with all the available information, with unlimited time and displaying no bias (Fiske, 2004).

Research into sources of error and bias seems to provide a much more accurate account of how people *actually* make causal attributions. Zebrowitz (1990) defines sources of bias as 'the tendency to favour one cause over another when explaining some effect. Such favouritism may result in causal attributions that deviate from predictions derived from rational attributional principles, like covariation …'.

Even though almost all behaviour is the product of both the person and the situation, our causal explanations tend to emphasise one or the other. According to Jones and Nisbett (1971), we all want to see ourselves as competent interpreters of human behaviour, and so we naïvely assume that simple explanations are better than complex ones. To try to analyse the interactions between personal and situational factors would take time and energy, and we seldom have all the relevant information at our disposal.

One kind of bias is the uneven use of different kinds of causal information that relate to Kelley's covariation model. Although all three types have some influence on attributions (thus supporting the broad outline of Kelley's model), we noted above that they're not used to an equal extent.

The time (and information) we had this morning to make attributions about Mr Inman's behaviour was certainly limited (especially in the case of the CN). This isn't unusual, especially in acute situations.

THE FUNDAMENTAL ATTRIBUTION ERROR (FAE)

The *fundamental attribution error* (FAE) refers to the general tendency to overestimate the importance of personal/dispositional factors relative to situational/environmental factors as causes of behaviour (Ross, 1977). This will tend to make others' behaviour seem more predictable, which, in turn, enhances our sense of control over the environment.

Heider (1958) believed that behaviour represents the 'figure' against the '(back)ground', comprising context, roles, situational pressures, and so on. In other words, behaviour is conspicuous, and situational factors are less easily perceived (see Gross, 2005).

For Zebrowitz (1990):

> … the fundamental attribution error is best viewed as a bias towards attributing an actor's behaviour to dispositional causes rather than as an attribution error. This bias may be limited to adults in Western societies and it may be most pronounced when they are constrained to attribute behaviour to a single cause …

Sayer (1992) gives the example of a male patient in an A&E department who's being verbally abusive. Staff may label him as an aggressive person (a correspondent inference), failing to realise that it is perhaps anxiety that is causing the aggression. Similarly, we may regard the victims of violence as somehow bringing an attack on themselves, either through something they do or a personal disposition. At a time when violence against nurses and other health professionals is increasing, this kind of FAE is particularly dangerous, because it can lead to victim-blaming. As a result, employers may fail to implement policies that deal adequately with such incidents, and victims can be left without support and feeling guilty that they're somehow responsible.

In the case of the aggressive male patient, his behaviour is 'figure' (i.e. it's what's most visible), while the '(back)ground' behaviour of staff may not have been witnessed by those judging him or is less obvious. For example, his aggression may have been triggered by staff who responded in a patronising and offhand way to what he considered a reasonable request (Sayer, 1992).

When assessing a patient, the nurse may fail to recognise the role played by external forces in shaping behaviour, resulting in the FAE of assuming that it's the patient's own fault they are ill. On admission to the ward, the nurse sees only the patients and their health problems, not their background and life experiences. Community nurses may be less likely to make this error, as they see patients in their home environment (Walsh, 1995).

I should have remembered what my community placement taught me! For us, Mr Inman's behaviour was the 'figure' against the familiar '(back)ground' of the ward that morning. A sudden perceptual flip shows me the ward as it must have appeared to him: it was hectic, all of us preoccupied with our own tasks – an alien environment.

The FAE and the just world hypothesis (JWH)

Related to the FAE, but not usually cited as an example of an attribution error, is the *just world hypothesis* (JWH) (Lerner, 1965, 1980). According to this, 'I am a just person living in a just world, a world where people get what they deserve'. When 'bad' things happen to people, we believe it's because they're in some way 'bad' people, so that they have at least partly 'brought it on themselves'. This can help explain the phenomenon of 'blaming the victim'. In rape cases, for example, the woman is often accused of having 'led the man on' or giving him the sexual 'green light' before changing her mind.

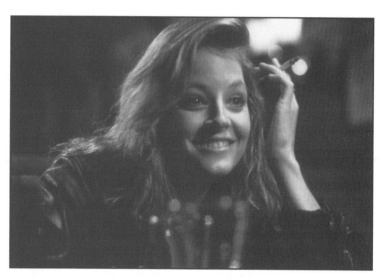

Jodie Foster, in *The Accused*, victim of gang-rape. Defence lawyers accused her of being of 'questionable character'

Believing in a just world gives us a sense of being in control: so long as we're 'good', only 'good' things will happen to us. By seeing failings and problems as the individual's own fault, we can preserve our belief in a just world. We then believe that it's not the fault of the NHS or nurses when things go wrong. Rather, it's the patient's own fault for engaging in unhealthy behaviour that any sensible person would avoid (Walsh, 1995).

*Until now, I never thought about it being the **nurses'** behaviour that contributed to Mr Inman leaving. Did we all blame Mr Inman?*

THE ACTOR–OBSERVER EFFECT (AOE)

Related to the FAE is the tendency for actors and observers to make different attributions about the same event. This is called the *actor–observer effect* (AOE) (Jones and Nisbett, 1971; Nisbett *et al.*, 1973):

◎ actors usually see their own behaviour as primarily a response to the situation and therefore as quite *variable* from situation to situation (the cause is *external*)

◎ the observer typically attributes the same behaviour to the actor's intentions and dispositions, and therefore as being quite *consistent* across situations (the cause is *internal*); the observer's attribution to internal causes is, of course, the FAE.

This is so uncomfortably accurate! From his point of view, Mr Inman behaved quite rationally: he was getting out of our way; I saw it as a fault in him.

One explanation for the AOE is that what's *perceptually salient* or vivid for the actor is different from what's perceptually salient or vivid for the observer (this is the figure–(back)ground explanation we noted when discussing the FAE). An important study by Storms (1973) supports this perceptual salience explanation of the AOE.

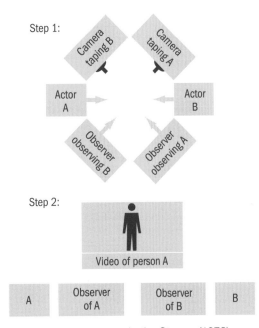

Figure 9.1 Diagram depicting the arrangement in the Storms (1973) experiment

KEY STUDY 9.1 Videotape and the attribution process (Storms, 1973)

- Two actor participants at a time engaged in a brief, unstructured conversation, while two observers looked on.
- Later, a questionnaire was used to measure the actors' attributions of their own behaviour in the conversation, and the observers' attributions of the behaviour of one of the two actors to whom they'd been assigned.
- Visual orientation was manipulated by the use of videotapes of the conversation so that:

  (a) the *no video* (control) group simply completed the questionnaire

  (b) the *same orientation* group simply saw a video of what they saw during the original conversation (before completing the questionnaire)

(c) the *new orientation* group saw a video which reversed the original orientation – actors saw themselves and observers saw the other actor (again, before completing the questionnaire).

- As predicted, in the first two groups the usual AOE was found. But, also as predicted, the AOE was reversed in the third group: actors made more dispositional attributions than did observers.

As we noted above, the aggressive patient in A&E may have attributed his behaviour to the attitude of the staff (an *external* cause). After waiting a long time to be seen, aggression may be more likely in anyone – not just those with an aggressive disposition.

House *et al.* (1986, in Knight, 1995) found that while doctors were more likely to view their diabetic patients' difficulties with their diet as due to motivational problems in the patient, the patients themselves were more likely to cite external causes.

Mr Inman, as the actor, would attribute his behaviour to his situation; I, as an observer, to his character.

THE SELF-SERVING BIAS (SSB)

Several studies have found that the AOE is most pronounced when judging *negative* behaviours, and may be absent or even reversed for positive ones.

ASK YOURSELF ...
- How might you explain this finding?

Naturally, no one wants to admit to being incompetent, so we're more likely to 'blame' our failures on something external to ourselves. This is the *self-protecting bias*, which protects our self-esteem. However, we're quite happy to take the credit for our successes. This is the *self-enhancing bias*, which enhances our self-esteem. Together, they constitute the *self-serving bias* (SSB) (Miller and Ross, 1975).

Marteau and Johnson (1986, in Knight, 1995) studied doctors' explanations of their failure to collect blood samples from diabetic children; 84 per cent of the attributions cited some feature of the child as the reason for failure. Similarly, doctors and nurses were more likely to attribute good diabetic control to medical intervention and poor control to the patient (Gamsu and Bradley, 1987, in Knight, 1995).

There's some evidence that positively valued outcomes (e.g. altruism) are more often attributed to people, and negatively valued outcomes (e.g. being late) to situational factors, regardless of who committed them. However, when either the self or someone closely associated with the self has committed the action, credit for positive events and denial of responsibility for negative ones are even stronger.

Putting myself in his place, I can see Mr Inman must have felt 'ejected' from his bed space and ignored when he tried to inform the CN he was going. He thought the injection of DDAVP he'd had before his operation was all he needed. His leaving was a negative outcome for the staff, so we would not have wanted to feel responsible for it. Looking back at my earlier comments, I see I've made the fact that we were all busy (i.e. blaming the situation) an explanation for none of us noticing him.

CRITICAL DISCUSSION 9.1 Cultural differences in attributional errors and biases

- Although the FAE has been assumed to be universal, more recent research suggests it may actually be specific to *individualist* (predominantly western) cultures (Fiske *et al.*, 1998; see Gross, 2005).

- In *collectivist* (mainly non-western) cultures, people are more likely to attribute someone's behaviour to situational factors as opposed to personality characteristics. They don't expect people to be consistent in their behaviour: different behaviours may be required when the situation calls for it (Nagayama Hall and Barongan, 2002).

- English-language newspapers reporting murders emphasise dispositional causes (such as a deeply disturbed, driven personality, very bad temper/'short fuse'), while Chinese-language papers reporting the same crime emphasise situational causes (relationships, rivalry and isolation, the social availability of guns, achievement pressure and the immediate context, such as recently being sacked) (Morris and Peng, 1994).

- The SSB isn't found among Asians, who are more likely to attribute their successes to external factors (such as luck) and their failures to internal factors (such as lack of effort) (Kitayama and Markus, 1995). This, in turn, reflects a bias towards *self-effacement*, which is more likely to maintain one's self-esteem in a collectivist culture (where the achievements of the individual are minimised).

- This strategy for maintaining self-esteem is also often used by women in individualist cultures 'whose belief system can also be characterized as collectivist in nature, in that they value relationships, put other people's needs before their own, and define themselves in terms of their connectedness to others ...' (Nagayama Hall and Barongan, 2002).

Being female, having Asian parents and my experiences in the community should have led me to make a situational attribution. I'm afraid, in spite of all that, I assumed it was something in Mr Inman's personality that made him leave as he did!

THE IMPORTANCE OF THE CONSEQUENCES

The more serious the consequences of the actor's behaviour, the more likely the FAE is to be made: the more serious the outcome, the more likely we are to judge the actor as responsible, regardless of his/her perceived intentions (e.g. Walster, 1966).

If more serious consequences can result in greater blame and responsibility, can the reverse inference occur – that is, can belief that an act is intentional affect perception of the seriousness of the consequences? Darley and Huff (1990) found that judgements of the damage caused by an action depended on whether participants believed it was done intentionally, through negligence or accidentally. Although the damage done was described in an identical way, those who read that the act was done intentionally inflated their estimation of the amount of damage done, compared with those who believed the damage was caused unintentionally (either through negligence or accident).

Another facet of the consequences of behaviour is how they affect us personally (*personal* or *hedonic relevance*): the more they affect us (the greater the hedonic relevance), the more likely we are to hold the actor responsible. Going one step further, *personalism* is the perceiver's belief that the actor intended to harm the perceiver. In terms of Jones and Davis's theory, this increases the chances of making a *correspondent inference*.

ASK YOURSELF ...
- Can you think of nursing situations (both actual and hypothetical) in which this source of error/bias has played a part?

173

Mr Inman's 'disappearance' created a panic. The trained staff were cross because they knew – as I do now – that they had a 'duty of care' to Mr Inman until he was properly discharged. If he'd had an internal bleed, all the attributions made (perhaps wrongly) would be more significant. As it was, he came back for his blood test and injection, and all was well.

CONCLUSIONS

All these errors and biases fall under the heading of *descriptive models*. They emphasise what people actually do when observed directly. What people 'ought' to do (according to normative models) if they're being completely rational is often *not* what they actually do. According to Fiske (2004):

> ... The descriptive models, by documenting biases, capture that discrepancy. In the case of ordinary personology, people ignore the hidden power of situations and focus on other people's dispositions more than they should, and people attribute more personal responsibility to themselves for good events than they should.

One of the reasons for assessment as the first stage of the nursing process is to establish baselines; it is much more difficult to establish a 'psychological baseline' than a physiological one. Fiske (2004) says we decide intuitively why people do things and only through systematic reflection can we understand how we came to those decisions (a very familiar principle!).

Reflecting on this experience in the light of attribution theory has shown that Mr Inman's actions were the consequence of his view of the situation (external), not his disposition (internal). It has also reminded me of the importance of clear communication with patients and that each patient interprets our routine behaviour from their own perspective.

In future I'll try to resist intuitive inclination and find out the facts about others' behaviour before making assumptions – even when in a hurry.

(And I discovered I was wrong about CN too – he was worried, not grumpy!)

CHAPTER SUMMARY

◎ **Attribution theory** refers to psychologists' attempts to explain the **attribution process**.

◎ Heider's 'common-sense' psychology sees people as **naïve scientists**, inferring unobservable causes (or meaning) from observable behaviour. In western culture, behaviour is explained in terms of both **personal** (**dispositional/internal**) and **situational** (**environmental/external**) factors.

◎ Jones and Davis were concerned with explaining how we make **correspondent inferences** about people's dispositions. One way of looking for dispositions that could have caused behaviour is through the **analysis of uncommon effects**.

◎ The likelihood of making dispositional attributions is influenced by **free choice**, **social desirability**, **roles** and **prior expectations**.

◎ Kelley's **covariation model** is concerned with the processes by which we make internal and external attributions for the causes of behaviour. Attributions about some effect/behaviour depend on the extent of its covariation with causal information regarding **consensus**, **consistency** and **distinctiveness**.

◎ Kelley's **configuration model** tries to account for 'single event attributions' in terms of **multiple necessary** and **multiple sufficient causal schemata**. The latter are associated with the **augmenting principle**, and we choose between two or more possible causes by using the **discounting principle**.

◎ People are actually less rational and scientific than Jones and Davis's, and Kelley's **normative** models require. A more accurate account of the attribution process involves looking at **systematic biases** in the attribution of cause.

◎ The **fundamental attribution error** (FAE) is the tendency to exaggerate the importance of internal/dispositional factors relative to external/situational factors. The likelihood of making it depends on the seriousness/importance of the **consequences** of behaviour, and **personal/hedonic relevance**.

◎ In the **actor–observer effect** (AOE), **actors** see their behaviours as responses to **situational factors**, whereas **observers** explain the same behaviours in **dispositional** terms.

◎ The AOE is most pronounced when one explains one's own negative behaviour (**self-protecting bias**). Personal successes tend to be explained in dispositional ways (**self-enhancing bias**). Together, they comprise **the self-serving bias** (SSB).

◎ There are important **cultural differences** with regard to the FAE and SSB in particular. These are related to **individualist** and **collectivist** cultures.

ATTITUDES AND ATTITUDE CHANGE

10

INTRODUCTION AND OVERVIEW

According to Gordon Allport (1935), 'The concept of attitudes is probably the most distinctive and indispensable concept in contemporary American social psychology ...'. More than 50 years later, Hogg and Vaughan (1995) claim that, 'Attitudes continue to fascinate research workers and remain a key, if controversial, part of social psychology.'

However, the study of attitudes has undergone many important changes during that time, with different questions becoming the focus of theory and research. According to Stainton Rogers *et al.* (1995), psychologists have tried to answer the following fundamental questions over the last 70 years:

1. Where do attitudes come from? How are they moulded and formed in the first place?
2. How can attitudes be measured?
3. How and why do attitudes change? What forces are involved and what intrapsychic mechanisms operate when people shift in their opinions about particular 'attitude objects'?
4. How do attitudes relate to behaviour? What is it that links the way people think and feel about an attitude object and what they do about it?

In this chapter, the emphasis is on some of the answers that have been offered to questions 3 and 4. This discussion is also relevant to prejudice, considered as an extreme attitude (see Chapter 11).

During the 1940s and 1950s, the focus of research was on attitude change, in particular *persuasive communication*. Much of the impetus for this came from the use of propaganda during the Second World War, as well as a more general concern over the growing influence of the mass media, especially in the USA. This period also saw the birth of a number of theories of attitude change, the most influential of these being Festinger's *cognitive dissonance theory*.

The 1960s and 1970s was a period of decline and pessimism in attitude research, at least partly due to the apparent failure to find any reliable relationship between measured attitudes and behaviour (Hogg and Vaughan, 1995). However, the 1980s saw a revival of interest, stimulated largely by the cognitive approach, so attitudes represent another important aspect of *social cognition* (see Chapter 8).

From my diary (18): Year 2/Surgical Ward

We had a termination of pregnancy on the theatre list today. Janet, 42, had an amniocentesis, which showed slightly raised Alpha-protein levels and a small risk her baby would have Down's syndrome. She had elected to have an abortion. Just before she was due for discharge, I found her crying in the bathroom. Eventually she calmed down and I asked if she was sad at 'losing' a baby. She said that was the trouble – she wasn't, but felt guilty. I tried to reassure her that, too, was a natural part of the grief reaction (see Chapter 20), but she said no, that wasn't it. She then told me that since her divorce she'd gone back to full-time work as a hairdresser and begun a new relationship, which had led to this 'slip-up'. Her children were 10 and 13 and she just didn't want another baby at her age; she'd used the Down's syndrome threat as an excuse. Now she felt what she'd done was wrong. I tried to comfort her and then reported it to Sister, who explained Janet's follow-up appointment would include an opportunity for counselling.

WHAT ARE ATTITUDES?

Allport (1935) regarded the study of attitudes as the meeting ground for the study of social groups, culture and the individual. Festinger (1950) also emphasised the integral interdependence of individual and group. But, with a few notable exceptions, attitude research has focused on *internal* processes, ignoring the influence of groups on attitude formation and change (Cooper *et al.*, 2004). Even Allport's (1935) definition reflects this bias: 'An attitude is a mental and neural state of readiness, organised through experience, exerting a directive or dynamic influence upon the individual's response to all objects and situations with which it is related.'

Warren and Jahoda's (1973) definition is probably the most 'social': '… attitudes have social reference in their origins and development and in their objects, while at the same time they have psychological reference in that they inhere in the individual and are intimately enmeshed in his behaviour and his psychological make-up.'

According to Zimbardo and Leippe (1991), 'An attitude is an evaluative disposition toward some object. It's an evaluation of something or someone along a continuum of like-to-dislike or favourable-to-unfavourable …'

According to Rosenberg and Hovland (1960), attitudes are 'predispositions to respond to some class of stimuli with certain classes of response'. These classes of response are:

◎ *affective*: what a person feels about the attitude object, how favourably or unfavourably it's evaluated.
◎ *cognitive*: what a person believes the attitude object is like, objectively.
◎ *behavioural* (sometimes called the '*conative*'): how a person actually responds, or intends to respond, to the attitude object.

This *three-component model*, which is much more a model of attitude structure than a simple definition (Stahlberg and Frey, 1988), is shown in Figure 10.1. It sees an attitude as an intervening/mediating variable between observable stimuli and responses, illustrating the influence that behaviourism was still having, even in social psychology, at the start of the 1960s. A major problem with this multi-component model is the assumption that the three components are highly correlated (see below, pages 181–184).

ATTITUDES, BELIEFS AND VALUES

An attitude can be thought of as a blend or integration of beliefs and values. Beliefs represent the knowledge or information we have about the world (although these may be inaccurate or incomplete) and, in themselves, are *non-evaluative*. To convert a belief

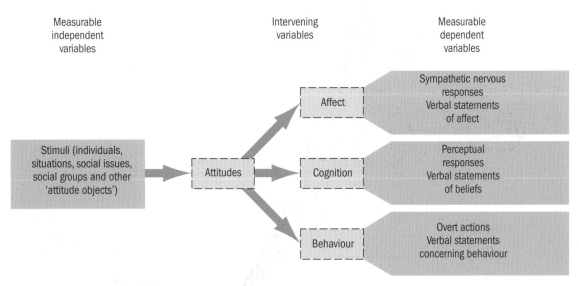

Figure 10.1 Three-component view of attitudes (Rosenberg & Hovland, 1960). From Stahlberg, D. & Frey, D. (1988) 'Attitudes 1: Structure, measurement and functions'. In Hewstone, M. *et al.* (eds) *Introduction to Social Psychology*. Oxford: Blackwell.

into an attitude, a 'value' ingredient is needed. Values refer to an individual's sense of what is desirable, good, valuable, worthwhile, and so on. While most adults will have many thousands of beliefs, they have only hundreds of attitudes and a few dozen values.

I thought I was quite clear what my attitude to abortion was – that in the circumstances outlined in the Abortion Act 1967 (and 1990 amendments), it is acceptable. I feel uncomfortable at the idea of it, but I can understand perfectly Janet's reasons for not wanting another baby. Behaviourally, I think I would have an abortion if the circumstances merited it. But at handover this morning, Bridie, an Irish student and a practising Catholic, also on placement on the ward, made her disapproval clear and asked not to be involved in Janet's care.

ASK YOURSELF ...
- Try to identify some of your most cherished values (there should be a relatively small number of these).

- Then try to identify some related attitudes, which are less abstract than values.

WHAT ARE ATTITUDES FOR?

According to Hogg and Vaughan (1995):

> ... attitudes are basic and pervasive in human life ... Without the concept of attitude, we would have difficulty construing and reacting to events, trying to make decisions, and making sense of our relationships with people in everyday life ...

In other words, attitudes provide us with ready-made reactions to, and interpretations of, events, just as other aspects of our cognitive 'equipment' do, such as stereotypes (see Chapters 8 and 11). Attitudes save us energy, since we don't have to work out how we feel about objects or events each time we come into contact with them.

However, not all attitudes serve the same function. Katz (1960), influenced by Freud's psychoanalytic theory, believes that attitudes serve both conscious and unconscious motives. He identified four major functions of attitudes (see Table 10.1).

179

Table 10.1 Four major functions of attitudes (based on Katz, 1960)

Knowledge function	We seek a degree of predictability, consistency and stability in our perception of the world. Attitudes give meaning and direction to experience, providing frames of reference for judging events, objects and people.
Adjustive (instrumental or utilitarian) function	We obtain favourable responses from others by displaying socially acceptable attitudes, so they become associated with important rewards (such as others' acceptance and approval). These attitudes may be publicly expressed, but not necessarily believed, as is the case with *compliance* (see Chapter 12).
Value-expressive function	We achieve self-expression through cherished values. The reward may not be gaining social approval, but confirmation of the more positive aspects of our self-concept, especially our sense of personal integrity.
Ego-defensive function	Attitudes help protect us from admitting personal deficiencies. For example, *prejudice* helps us to sustain our self-concept by maintaining a sense of superiority over others. Ego defence often means avoiding and denying self-knowledge. This function comes closest to being unconscious in a Freudian sense (see Chapters 2 and 6).

Katz's functional approach implies that some attitudes will be more resistant to efforts to change them than others – in particular, those that serve an ego-defensive function. This is especially important when trying to account for prejudice and attempts to reduce it (see Chapter 11).

My attitude was that there is nothing ethically wrong in terminating a pregnancy if there is good reason, so I was accepting of Janet's decision. I'm wondering now if that is serving an adjustive function. It must have taken a bit of courage (a value-expressive function) for Bridie to speak out in front of the staff; obviously she felt very strongly about it. She later argued I was rationalising what is, essentially, murder!

THE MEASUREMENT OF ATTITUDES

An attitude cannot be measured directly, because it's a *hypothetical construct*. Consequently, it's necessary to find adequate attitude indicators, and most methods of attitude measurement are based on the assumption that they can be measured by people's beliefs or opinions about the attitude object (Stahlberg and Frey, 1988). Most attitude scales rely on verbal reports, and usually take the form of standardised statements that clearly refer to the attitude being measured. Such scales make two further assumptions:

1. the same statement has the *same meaning* for all respondents and, more fundamentally,
2. subjective attitudes, when expressed verbally, can be *quantified* (represented by a numerical score).

One of the most widely used scales is the Likert scale (1932), which, applied to abortion, would require the participant to indicate how much s/he agrees or disagrees with the following statement:

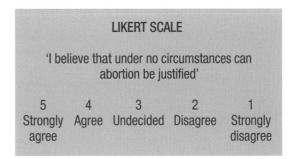

LIKERT SCALE

'I believe that under no circumstances can abortion be justified'

5	4	3	2	1
Strongly agree	Agree	Undecided	Disagree	Strongly disagree

(For a more detailed account of this and other scales, see Gross (2005).)

On this scale I would have ticked 1 or 2; Bridie, I think, would have ticked 5.

THE RELATIONSHIP BETWEEN ATTITUDES AND BEHAVIOUR

Once we've established people's attitudes, can we then accurately predict how they'll behave? Rosenberg and Hovland's (1960) three-components model (see page 179) implies that the behavioural component will be highly correlated with the cognitive and affective components.

An early study that shows the *inconsistency* of attitudes and behaviour is that of LaPiere (1934).

ASK YOURSELF ...
- Do people's expressed attitudes (cognitive and affective components) necessarily coincide with their overt actions (behavioural component)?
- Do we always act in accordance with our attitudes?

ASK YOURSELF ...
- Try to account for LaPiere's findings.

KEY STUDY 10.1 Some of my best friends are Chinese ... (LaPiere, 1934)

- Beginning in 1930 and for the next two years, LaPiere travelled around the USA with a Chinese couple (a young student and his wife), expecting to encounter anti-Oriental attitudes that would make it difficult for them to find accommodation.

- But in the course of 10,000 miles of travel, they were discriminated against only once and there appeared to be no prejudice. They were given accommodation in 66 hotels, auto-camps and 'tourist homes' and refused at only one. They were also served in 184 restaurants and cafés and treated with 'more than ordinary consideration' in 72 of them.

- However, when each of the 251 establishments visited was sent a letter six months later asking: 'Will you accept members of the Chinese race as guests in your establishment?', 91 per cent of the 128 that responded gave an emphatic 'No'. One establishment gave an unqualified 'Yes' and the rest said 'Undecided: depends upon circumstances'.

INFLUENCES ON BEHAVIOUR

It's generally agreed that attitudes form only one determinant of behaviour. They represent *predispositions* to behave in particular ways, but how we actually act in a particular situation will depend on the immediate consequences of our behaviour, how we think others will evaluate our actions, and habitual ways of behaving in those kinds of situations. In addition, there may be specific *situational factors* influencing behaviour. For example, in the LaPiere study, the high quality of his Chinese friends' clothes and luggage, and their politeness, together with the presence of LaPiere himself, may have made it more difficult to show overt prejudice. Thus, sometimes we experience a conflict of attitudes, and behaviour may represent a compromise between them.

I've said I could make the decision to terminate a pregnancy if necessary – but would I do it if it meant being socially ostracised/vilified as a result?

Compatibility between attitudes and behaviour

The same attitude may be expressed in a variety of ways. For example, having a positive attitude towards the Labour Party doesn't necessarily mean that you actually become a member or that you attend public meetings. But if you don't vote Labour in a general or local election, people may question your attitude. In other words, an attitude should predict behaviour to some extent, even if this is extremely limited and specific.

Indeed, Ajzen and Fishbein (1977) argue that attitudes can predict behaviour, provided that both are assessed at the same level of generality: there needs to be a high degree of *compatibility* (or *correspondence*) between them. They argue that much of the earlier research (LaPiere's study included) suffered from either trying to predict specific behaviours from general attitudes, or vice versa, and this accounts for the generally low correlations. A study by Davidson and Jaccard (1979) tried to overcome this limitation.

Ajzen and Fishbein (1977) are saying that, in spite of my expressed attitude, trying to predict whether I would have an abortion without knowing the specific circumstances would be difficult.

> **KEY STUDY 10.2 Attitudes can predict behaviour if you ask the right questions (Davidson and Jaccard, 1979)**
>
> - Davidson and Jaccard analysed correlations between married women's attitudes towards birth control and their actual use of oral contraceptives during the two years following the study.
> - When 'attitude towards birth control' was used as the attitude measure, the correlation was 0.08. Clearly, the correspondence here was very low.
> - But when 'attitudes towards oral contraceptives' were measured, the correlation rose to 0.32, and when 'attitudes towards using oral contraceptives' were measured, the correlation rose still further, to 0.53.
> - Finally, when 'attitudes towards using oral contraceptives during the next two years' was used, it rose still further, to 0.57. Clearly, in the last three cases, *correspondence* was much higher.

> *ASK YOURSELF ...*
> - Do you believe it is right for nurses and other health professionals to take industrial action, even if this is aimed at improving patient care?

According to Ajzen and Fishbein, every single instance of behaviour involves four specific elements:

1. a specific action
2. performed with respect to a given target
3. in a given context
4. at a given point in time.

According to the *principle of compatibility*, measures of attitude and behaviour are compatible to the extent that the target, action, context and time element are assessed at identical levels of generality or specificity (Ajzen, 1988).

For example, a person's attitude towards a 'healthy lifestyle' specifies only the target, leaving the other three unspecified. A behavioural measure that would be compatible with this global attitude would have to aggregate a wide range of health behaviours across different contexts and times (Stroebe, 2000).

In general, Janet seemed to be anti-abortion, but (reflecting Ajzen and Fishbein's four elements, above) she had an abortion (1) in order to keep on working, as she was a single mother of two older children (2), had a new career (3), and felt too old at 42 to have another baby (4). If she hadn't needed to work, had been happily married, or been younger she may have decided differently, although her attitude to abortion was the same.

The reliability and consistency of behaviour

Many of the classic studies that failed to find an attitude–behaviour relationship assessed just single instances of behaviour (Stroebe, 2000). As we noted earlier when discussing the LaPiere study, behaviour depends on many factors in addition to the attitude. This makes a single instance of behaviour an unreliable indicator of an attitude (Jonas *et al.*, 1995). Only by sampling many instances of the behaviour will the influence of specific factors 'cancel out'. This *aggregation principle* (Fishbein and Ajzen, 1974) has been demonstrated in a number of studies.

According to Hogg and Vaughan (1995), what emerged in the 1980s and 1990s is a view that attitudes and overt behaviour aren't related in a simple one-to-one fashion. In order to predict someone's behaviour, it must be possible to account for the interaction between attitudes, beliefs and behavioural intentions, as well as how all of these connect with the later action. One attempt to formalise these links is the *theory of reasoned action* (TRA) (Ajzen and Fishbein, 1970; Fishbein and Ajzen, 1975; see Chapter 4).

Janet's decision to terminate this particular pregnancy might indeed indicate a very different attitude to abortion than her willingness to repeat the experience. The TRA emphasises the importance of subjective norms derived from our social context (see Chapter 4). Bridie is a Catholic brought up in Ireland, whereas although my parents are Asian, they, and I, have been brought up in London; our very different norms are likely to affect our intentions and behaviour.

The strength of attitudes

Most modern theories agree that attitudes are represented in memory and that an attitude's *accessibility* can exert a strong influence on behaviour (Fazio, 1986). By definition, strong attitudes exert more influence over behaviour, because they can be *automatically activated*. According to the MODE model – 'motivation and opportunity as determinants' (Fazio, 1986, 1990) – spontaneous/automatic attitude–behaviour links occur when people hold highly accessible attitudes towards certain targets. These spontaneously guide behaviour, partly because they influence people's selective attention and perceptions of a particular target or situation.

So are they a shortcut to decision-making – like stereotypes? I didn't have to consider my reaction to Janet's operation; I read her notes and assumed it reasonable, until Bridie challenged me.

One factor that seems to be important is *direct experience*. For example, Fazio and Zanna (1978) found that measures of students' attitudes towards psychology experiments were better predictors of their future participation if they'd already taken part in several experiments than if they'd only read about them.

MODE acknowledges that, in some situations, people engage in *deliberate, effortful* thinking about their attitudes when deciding how to act (forming behavioural intentions). For example, a student deciding which university to go to will probably scrutinise his/her attitudes before making a choice. But research conducted under MODE focuses on automatic processing (Cooper *et al.*, 2004). The *theory of planned behaviour* (TPB: Ajzen, 1991), which built on the TRA (see above), was designed to explain the relationship between attitudes and behaviour when deliberate, effortful processing is required. According to TPB, it's behavioural *intentions*, rather than attitudes, that directly influence behaviour (again, see Chapter 4).

The TPB sees intentions as strategies to achieve particular goals. While upset, Janet confessed to me she had agonised about her decision to have a termination, but having invested so much time and effort in a better future for her children and herself, she felt she couldn't jeopardise it.

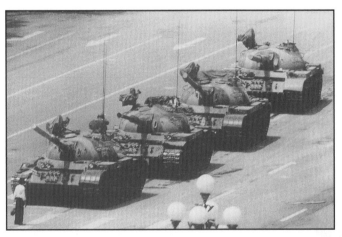

A demonstration of attitude–behaviour consistency that amazed the world; a pro-democracy Chinese student stands up for his convictions and defies tanks sent in against fellow rebels in Tiananmen Square, Beijing, China. Some 2000 demonstrators died in the subsequent massacre and the student was tried and shot a few days later

SOCIAL INFLUENCE AND BEHAVIOUR CHANGE

PERSUASIVE COMMUNICATION

According to Laswell (1948), in order to understand and predict the effectiveness of one person's attempt to change the attitude of another, we need to know 'who says what in which channel to whom and with what effect'. Similarly, Hovland and Janis (1959) say that we need to study:

◎ *the source* of the persuasive communication – that is, the communicator (Laswell's 'who')
◎ *the message* itself (Laswell's 'what')
◎ *the recipient* of the message or the audience (Laswell's 'whom'), and
◎ the *situation* or *context*.

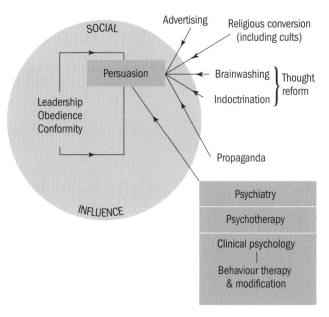

Figure 10.2 Different kinds of attempt to change people's attitudes and behaviour. These range from professional help for emotional and behavioural problems, through inevitable features of social interaction/social influence, to deliberate attempts to manipulate and control others for the benefit of the manipulator

Bridie had a religious motive for her message, which was quite clear: abortion is sin. The nursing staff, used to terminations, were not receptive to the message: one staff nurse said dismissively, 'Well, you would think that, wouldn't you?'

The basic paradigm in laboratory attitude–change research involves three steps or stages:

1. measure people's attitude towards the attitude object (*pre-test*)
2. expose them to a *persuasive communication* (manipulate a source, message or situational variable, or isolate a recipient-variable as the independent variable)
3. measure their attitudes again (*post-test*).

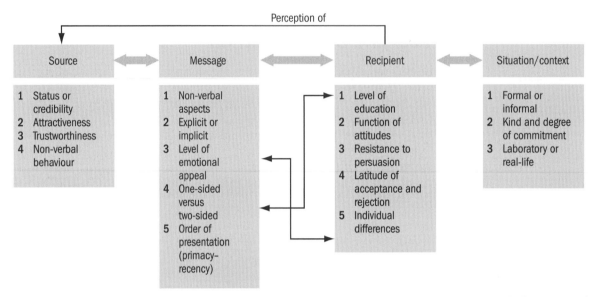

Figure 10.3 The four major factors involved in persuasive communication (arrows between boxes indicate examples of interaction between variables)

If there's a difference between pre- and post-test measures, then the persuasive communication is judged to have 'worked'.

If Bridie and I had done the Likert scale test (see page 181) before and after our discussion, I believe my attitude score would have shifted towards uncertainty, but I suspect Bridie's wouldn't have moved at all.

Theories of persuasion

The early research into persuasive communication was conducted for the US War Department's Information and Education Department. This largely pragmatic approach is known as the *Yale approach*, with Hovland being one of its leading figures. It told us a great deal regarding *when* attitude change is most likely to occur, and *how*, in practical terms, it can be produced. But it told us less about *why* people change their attitudes in response to persuasive messages.

Theories of systematic processing

According to *theories of systematic processing*, what's important is that the recipient processes the message content in a detailed way. This approach began with Hovland *et al.*'s (1953) proposal that the impact of persuasive messages can be understood in terms of a sequence of processes:

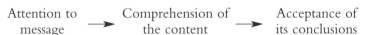

| Attention to message | → | Comprehension of the content | → | Acceptance of its conclusions |

If any of these fails to occur, persuasion is unlikely to be achieved.

McGuire (1969) proposed a longer chain of processes. We should ask if the recipient: (i) attended to the message; (ii) comprehended it; (iii) yielded to it (accepted it);

(iv) retained it; and (v) acted as a result. As with Hovland *et al.*'s theory, the failure of any one of these steps will cause the sequence to be broken.

I attended to Bridie's arguments, understood them and her reasons for making them. But I couldn't wholly accept them, which 'broke the sequence' and means she failed to radically change, although she might have affected my attitude.

Dual process/cognitive models

According to the *dual-process* or *cognitive perspective* (e.g. Chaiken, 1987), the key questions are as follows.

◎ What cognitive processes determine whether someone is actually persuaded?
◎ What do people think about when exposed to persuasive appeals?
◎ How do their various cognitive processes determine whether and to what extent they experience attitude changes (Baron and Byrne, 1991)?

Chaiken's (1987) answer to these questions is in the form of his *heuristic model of persuasion*. (Heuristics are rules of thumb or mental shortcuts, which we use in processing social or any other kind of information: stereotypes represent a major form of mental shortcut (see Chapter 8).)

When a situation is personally involving or salient, careful, cognitive analysis of the input occurs. The degree of attitude change depends largely on the quality of the arguments presented. However, when personal involvement is low, individuals rely on various heuristics to determine whether to change their attitudes. Much of the Yale approach, in fact, deals with the content of these heuristics. For example we are more easily persuaded by:

◎ experts than non-experts
◎ likeable sources than non-likeable
◎ a greater number of arguments backed up by statistics than a smaller number
◎ 'if other people think something is right (or wrong), then I should too'.

These are essentially peripheral, non-content issues.

We consider doctors are experts and, as professionals, they demand our respect if not our liking. Statistically, the act of abortion is common now. In England and Wales, 185,375 legal abortions were carried out in 2000 – it is estimated that 17 in 1000 women of reproductive age have an abortion (Graig, 2001, in Tschudin, 2003). Abortion is considered 'right' by law and accepted by the ward staff. I can see that all of these played a part in forming my attitude to abortion. However, I'm now seeing it as a much more complex and emotive issue, so I don't think heuristics are enough to make a judgement.

An evaluation of heuristic models

It's assumed that attitudes formed or changed on the basis of heuristic processing will be less stable, less resistant to counter-arguments, and less predictive of subsequent behaviour than those based on systematic processing. Several studies have shown that attitude change accompanied by high levels of issue-relevant cognitive activity are more persistent than those accompanied by little such activity (Stroebe, 2000).

Fear and persuasion

A famous early attempt to induce attitude change through the manipulation of fear was made by Janis and Feshbach (1953).

KEY STUDY 10.3 Fear of the dentist as a means to healthier teeth (Janis and Feshbach, 1953)

- Janis and Feshbach randomly assigned American high-school students to one of four groups (one control and three experimental).

- The message was concerned with dental hygiene, and degree of fear arousal was manipulated by the number and nature of consequences of improper care of teeth (which were also shown in colour slides). Each message also contained factual information about the causes of tooth decay, and some advice about caring for teeth.

- The *high fear condition* involved 71 references to unpleasant effects (including toothache, painful treatment and possible secondary diseases, such as blindness and cancer). The *moderate fear condition* involved 49 references, and the *low fear condition* just 18. The control group heard a talk about the eye.

- Before the experiment, participants' attitudes to dental health, and their dental habits, were assessed as part of a general health survey. The same questionnaire was given again immediately following the fear-inducing message, and one week later.

- The results show that the stronger the appeal to fear, the greater their anxiety (an index of attitude change). But as far as actual changes in dental *behaviour* were concerned, the high fear condition proved to be the least effective. Eight per cent of the high fear group had adopted the recommendations (changes in tooth brushing and visiting the dentist in the weeks immediately following the experiment), compared with 22 per cent and 37 per cent in the moderate and low fear conditions respectively.

Similar results were reported by Janis and Terwillinger (1962), who presented a mild and strong fear message concerning the relationship between smoking and cancer.

These studies suggest that, in McGuire's terms, you can frighten people into attending to a message, comprehending it, yielding to it and retaining it, but not necessarily into acting upon it. Indeed, fear may be so great that action is *inhibited* rather than facilitated. However, if the audience is told how to avoid undesirable consequences and believes that the preventative action is realistic and will be effective, then even high levels of fear in the message can produce changes in behaviour. The more specific and precise the instructions, the greater the behaviour change (the *high availability factor*).

'One certain reason for the increase in abortion is that women use less hormonal contraception than they used to and lack the knowledge to use barrier methods effectively. Media myths about contraceptives can frighten people and they lose confidence in their use' (Tschudin, 2003: 125). It may be that for some women the fear of hormonal contraception is greater than the fear of getting pregnant; if abortion were still illegal, perhaps more women would risk hormonal contraception?

According to Stroebe (2000), mass-media campaigns designed to change some specific health behaviour should use arguments aimed mainly at changing beliefs relating to that *specific* behaviour – rather than focusing on more general health concerns. This is another example of the compatibility principle. For example, to persuade people to lower their dietary cholesterol, it wouldn't be very effective merely to point out that coronary heart disease is the major killer and/or that high levels of saturated fat are bad for one's heart. To influence diet, it would have to be argued that very specific dietary

ASK YOURSELF ...
- Can you relate the high availability factor to one of the principles we identified when discussing the measurement of attitude–behaviour correlations?

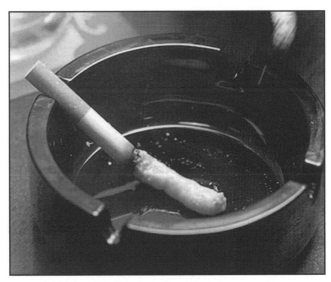

Part of an anti-smoking commercial based on the appeal to fear

changes, such as eating less animal fat and red meat, would have a positive impact on blood cholesterol levels, which, in turn, should reduce the risk of developing CHD.

To persuade Janet to use more reliable contraception it wouldn't be much use merely to point out that unprotected sex can lead to pregnancy and/or sexually transmitted disease (STD). It would be more effective to discuss specific contraceptive methods, and specify where and how they can be obtained. (This is something that will be discussed at Janet's follow-up appointment.)

In situations of minimal or extreme fear, the message may fail to produce any attitude change, let alone any change in behaviour. According to McGuire (1968), there's an inverted U-shaped curve in the relationship between fear and attitude change (as shown in Figure 10.4).

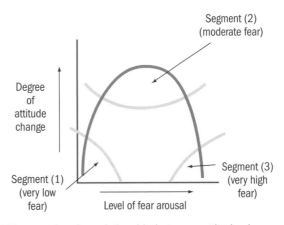

Figure 10.4 Inverted U curve showing relationship between attitude change and fear arousal (based on McGuire, 1968)

In segment 1 of the curve, the participant isn't particularly interested in (aroused by) the message: it's hardly attended to and may not even register. In segment 2, attention and arousal increase as fear increases, but the fear remains within manageable proportions. In segment 3, attention will decrease again, but this time because defences are being used to deal with extreme fear: the message may be denied ('it couldn't happen to me' – see Chapter 4) or repressed (see Chapter 6). Despite evidence of defensive processing, Stroebe (2000) maintains that:

> ... the overwhelming majority of studies on fear appeals has found that higher levels of threat resulted in greater persuasion than did lower levels. However, the effectiveness of high-fear messages appeared to be somewhat reduced for respondents who feel highly vulnerable to the threat ...

Despite the millions of pounds spent by the UK Government in 2005 on hard-hitting campaigns (such as that pictured on page 189) aimed at reducing smoking rates to under 21 per cent by 2010, the proportion of adults who smoke fell just 3 per cent (to 25 per cent) between 1998 and 2004. And rates among younger age groups, considered to be more susceptible to such advertising campaigns, have *risen* (Frith, 2006). At the Royal College of Nursing's (RCN) 2006 annual conference, a resolution was debated suggesting that this money has been wasted. Instead, funds would be better spent on treating patients and targeting the most at-risk groups.

... such as providing contraceptive information (see my diary entry on page 323) and free condoms for teenagers as they did at Josh's school – one way to target that particular 'at-risk' group.

The importance of feeling vulnerable

In order to arouse fear, it isn't enough that a health risk has serious consequences: the individual must also feel personally at risk (i.e. vulnerable). There's some evidence that unless individuals feel vulnerable to a threat, they're unlikely to form the intention to act on the recommendations in the message (Kuppens *et al.*, 1996).

Feeling vulnerable relates to what McGuire calls the *initial level of concern*. Clearly, someone who has a high level of initial concern will be more easily pushed into segment 3 of the curve than someone with a low level. The former may be overwhelmed by a high-fear message (in which case defences are used against it), while the latter may not become interested and aroused enough for the message to have an impact.

Janet, who's already had an abortion, probably does feel vulnerable and have a higher initial level of concern.

Fear appeals are also most likely to be effective for individuals who are unfamiliar with a given health risk. For example, when the dangers involved in unprotected anal intercourse among homosexuals became known in the early 1980s, the information appeared to produce an enormous reduction in such practices. But there was a hard core of men who were unaffected by the information, illustrating that simply repeating the dangers of HIV infection doesn't achieve risk reduction with such individuals (Stroebe, 2000; see also Chapter 4).

These men are either using defences against a high level of fear – or might they be unconcerned about the consequences?

THEORIES OF ATTITUDE CHANGE

The most influential theories of attitude change have concentrated on the principle of *cognitive consistency*. Human beings are seen as internally active information processors, who sort through and modify a large number of cognitive elements in order to achieve some kind of cognitive coherence. This need for cognitive consistency means that theories such as Festinger's *cognitive dissonance theory* (1957) aren't just theories of attitude change, but are also accounts of human motivation (see Gross, 2005).

COGNITIVE DISSONANCE THEORY (CDT)

ASK YOURSELF ...
• How might someone who smokes try to reduce dissonance?

According to *cognitive dissonance theory* (CDT), whenever we simultaneously hold two cognitions that are psychologically inconsistent, we experience *dissonance*. This is a negative drive state, a state of 'psychological discomfort or tension', which motivates us to reduce it by achieving consonance. Attitude change is a major way of reducing dissonance. Cognitions are 'the things a person knows about himself, about his behaviour and about his surroundings' (Festinger, 1957), and any two cognitions can be consonant (A implies B), dissonant (A implies not-B) or irrelevant to each other.

Janet was in a state of cognitive dissonance; her true attitude to abortion was that it was wrong, so she had done something she didn't approve of.

To give another example, the cognition 'I smoke' is psychologically inconsistent with the cognition 'smoking causes cancer' (assuming that we don't wish to get cancer).

Perhaps the most efficient (and certainly the healthiest!) way to reduce dissonance is to stop smoking, but many people will work on the other cognition. For example, they might:

◎ belittle the evidence about smoking and cancer (e.g. 'The human data are only correlational')
◎ associate with other smokers (e.g. 'If so-and-so smokes, then it can't be very dangerous')
◎ smoke low-tar cigarettes
◎ convince themselves that smoking is an important and highly pleasurable activity.

These examples illustrate how CDT regards human beings as *rationalising* (not rational) creatures: attempting to *appear* rational, both to others and to oneself.

Janet used the fact there was a risk of a Down's syndrome baby to rationalise, or justify, her decision to herself.

Dissonance following a decision

If we have to choose between two equally attractive objects or activities, then one way of reducing the resulting dissonance is to emphasise the undesirable features of the one we've rejected. This adds to the number of consonant cognitions and reduces the number of dissonant ones.

This was demonstrated in a study by Brehm (1956). Female participants had to rate the desirability of several household appliances on an eight-point scale. They then had to choose between two of the items (their reward for participating). For one group the items were ½ to 1½ points apart on the scale (*high dissonance condition*), while for a second group they were a full three points apart (*low dissonance condition*). When they were asked

191

to re-evaluate the items they'd chosen and rejected, the first group showed increased liking for the chosen item and decreased liking for the rejected one.

CDT also predicts that there'll be *selective exposure* to consonant information: seeking consistent information that isn't present at the time. However, selective perception also includes *selective attention* (looking at consistent information that is present) and *selective interpretation* (perceiving ambiguous information as being consistent with our other cognitions). According to Fiske and Taylor (1991), the evidence overall is stronger for selective attention and interpretation than for selective exposure.

For Janet, a severe risk of Down's syndrome would have been a low dissonance condition – a mild threat of it produced a high dissonance condition. This explains her telling me other reasons for her decision – her age increased her risk, and she'd discovered that Down's babies might have lots of other problems as well. It was as if she had to convince me of a legitimate reason for her termination, even though I fully accepted it.

Dissonance resulting from effort

KEY STUDY 10.4 Preferring things that turn out for the worst (Aronson and Mills, 1959)

- Female college students volunteered for a discussion on the psychology of sex, with the understanding that the research was concerned with the dynamics of group discussion. Each student was interviewed individually and asked if she could participate without embarrassment; all but one said yes.

- If a student had been assigned to the *control condition*, she was simply accepted. But for acceptance to the *severe embarrassment condition*, she had to take an 'embarrassment test' (reading out loud to a male experimenter a list of obscene words and some explicit sexual passages from modern novels). For acceptance to the *mild embarrassment condition*, she had to read aloud words like 'prostitute' and 'virgin' (remember the year was 1959!).

- They then all heard a tape recording of an actual, extremely dull, discussion (by a group, which they believed they'd later join) about sex in lower animals.

- They then had to rate the discussion, and the group members, in terms of how interesting and intelligent they found them.

- As predicted, the *severe embarrassment group* gave the *most positive* ratings – because they'd experienced the greatest dissonance!

When a voluntarily chosen experience turns out badly, the fact that we chose it motivates us to try to think that it actually turned out well. The greater the sacrifice or hardship associated with the choice, the greater the dissonance and, therefore, the greater the pressure towards attitude change (the *suffering-leads-to-liking effect*).

Janet's termination didn't 'turn out badly' in the sense that anything went wrong – but she obviously had a feeling of regret and perhaps grief. She kept saying, 'I know I did the right thing', which was presumably her way of convincing herself it was and reducing her dissonance. These were all ways of rationalising her behaviour, which didn't match the cognitive and affective components of her attitude.

Engaging in counter-attitudinal behaviour

This aspect of CDT is of most relevance to our earlier discussion of the relationship between attitudes and behaviour.

ASK YOURSELF ...
- How would CDT explain these findings? (You first need to ask yourself who experienced the greater dissonance.)

> **KEY STUDY 10.5 The '1 dollar/20 dollar' experiment (Festinger and Carlsmith, 1959)**
>
> - College students were brought, one at a time, into a small room to work for 30 minutes on two extremely dull and repetitive tasks (stacking spools and turning pegs).
> - Later, they were offered either 1 dollar or 20 dollars to try to convince the next 'participant' (in fact, a female stooge) that the tasks were interesting and enjoyable.
> - Common sense would predict that the 20-dollar students would be more likely to change their attitudes in favour of the tasks (they had more reason to do so), and this is also what *reinforcement/incentive theory* (Janis *et al.*, 1965) would predict (the greater the reward/incentive, the greater the attitude change).
> - However, as predicted by CDT, it was in fact the 1-dollar group that showed the greater attitude change (the *less-leads-to-more effect*).

The large, 20-dollar incentive gave those participants ample justification for their counter-attitudinal behaviour, and so they experienced very *little* dissonance. But the 1-dollar group experienced considerable dissonance: they could hardly justify their counter-attitudinal behaviour in terms of the negligible reward (hence, the change of attitude to reduce the dissonance).

Festinger and Carlsmith's findings have been replicated by several studies in which children are given either a mild or a severe threat not to play with an attractive toy (Aronson and Carlsmith, 1963; Freedman, 1965). If children obey a *mild* threat, they'll experience *greater* dissonance, because it's more difficult for them to justify their behaviour than for children given a severe threat. So, the mild threat condition produces greater reduction in liking of the toy.

However, dissonance occurs only when the behaviour is *volitional* (voluntary) – that is, when we feel we've acted of our own free will. If we believe we had no choice, there's no dissonance, and hence no attitude change. A study by Freedman (1963) shows that dissonance theory and reinforcement theory aren't mutually exclusive; instead, they seem to apply to voluntary and involuntary behaviour respectively.

SELF-PERCEPTION THEORY (SPT)

According to Bem's *self-perception theory* (SPT) (1965, 1967), the concept of dissonance is both unnecessary and unhelpful. Any self-report of an attitude is an *inference* from observation of one's own behaviour and the situation in which it occurs. This is because we don't have 'privileged access' to our own thoughts and feelings, but find out about them in the same way as we learn about other people's. (Bem was a behaviourist: see Chapter 2.)

If the situation contains cues (such as the offer of a large, 20-dollar incentive) which imply that we might have behaved that way regardless of how we personally felt (we lie about the task being interesting even though it was boring), then we don't infer that the behaviour reflected our true attitudes. But in the absence of obvious situational pressures (the 1-dollar condition), we assume that our attitudes are what our behaviour suggests they are.

This theory says that If Janet could have attributed her action unequivocally to the situation, she would not have thought it reflected her true attitude (anti-abortion). But not having the 'excuse' of the situation, she would attribute the cause to her own desires and so feel guilty?

In attributional terms, the 20-dollar group can easily make a *situational attribution* ('I did it for the money'), whereas the 1-dollar group had to make a *dispositional attribution* ('I did it because I really enjoyed it'). Bem combined attributional principles with his basic behaviourist beliefs.

Janet definitely used a situational attribution to justify her decision. But her feeling of guilt seemed to indicate it wasn't enough to justify acting against her true attitude.

If there was no dissonance then she would not have needed to justify her decision by blaming the situation.

An evaluation of CDT and SPT

◎ Eiser and van der Pligt (1988) believe that, conceptually, it's very difficult to distinguish between the two theories. Perhaps, as with CDT and incentive theories, both processes operate but to different extents under different circumstances. Fazio *et al.* (1977), for example, argue that dissonance may apply when people behave in a way that is contrary to their initial attitude (*counter-attitudinal behaviour*), while self-perception may apply better where their behaviour and initial attitude are broadly consistent (*attitude-congruent behaviour*). According to Fiske (2004), Bem's theory best accounts for those circumstances where we don't know our own mind or attitudes ahead of time.

◎ Zanna and Cooper's (1974) experiment provides support for *both* CDT and SPT.

KEY STUDY 10.6 Is there a dissonance-reduction pill? (Zanna and Cooper, 1974)

• Zanna and Cooper had participants write an essay supporting attitudes opposed to their own. The instructions implied either high or low freedom of choice (they believed either that they were free to express their true opinions or they weren't).

• Consistent with previous findings, the prediction that high-freedom-of-choice participants change their opinions more than low-freedom-of-choice participants was confirmed.

• The novel feature of the experiment was that participants were also given a placebo pill; they were either told it would make them feel tense, or relaxed, or told nothing about it at all.

• The dissonance theory prediction was upheld when participants were given no information about the pill, and even more strongly when they were told it would relax them.

• But when they were told it would make them feel tense, no difference between the high- and low-choice conditions was found.

ASK YOURSELF ...
• How can you explain these findings?

◎ If participants believe the pill will either relax them or have no effect, and they also believe they're acting of their own free will, they change their opinions, presumably because they experience an internal state of dissonance. But if told the pill will make them tense, they will (mis)attribute their tension to the pill, and so little attitude change will occur (as is also true of low-freedom-of-choice participants). This attributional explanation is consistent with SPT, and so the Zanna and Cooper experiment offers support for both Festinger and Bem.

◎ Fiske (2004) believes that one of the most provocative lines of research to have emerged from SPT is the *overjusitification effect*. If one has a situational justification for one's behaviour (such as an external reward), then one doesn't need to make a dispositional attribution for it. For example, if a child enjoys reading and receives a gold star for each book completed, s/he may infer that the reading is motivated by the reward. If the rewards are discontinued, the reading may be too (the opposite effect to what was intended).

◎ Conflict or inconsistency often arises between two attitudes, rather than between an attitude and behaviour. Both situations can be explained by CDT. But because SPT is based on attribution principles, it requires some overt behaviour from which we then make an inference about our attitudes.

I did experience a degree of cognitive dissonance about abortion because of my discussion with Bridie, but Janet's distress arose because she perceived her behaviour as counter-attitudinal.

◎ According to some *impression management theorists* (e.g. Schlenker, 1982; Tedeschi and Rosenfield, 1981; see also Chapter 8), many dissonance experiments might not reflect genuine cases of 'private' attitude change (a drive to be consistent). Rather, they reflect the need to *appear* consistent, and hence to avoid social anxiety and embarrassment, or to protect positive views of one's own identity. So, the 1-dollar group's attitude change is genuine, but is motivated by *social* (rather than *cognitive*) factors.

I have to admit – reluctantly – that any attitude change I may privately undergo following this experience and reflection will remain private at work. I'm more concerned with social norms (I'm high self-monitoring – see Chapter 8) than Bridie is, apparently.

CRITICAL DISCUSSION 10.1 Are theories of attitude change culturally biased?

• Although lying to another 'participant' (as in the 1-dollar/20-dollar experiment) may contravene the norms of many cultures, other commonly used dissonance paradigms may *not* induce the same level of dissonance in all cultures (Cooper *et al.*, 2004).

• For example, Heine and Lehman (1997) used the 'free-choice' method used by Brehm (1956; see above). Japanese and Canadian participants were asked to rate a selection of western rock and pop CDs, then asked to choose between two that they'd rated similarly. The Canadians showed the usual dissonance effect, but the Japanese didn't. Heine and Lehman concluded that Japanese people may not be as concerned about the inconsistency that arises when they 'lose' the positive aspect of the unchosen option and 'accept' the negative aspects of the chosen option.

- The tendency to change one's attitude or behaviour in order to be more consistent (and so reduce dissonance) reflects a need to view behaviour as driven by *internal* factors. But members of *collectivist* cultures don't demonstrate these tendencies. They're willing to sacrifice consistency to maintain a sense of harmony with others (Nagayama Hall and Barongan, 2002). It may even be considered selfish to act according to one's own desires, or to express one's attitudes, if they make others feel uncomfortable (Fiske *et al.*, 1998).

- The evidence for the overjustification effect is strong in the USA, but it rests on that culture's bias towards individual autonomy and perceived choice (Fiske, 2004). In more *interdependent* (i.e. collectivist) cultures, children's intrinsic motivation increases when choices are made *for them* by trusted authorities and peers (Iyengar and Lepper, 1999).

◎ Despite these and other challenges and reconceptualisations, Hogg and Vaughan (1995) maintain that:

> … cognitive dissonance theory remains one of the most widely accepted explanations of attitude change and many other social behaviours. It has generated over one thousand research studies and will probably continue to be an integral part of social psychological theory for many years …

The experience of being so involved in Janet's care (although inadvertently) has made me scrutinise my attitude more closely. I realise my own feelings of discomfort indicate a degree of cognitive dissonance in my attitude to abortion; I need to work out why.

Rosenberg and Hovland's (1960) 'classes of response' model of attitude helps me analyse my own attitude to abortion rather than accept it on the basis of its legality. Ajzen and Fishbein's (1977) view on predicting behaviour helps me understand that Janet's decision to have a termination didn't necessarily reflect her attitude. Consistency of behaviour (avoiding the necessity for termination in future) would lead to a more accurate prediction.

Chaiken's (1987) heuristics model of persuasion and the Yale approach will make me more critically aware of why and how I'm being persuaded into a point of view in future.

On that theme – I wonder if McGuire's 1969 'chain of processes' might be useful in analysing patients' adherence to prescribed treatment or advice?

CHAPTER SUMMARY

◎ The **three-component model** of attitude structure sees attitudes as comprising **affective**, **cognitive** and **behavioural** components. Attitudes have much in common with beliefs and values, but they need to be distinguished.

◎ Katz identifies the **knowledge**, **adjustive**, **value-expressive** and **ego-defensive functions** of attitudes.

◎ Early research into the **relationship between attitudes and behaviour** showed that attitudes are very poor predictors of behaviour. But attitudes represent only one of several determinants of behaviour, including situational factors.

◎ Attitudes can predict behaviour, provided there's a close correspondence between the way the two variables are defined and measured (the **principle of compatibility**). Also, measures of a representative sample of behaviours relevant to the attitude must be made (the **aggregation principle**).

◎ **Persuasive communication** has traditionally been studied in terms of the influence of four interacting factors: the **source** of the persuasive message, the **message** itself, the **recipient** of the message, and the **situation/context**.

◎ **Theories of systematic processing** see the impact of persuasive messages as dependent on a sequence of processes, including **attending** to the message, **comprehending** it, **accepting** its conclusions, **retaining** it, and **acting** as a result.

◎ The more recent **cognitive perspective** focuses on **why** people change their attitudes, not merely **when** and **how** it's likely to happen. The **heuristic model of persuasion**, for example, explains why we're more likely to be persuaded when the situation isn't personally involving or if the arguments are convincing.

◎ People can be frightened into attending to, comprehending, accepting and retaining a message, but the **high availability factor** is necessary for any behaviour change to take place.

◎ People also need to feel personally **vulnerable** if fear appeals are to have any impact. There appears to be an inverted U-shaped curve in the relationship between fear and attitude change.

◎ The major theories of attitude change share the basic principle of **cognitive consistency**. The most influential of these is Festinger's **cognitive dissonance theory** (CDT).

◎ **Dissonance** is most likely to occur after making a very **difficult choice/decision**, when putting ourselves through **hardship** or making a **sacrifice** only to find it was for nothing, or when engaging **voluntarily** in **counter-attitudinal behaviour**.

◎ Bem's **self-perception theory** (SPT) explains the results of dissonance experiments in terms of **attributional principles**. Dissonance theory may apply under conditions of 'true' counter-attitudinal behaviour, while self-perception theory applies to attitude-congruent behaviour.

◎ **Impression management theory** stresses the **social** rather than the **cognitive** motivation underlying attitude change.

◎ Like most western psychology, theories of attitude change are **culturally biased**.

PREJUDICE AND DISCRIMINATION 11

INTRODUCTION AND OVERVIEW

While genocide – the systematic destruction of an entire cultural, ethnic or racial group – is the most extreme form of discrimination, the prejudice that underlies it is essentially the same as that which underlies less extreme behaviours. Prejudice is an *attitude* that can be expressed in many ways, or that may not be overtly or openly expressed at all. Like other attitudes, prejudice can be regarded as a *disposition* to behave in a prejudiced way (to practise *discrimination*). So, the relationship between prejudice and discrimination is an example of the wider debate concerning the attitude–behaviour relationship (see Chapter 10).

Theories of prejudice and discrimination try to explain their origins: how do people come to be prejudiced and to act in discriminatory ways? Answers to these questions potentially answer the further question: how can they be reduced or even prevented altogether? This, of course, has much greater practical significance for people's lives. Perhaps for nurses and other health professionals, the key issues are:

◎ being aware of their own (often unconscious) prejudices, and
◎ recognising how this may affect their professional practice (again, something that often goes unnoticed by the professionals themselves).

Patients may be from a different ethnic/cultural background to the nurse, they may be gay or lesbian, they may have HIV/AIDS (see George, 1995; McHaffie, 1994), they may be transsexual (see Rees, 1993; Thomas, 1993), or obese (see Whyte, 1998), or even the victim of rape (see Donnelly, 1991). In all these cases, they may become the victims of the nurse's prejudice and discrimination.

People's personal belief systems differ, creating the potential for conflict between health professionals and consumers. But factors such as race, class and culture can increase the depth of these differences.

From my diary (9): Year 1/Orthopaedic Ward

A patient made me angry today. Mrs Maitland (she declined to be called by her first name) – a rather overweight, 64-year-old woman – had been admitted for internal fixation of neck of femur following an accident. When Rasheed, the Asian anaesthetist, came to see her prior to operation. Mrs M hardly answered him. Afterwards I asked her if she was happy with everything she'd been told. Sounding very disparaging, she said she didn't know what she'd been told, she couldn't understand a word Rasheed had been saying. Then she looked anxious and asked if the 'other nice doctor' (a medical student) would be giving her the anaesthetic. I explained Rasheed was a highly experienced *anaesthetist and went over what he'd said. I then tried to help her get into her theatre gown. She said she could manage, although I could see she was in pain. Minutes later, I saw a (white) HCA, Rachel, was helping her. I wondered what she'd say if she knew Rachel was gay!*

PREJUDICE AS AN ATTITUDE

As an *extreme* attitude, prejudice comprises the three components common to all attitudes:

1. the *cognitive* component is the *stereotype* (see Chapter 8)
2. the *affective* component is a *strong feeling of hostility*
3. the *behavioural* component can take different forms.
   Allport (1954) proposed five stages of this component:
1. *antilocution* – hostile talk, verbal denigration and insult, racial jokes
2. *avoidance* – keeping a distance but without actively inflicting harm
3. *discrimination* – exclusion from housing, civil rights, employment
4. *physical attack* – violence against the person and property
5. *extermination* – indiscriminate violence against an entire group (including genocide).

Mrs M's disparaging remarks aren't exactly antilocution, nor is her not wanting me to help actually avoidance. They are milder forms of discrimination but they still reveal the attitude underneath.

'Discrimination' is often used to denote the behavioural component, while 'prejudice' denotes the cognitive and affective components. But just as the cognitive and affective components may not necessarily be manifested behaviourally, so discrimination doesn't necessarily imply the presence of cognitive and affective components. People may discriminate if the prevailing social norms dictate that they do so, and if their wish to become or remain a member of the discriminating group is stronger than their wish to be fair and egalitarian (see below). According to Fiske (2004), the affective component is crucial. This is illustrated by the findings that individual differences in emotional prejudice correlate with discrimination better than stereotypes do (Dovidio *et al.*, 1996), and affective reactions to gay men predict discrimination far better than stereotypes do (Talaska *et al.*, 2003, in Fiske, 2004).

Although the relationship between prejudice and discrimination is moderate, it's comparable to the general attitude–behaviour relationship (Fiske, 2004; see also Chapter 10).

DEFINITIONS OF PREJUDICE

Most definitions of prejudice stress the hostile, negative kind of prejudice (it can also be positive), as does the research that tries to identify how prejudice arises and how it might be reduced.

Again, Mrs M didn't articulate negative feelings, but she was revealing a preference to be treated by a white 'doctor'. Because she couldn't understand easily what Rasheed was saying (his English is excellent but he has an accent), she assumed he wasn't capable of managing her anaesthetic. (I think this is an example of the halo effect.) I perceived her refusal of help from me, then accepting it from someone else, as discriminatory.

Table 11.1 Some definitions of prejudice and discrimination

'… an antipathy based on faulty and inflexible generalisation directed towards a group as a whole or towards an individual because he is a member of that group. It may be felt or expressed' (Allport, 1954)

'Prejudice is an attitude (usually negative) toward the members of some group, based solely on their membership in that group …' (Baron and Byrne, 1991)

'Prejudice is a learned attitude towards a target object that typically involves negative affect, dislike or fear, a set of negative beliefs that support the attitude and a behavioural intention to avoid, or to control or dominate, those in the target group … Stereotypes are prejudiced beliefs … when prejudice is acted out, when it becomes overt in various forms of behaviour, then discrimination is in practice …' (Zimbardo and Leippe, 1991)

The definitions in Table 11.1 locate prejudice squarely *within the individual* – it's an attitude that represents one aspect of social cognition. However, Vivian and Brown (1995) prefer to see prejudice as a special case of *intergroup conflict*, which occurs when 'people think or behave antagonistically towards another group or its members in terms of their group membership and seem motivated by concerns relating to those groups'.

Defining prejudice in terms of intergroup conflict 'lifts' it to the social plane. Consistent with this is Fernando's (1991) distinction between 'racial prejudice' and 'racism': the former denotes an attitude possessed by an individual, while the latter refers to a political and economic ideology, which is a characteristic of society. Strictly, then, it is societies (or institutions, such as the police or the armed forces) that are racist and individuals who are racially prejudiced.

Mrs M's attitude suggested she was racially prejudiced towards Rasheed and me. When I discussed it with Maggie, my mentor, she said we can't control patients' attitudes, but the NHS couldn't allow discrimination. If it did, it would be a racist institution.

Until quite recently, most of the theory and research into prejudice and discrimination was concerned with racism, 'the quite specific belief that cultural differences between ethnic groups are of biological origin and that groups should be ranked in worth' (Littlewood and Lipsedge, 1989). However, gender (as in *sexism* – see Gross, 2005), sexual orientation or preference (as in *heterosexism* – see below) and age (as in *ageism* – see Chapter 19) can all be targets for hostility and discrimination. Other examples include *sizeism* (hostility and discrimination against people who are obese – see below) and '*HIV/AIDS-ism*' (independently of the perceived link with homosexuality – see below).

ASK YOURSELF …
• Apart from racism, what other 'isms' are there that meet these criteria for being social, rather than individual, phenomena?

My first reaction to Mrs M was anger. As I walked away I thought to myself – if you weren't so fat you probably wouldn't have fallen over and broken your leg! When I'd calmed down I was ashamed I'd allowed anger to trigger an aggressive attitude in me; I should now know better. It revealed my 'sizeist' prejudice, didn't it?

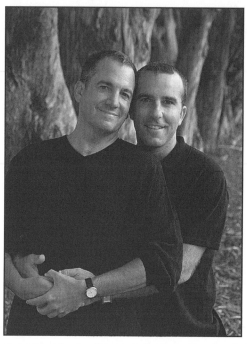

Sexual orientation is a target for hostility and discrimination in a heterosexist society

ASK YOURSELF ...

• Are you a racist?

• While most people would automatically say 'no', the question isn't as simple as it seems. Racism can stem from ignorance, both of what it is and what can be done to combat it.

• A questionnaire (Nursing Times, 1990) aimed to help nurses explore how much they really know about racial discrimination in the workplace.

1. The Race Relations Act 1976 outlawed discrimination in the workplace against anyone on racial grounds. But what do you understand by the term 'racial grounds'? Does it refer to (a) colour; (b) nationality; (c) ethnic or national origin; (d) race?

2. Direct discrimination in the workplace occurs when a person treats another person less favourably on racial grounds. Which of the following scenarios do you think are examples of direct discrimination?

   (a) Hospital management decides not to promote a nurse because 'the consultant won't work with an Asian ward sister'.

   (b) An inner-city mental health team advertises for an Afro-Caribbean RMN to work with the Afro-Caribbean clients.

   (c) A Turkish applicant for a staff nurse post is rejected because the previous year there was a Turkish nurse in the ward who was constantly taking time off work because of her children.

   (d) A Nigerian auxiliary (health care assistant/HCA) is dismissed for theft of hospital property.

3. Indirect discrimination is more insidious. It refers to the way in which health authority policies on such issues as recruitment and advertising for promotion discriminate, possibly inadvertently, against people from different racial groups. Which of the following might constitute examples of indirect discrimination?

(a) Refusing to employ a Pakistani nurse who, because of her Muslim beliefs, will not wear a nurse's uniform – although she offers to wear matching trousers and top.

(b) A job advertisement which requires that English must be the applicant's mother tongue.

(c) An applicant for an auxiliary (HCA) post is turned down on the grounds that she has been unemployed for over two years. The management argues that it would be difficult to obtain references in such a case.

(d) A young Kenyan girl is refused entry for Registered Nurse training because she doesn't have five GCSEs.

1. 'Racial grounds' includes all of these (Commission for Racial Equality/CRE, 1983).

2. Both (a) and (c) constitute direct discrimination (CRE, 1989).

3. Both (b) and (c) constitute indirect discrimination (CRE, 1985, 1989). Neither (a) nor (d) is clear-cut (see Nursing Times, 1990).

PREJUDICE AND DISCRIMINATION IN HEALTH CARE

Institutionalised racism within the NHS

If this truly exists, then both nurses themselves and patients can become victims. According to Kroll (1990):

> ... The NHS was created with the philosophy of providing care for all, irrespective of race, colour or creed. It is assumed that NHS staff are free from prejudice and knowledgeable about the needs of a multiracial society. However, most experts believe that racism is embedded in the organisational culture of the NHS, which is run predominantly by white, middle-class professionals.

We're taught to care for all patients as individuals. The Roper-Logan-Tierney model of nursing has five components, the first of which is 'activities of living'. Included in this is a socio-cultural factor, which influences the way individual patients perform those activities. So consideration of ethnic differences should be an essential part of nursing assessment (Roper et al., 1996, in Alexander et al., 2006).

Black and minority ethnic nurses account for about 20 per cent of the UK nursing profession, but new figures indicate that they experience disturbing levels of bullying and racism. A survey of 9000 RCN members working in the NHS and the independent sector revealed that 45 per cent of Afro-Caribbean nurses had been bullied or harassed in the previous year (2005, in Staines, 2006). Of these, 61 per cent said the bullying was racially motivated and 43 per cent that it was linked to their nationality. This contrasted with just 21 per cent of the white British and 24 per cent of the Asian nurses who responded. Perhaps most disturbing of all is the finding that 30 per cent of the bullying came from other nursing colleagues and 45 per cent from supervisors or senior managers.

The CRE is keen to dispel the myth that racism is just about colour prejudice. Snell (1997) describes claims of discrimination against Irish nurses, who make up the largest group in Europe applying to go on the UKCC register.

As far as I know I haven't experienced bullying, but maybe I haven't recognised it as such. According to 'Bully OnLine', the website of the UK National Workplace Bullying Advice Line, bullying includes: constant taunting, teasing, discrimination, damage to property, racist slurs and name-calling.

According to Kroll (1990), racism is endemic in midwifery. She identifies four major features of antenatal clinics that may make them seem alienating, racially prejudiced places to women from non-white ethnic groups:
◎ the language barrier
◎ lack of awareness by ethnic minorities of the availability of certain services (for example, most Afro-Caribbean women still know very little about sickle-cell anaemia)
◎ midwives know very little about the spiritual beliefs and customs of the different cultural groups within their health authorities
◎ midwives rarely consult the groups and advisory centres that exist in the various ethnic communities.

On a post-natal ward, Asian Muslim women couldn't eat the food provided because they observed strict dietary laws and the ward staff wouldn't let their families bring them in cooked food. The fact that other women had take-away burgers and chips brought in for them wasn't noticed or perhaps overlooked, until a Muslim midwife joined the staff and pointed out the inconsistency (Schott and Henley, 1999). This is an example of discrimination.

Anti-gay and lesbian prejudice and discrimination

According to Rose and Platzer (1993), the attitudes of many nurses are grounded in their assumptions about people's heterosexual nature and their lack of knowledge about different lifestyles and how these affect people's health. Ignorance about how lesbians and gay men live can lead nurses to ask inappropriate questions during assessments, resulting in mistaken judgements.

For example, one lesbian patient who was receiving a cervical smear test was asked if she was sexually active. After saying she was, she was asked what contraceptive she used and replied 'none'. She was then asked if she was trying to become pregnant, which she wasn't. She had to disclose her lesbianism in order to ensure that health professionals didn't make incorrect assumptions about her, which could have led to an incorrect diagnosis.

In another example, one patient's charts were labelled 'high risk'. These labels, which were clearly visible to other patients and members of staff, were there simply because he was gay and so was seen as being at risk of having HIV – the nurses simply assumed that gay men were likely to be HIV-positive and that heterosexual men weren't. Such assumptions are, of course, linked to stereotypes about what gay men do, rather than to a knowledge of sexual behaviours, which can differ widely regardless of sexual orientation.

James *et al.* (1994) cite several studies showing that many nurses and doctors are homophobic. The research also indicates that lesbians and gay men fear homophobia from health care providers, are anxious about the consequences of revealing their sexual orientation and breaches of confidentiality, and are concerned about facing hostility and even physical harm.

According to the UKCC Code of Professional Conduct (1992), nurses are required to respect patients or clients *unconditionally*. Homophobia is clearly a breach of this obligation. In describing the results of a survey of lesbian nurses, Rose (1993) states that nurses must also demonstrate this respect for each other. Nurses may believe that homosexuality is wrong, but when faced with working with openly gay colleagues, they may experience cognitive dissonance (see also Chapter 10).

I realise I've met some of these forms of prejudice, including, unfortunately, my own. Admitting a patient, I asked a woman who her next of kin was; she said 'my partner' and gave another woman's name. I put it down but felt flustered as I was surprised, which probably showed. Also, I didn't know if it was legal, so I asked for another next of kin.

> **ASK YOURSELF ...**
> • How might a homophobic nurse deal with such cognitive dissonance?

INSTITUTIONALISED PREJUDICE AND DISCRIMINATION

The discussion above illustrates that a great deal of prejudice and discrimination is unconscious, reflected in basic, stereotyped assumptions that we make about others. These assumptions influence our behaviour towards them, which may not necessarily be overtly hostile or 'anti'. It's this pervasive form of prejudice and discrimination that's perhaps the most difficult to break down, because we're unaware of it and because it reflects institutionalised heterosexism, racism, and so on.

Both Cochrane (1983) and Littlewood and Lipsedge (1989) show how ethnic minorities in England are more often hospitalised for mental illness than non-black English people. This is interpreted as reflecting an implicit, unwitting prejudice against minority groups that pervades the NHS as an institution. This definition of 'institutionalised racism' as 'unwitting' was included in the government report (1999) on the behaviour of the police in their investigation of the murder of the black London teenager, Stephen Lawrence (in Horton, 1999).

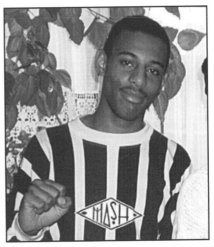

Stephen Lawrence

The concept of race

Underlying racism is the deep-seated and widely held belief that people resembling each other in obvious physical ways (such as skin colour and hair texture) belong to a 'race' that represents a genetically distinct human type. Anthropologists, biologists and medical people are all guilty of perpetuating the myth, despite the widely held belief that 'race' has ceased to have a scientific meaning.

Wetherell (1996) argues that 'race' is a *social* as opposed to a natural (biological) phenomenon, 'a process which gives significance to superficial physical differences, but where the construction of group divisions depends on … economic, political and cultural processes'.

She points out that many writers prefer to put quotation marks around the word 'race' to indicate that we're dealing with one possible social classification of people and groups, rather than an established biological or genetic reality.

Does reliance on classification, whether social or biological, threaten our perception of people as individuals?

THEORIES OF PREJUDICE AND DISCRIMINATION

Attempts to explain prejudice and discrimination fall into three broad categories:
1. those that see prejudice as stemming from *personality variables* and other aspects of the psychological make-up of individuals
2. those that emphasise the role of *environmental factors* (sometimes called the *conflict approach*)
3. those that focus on the effects of the mere fact of *group membership*.

Each approach may be important to a complete understanding of the causes of intergroup conflict and prejudice, and to their reduction (Vivian and Brown, 1995).

PREJUDICE AND PERSONALITY

The authoritarian personality

Adorno *et al.* (1950) proposed the concept of the *authoritarian personality* (in a book of the same name), someone who's prejudiced by virtue of specific personality traits that predispose them to be hostile towards ethnic, racial and other minority or outgroups.

Adorno *et al.* began by studying anti-Semitism in Nazi Germany in the 1940s, and drew on Freud's theories to help understand the relationship between 'collective ideologies' (such as fascism) and individual personality (Brown, 1985). After their emigration to the USA, studies began with college students and other native-born, white, non-Jewish, middle-class Americans (including school teachers, nurses, prison inmates and psychiatric patients). These involved interviews concerning their political views and childhood experiences, and the use of *projective tests* – in particular, the thematic apperception test/TAT (see Gross, 2005) – designed to reveal unconscious attitudes towards minority groups. In the course of their research, Adorno *et al.* constructed a number of scales:
◎ *Antisemitism (AS) scale*
◎ *Ethnocentrism (E) scale* (the term 'ethnocentrism' was first defined by Sumner (1906) as 'A view of things in which one's own group is the centre of everything, and all others are scaled and rated with reference to it … each group … boasts itself superior … and looks with contempt on outsiders. Each group thinks its own folkways the only right one …')

◎ *Political and Economic Conservatism (PEC) scale*

◎ *Potentiality for Fascism (F) scale* (according to Brown (1965), Adorno *et al.* never referred to the F scale as the authoritarianism scale. But since it's supposed to identify the kind of personality the book is talking about, it's reasonable to suppose that the scale could also correctly be called the authoritarianism scale (as it has been in many subsequent research reports). The F scale items don't refer directly to minority groups or politico-economic issues. It was intended to measure implicit authoritarian and antidemocratic trends in personality, making someone with such a personality susceptible to explicit fascist propaganda).

Adorno *et al.* concluded from the correlations between scores on the different scales that people who are anti-Semitic are also likely to be hostile towards 'Negroes', 'Japs' and any other minority group or 'foreigner' (all *outgroups*): the authoritarian personality is prejudiced in a very *generalised* way.

What's the authoritarian personality like?

Typically, authoritarians are hostile to people of inferior status, servile to those of higher status, and contemptuous of weakness. They're also rigid and inflexible, intolerant of ambiguity and uncertainty, unwilling to introspect feelings, and upholders of conventional values and ways of life (such as religion). This belief in convention and intolerance of ambiguity combine to make minorities 'them' and the authoritarian's membership group 'us'; 'they' are by definition 'bad' and 'we' are by definition 'good'.

Is Mrs Maitland authoritarian? We don't know her well enough to judge. She was conventional – she wanted to be addressed formally, and seemed intolerant of both Rasheed and me, to see us as 'them' (i.e. black). She thought the white medical student with a refined accent was the senior doctor – an assumption that black people aren't as able as white doctors? (The halo effect again!)

Evaluation of the authoritarian personality theory

◎ While some evidence is broadly consistent with the theory, there are a number of serious methodological and other problems that make it untenable. For example, if prejudice is to be explained in terms of individual differences, how can it then be manifested in a whole population, or at least a vast majority of that population (Brown, 1988)? In pre-war Nazi Germany, for example (and in many other places since), consistent racist attitudes and behaviour were shown by hundreds of thousands of people, who must have differed on most other psychological characteristics.

◎ It assumed that authoritarianism is a characteristic of the *political right*, implying that there's no equivalent authoritarianism on the left. According to Rokeach (1960), 'ideological dogmatism' refers to a relatively rigid outlook on life and intolerance of those with opposing beliefs. High scores on the *dogmatism scale* reveal: (i) closedness of mind; (ii) lack of flexibility; and (iii) authoritarianism, regardless of particular social and political ideology. Dogmatism is a way of *thinking*, rather than a set of beliefs (Brown, 1965).

Maggie pointed out that Mrs M's notes showed she'd always lived in a small Somerset village; coming into a multiracial city hospital might have made her very uncertain and apprehensive. Her reaction could be explained as an instinctive, 'prejudged' response to seeing people who were different.

Scapegoating: the frustration–aggression hypothesis

According to Dollard *et al.*'s (1939) *frustration–aggression hypothesis*, frustration always gives rise to aggression and aggression is always caused by frustration (see Gross, 2005). The source of frustration (whatever prevents us from achieving our goals) might often be seen as a fairly powerful threat (such as parents or employers) or may be difficult to identify. Drawing on Freudian theory, Dollard *et al.* claim that when we need to vent our frustration but are unable to do this directly, we do so *indirectly* by displacing it onto a substitute target (we find a *scapegoat*).

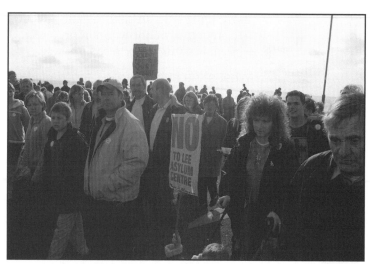

According to the frustration–aggression hypothesis, discrimination against outsiders (in this case eastern European asylum seekers) is a form of displaced aggression

I recognise displacement as one of Freud's defence mechanisms (see Chapter 2).

The choice of scapegoat isn't usually random. In England during the 1930s and 1940s, it was predominantly the Jews, who were replaced by West Indians during the 1950s and 1960s, and during the 1970s, 1980s and 1990s by Asians from Pakistan. In the southern USA, lynchings of blacks from 1880 to 1930 were related to the price of cotton: as the price dropped, so the number of lynchings increased (Hovland and Sears, 1940). While this is consistent with the concept of displaced aggression, the fact that whites chose blacks as scapegoats rather than some other minority group suggests that there are usually socially approved (legitimised) targets for frustration-induced aggression.

Limitations of the personality approach

◎ Several researchers (e.g. Billig, 1976; Brown, 1988; Hogg and Abrams, 1988) have argued that any account of prejudice and discrimination in terms of individuals (*intrapersonal behaviour*) is *reductionist*. In other words, the *social* nature of prejudice and discrimination requires a *social* explanation (in terms of *intergroup behaviour*).

◎ Adorno *et al.* (1950) imply that racism is the product of the abnormal personality of a small minority of human beings, rather than a social and political ideology. This distinction is of great practical as well as theoretical importance, because what's

ASK YOURSELF ...

• Can you see any connections between the frustration–aggression hypothesis and certain parts of Adorno *et al.*'s theory?

considered to be the cause of prejudice has very real implications for its reduction. Indeed, Adorno *et al.* (1950) recognised that *society* provides the content of attitudes and prejudice, and defines the outgroups.

◎ According to Brown (1985), 'cultural or societal norms may be much more important than personality in accounting for ethnocentrism, outgroup rejection, prejudice and discrimination'.

This explains why getting rid of an authoritarian leader (as in Iraq) doesn't stop intergroup conflict, which has become a 'way of life'.

THE ROLE OF ENVIRONMENTAL FACTORS

The impact of social norms: prejudice as conformity

Individual bigotry is only part of the explanation of racial discrimination. For example, even though overt discrimination has, traditionally, been greater in the southern USA, white southerners haven't scored higher than whites from the north on measures of authoritarianism (Pettigrew, 1959). So, clearly, *conformity to social norms* can prove more powerful as a determinant of behaviour than personality factors.

Pettigrew (1971) also found that Americans in the south are no more anti-Semitic or hostile towards other minority groups than those from the north (as the authoritarian personality explanation would require). In other words, prejudice *isn't* the generalised attitude that Adorno *et al.* claimed. According to Reich and Adcock (1976), the need to conform and not be seen as different may cause milder prejudices. But active discrimination against, and ill-treatment of, minorities reflects a prejudice that already exists and that is maintained and legitimised by conformity.

If the NHS is a racist institution, it reflects social norms that are accepted as legitimate. This makes another good reason why we are encouraged to challenge practice. But it's difficult to challenge a patient, a more senior nurse or a doctor.

REALISTIC GROUP CONFLICT THEORY (RGCT)

According to Sherif's (1966) *realistic group conflict theory* (RGCT), intergroup conflict arises as a result of a conflict of interests. When two groups want to achieve the same goal but cannot both have it, hostility is produced between them. Indeed, Sherif claims that conflict of interest (or competition) is a *sufficient* condition for the occurrence of hostility or conflict. He bases this claim on the 'Robber's Cave' experiment, which Brown (1986) describes as the most successful field experiment ever conducted on intergroup conflict (see Gross, 2005).

This experiment was about the hostility that developed between two groups of boys at a summer camp, who were 'set up' by experimenters to compete for prizes, which supports the 'competing for scarce resources' concept. It helps explain remarks like 'they come over here and take our jobs' – the reason given for dislike of 'foreign' workers in the NHS and elsewhere. But it doesn't explain prejudice against black people in general, or homosexuals, or religious groups.

An evaluation of RGCT

◎ According to Fiske (2004), RGCT is the most obvious explanation for prejudice and discrimination, but it has received only limited and inconsistent support, and the *perceived*, *symbolic threat* posed by outgroups matters more than any real or tangible threat. For this reason, the 'realistic' may as well be dropped from its name and the theory renamed 'perceived group conflict theory'.

◎ Perceived conflict *does* predict negative attitudes towards outgroups (Brown *et al.*, 2001; Hennessy and West, 1999), and conflict matters only when people identify with their ingroups. More importantly, ingroup identification *by itself* can account for intergroup hostility, even in the absence of competition (Brewer and Brown, 1998). Intangible outcomes (such as group recognition, status, prestige) produce conflict far more often than do tangible resources. Even when the conflict appears to involve resources, often the real pay-off is pride in one's own identification with a group capable of winning them. As Fiske (2004) says, 'Group conflict is an inherently social competition that goes beyond concrete self-interest. One result of the struggle for positive identity is bias against the outgroup …' This is related to *social identity theory* (see below, pages 211–212).

◎ It seems, then, that 'competition' may not be a sufficient condition for intergroup conflict and hostility after all. If we accept this conclusion, the question arises whether it's even a necessary condition. In other words, can hostility arise in the absence of conflicting interests?

White racists believe they are superior to black people, in any circumstances. However, prejudice exists also between Asian and Afro-Caribbean people, and what about the professional rivalry between health professionals – traditionally doctors and nurses?

THE INFLUENCE OF GROUP MEMBERSHIP

Minimal groups

According to Tajfel *et al.* (1971), the *mere perception* of another group's existence can produce discrimination. When people are arbitrarily and randomly divided into two groups, knowledge of the other group's existence is a sufficient condition for the development of pro-ingroup and anti-outgroup attitudes. These artificial groups are known as *minimal groups*.

Before any discrimination can occur, people must be categorised as members of an ingroup or an outgroup (making categorisation a *necessary* condition). More significantly, the very act of categorisation produces conflict and discrimination (making it also a *sufficient* condition).

Doesn't becoming a nurse, physiotherapist or radiologist give us a sense of professional 'belonging'?

An evaluation of minimal group experiments

◎ According to Brown (Brown, 1988), intergroup discrimination in this minimal group situation has proved to be a remarkably robust phenomenon. In more than two dozen independent studies in several different countries, using a wide range of experimental participants of both sexes (from young children to adults), essentially the same result has been found: the mere act of allocating people into arbitrary social categories is sufficient to elicit biased judgements and discriminatory behaviours.

◎ Wetherell (1982) maintains that intergroup conflict *isn't* inevitable. She studied white and Polynesian children in New Zealand, and found the latter to be much more generous towards the outgroup, reflecting cultural norms that emphasised cooperation.

◎ The minimal group paradigm has been criticised on several methodological and theoretical grounds, especially its artificiality and *meaninglessness* (e.g. Schiffman and Wicklund, 1992; see Gross, 2005). But Tajfel (1972) argues that it's precisely the need to find meaning in an 'otherwise empty situation' (especially for the *self*) that leads participants to act in terms of the minimal categories.

If culture can affect behaviour it means it's learned. In present nursing culture we're being taught not to 'prejudge' but Brown's (1988) research (and my own experience!) shows it's not easy to overcome such tendencies.

Social identity theory (SIT)

Tajfel (1978) and Tajfel and Turner (1986) explain the minimal group effect in terms of *social identity theory* (SIT). According to SIT, an individual strives to achieve or maintain a positive self-image. This has two components: *personal identity* (the personal characteristics and attributes that make each person unique) and *social identity* (a sense of who we are, derived from the groups we belong to).

In fact, each of us has several social identities, corresponding to the different groups with which we identify. In each case, the more positive the image of the group, the more positive will be our own social identity, and hence our self-image. By emphasising the desirability of the ingroup(s) and focusing on those distinctions that enable our own group to come out on top, we help to create for ourselves a satisfactory social identity. This can be seen as lying at the heart of prejudice.

Some individuals may be more prone to prejudice because they have an intense need for acceptance by others. Their personal and social identities may be much more interconnected than for those with a lesser need for social acceptance. Prejudice can be seen as an adjustive mechanism that bolsters the self-concept of individuals who have feelings of personal inadequacy – but with potentially undesirable social implications.

Evaluation of SIT

◎ While there's considerable empirical support for the theory, much of this comes from minimal group experiments. Not only have they been criticised (see above), but SIT was originally proposed to explain the findings from those experiments. So, there's a *circularity* involved, making it necessary to test SIT's predictions in other ways.

◎ SIT has been criticised on the grounds that it presents racism (and other forms of prejudice) as 'natural', helping to justify it. Stemming from Allport's (1954) claims that stereotypes are 'categories about people' and that 'the human mind must think with the aid of categories' (see Chapter 8), Tajfel (1969; Tajfel *et al.*, 1971) saw the process of *categorisation* as a basic characteristic of human thought. SIT implies that intergroup hostility is natural and built into our thought processes as a consequence of categorisation. If this is correct, then racism (conceived as a form of intergroup hostility or ingroup favouritism) may also be construed as natural. In terms of the distribution of resources, racism is thus justified as the norm ('charity begins at home') (Howitt and Owusu-Bempah, 1994). But, of course, Tajfel never intended SIT to be seen as a justification of racism (he was a life-long opponent of racism).

211

◎ Although there's abundant evidence of intergroup discrimination, this appears to stem from raising the evaluation of the ingroup, rather than denigrating the outgroup (Vivian and Brown, 1995). Indeed, SIT suggests that prejudice consists largely of liking 'us' more than disliking 'them': favouring the ingroup is the core phenomenon, *not* outgroup hostility (Brewer, 1999; Hewstone *et al.*, 2002). However, one form that ingroup favouritism can take is 'modern' or *symbolic* racism.

Using cognitive 'shortcuts' such as stereotyping doesn't justify denigrating other groups. Taking a pride in being a nurse doesn't mean devaluing other health professionals or accepting things I know are wrong.

Box 11.1 Modern (or symbolic) racism and subtle prejudice

- According to Fiske (2004), most estimates put 70–80 per cent of whites as relatively high on *modern/subtle* forms of racism; these are 'cool' and indirect, automatic, unconscious, unintentional, ambiguous and ambivalent. This is in sharp contrast with the crude and blatant racist abuse associated with Allport's 'antilocution' (see above).

- Subtle prejudice isn't a uniquely American, white-on-black phenomenon (Pettigrew, 1998; Pettigrew and Meertens, 1995). In Europe, there are French/North Africans, British/South Asians, Germans/Turks.

- Symptomatic of this form of racism (or perhaps a variety of it) is the belief that 'one is not a racist' while simultaneously engaging in racist talk. A classic recent example involved Ron Atkinson, an eminent ex-football manager and TV football pundit, who was heard to make 'old-fashioned' racist remarks about a black player when he thought the microphone was switched off. In his defence, he claimed, 'What I said was racist – but I'm not a racist. I am an idiot' (in Eboda, 2004). He was sacked from his job.

- In 2002, Pat Bottrill (MBE) resigned from her job as chair for the RCN's Governing Council after making a remark perceived as racist. She said,

    'Although I did not intend any offence, I am stepping down as a sign of my own and the RCN's commitment to tackling any form of racism . . . the RCN has stated that it will not tolerate racism – even if it is unintentional'.

  Dr Beverly Malone (the RCN's first black general secretary) commented, 'Pat has demonstrated that the RCN is committed to tackling institutional racism in all its forms'. (Craig Kenny, Nursing Times (20.8.2003) Vol 98, No 34 p. 8)

Mrs M would probably deny being racist too.

◎ The *authoritarian personality theory* implies that, by changing the personality structure of the prejudiced individual, the need for an ego-defensive 'prop' such as prejudice is removed. By its nature, this is practically very difficult to achieve, even if it is theoretically possible.

◎ According to the *frustration–aggression hypothesis*, preventing frustration, or providing people with ways to vent their frustration in less anti-social ways than discrimination, are possible solutions. However, this would involve putting the historical clock back, or changing social conditions in quite fundamental ways.

◎ RGCT makes it very clear that removing competition and replacing it with superordinate goals and cooperation will remove or prevent hostility (this is discussed further below).

◎ SIT implies that if intergroup stereotypes can become less negative and automatic, and if boundaries between groups can be made more blurred or more flexible, then group memberships may become a less central part of the self-concept, making positive evaluation of the ingroup less inevitable. We will return to this theme below.

We're unlikely to change Mrs M's personality, but by coming into this hospital a degree of social change has been imposed on her, however briefly.

THE CONTACT HYPOTHESIS

Probably the first formal proposal of a set of social–psychological principles for reducing prejudice was Allport's (1954) *contact hypothesis* (as it's come to be called), according to which:

> Prejudice (unless deeply rooted in the character structure of the individual) may be reduced by equal status contact between majority and minority groups in the pursuit of common goals. The effect is greatly enhanced if this contact is sanctioned by institutional supports (i.e. by law, custom or local atmosphere) and provided it is of a sort that leads to the perception of common interests and common humanity between members of the two groups.

Most programmes aimed at promoting harmonious relations between groups that were previously in conflict have operated according to Allport's 'principles', in particular *equal status contact* and the pursuit of *common (superordinate) goals*.

Equal status contact

When people are segregated, they're likely to experience *autistic hostility* – that is, ignorance of others, which results in a failure to understand the reasons for their actions. Lack of contact means there's no 'reality testing' against which to check our own interpretations of others' behaviour, and this in turn is likely to reinforce *negative stereotypes*. By the same token, ignorance of what 'makes them tick' will probably make 'them' seem more dissimilar from ourselves than they really are. Bringing people into contact with each other should make them seem more familiar, and at least offers the possibility that this negative cycle can be interrupted, and even reversed.

Related to autistic hostility is the *mirror-image phenomenon* (Bronfenbrenner, 1960), whereby enemies come to see themselves as being in the right (with 'God on our side') and the other side as in the wrong. Both sides tend to attribute to each other the same negative characteristics (the 'assumed dissimilarity of beliefs'). Increased contact provides the opportunity to disconfirm our stereotypes. The outgroup loses its strangeness, and group members are more likely to be seen as unique individuals, rather than an 'undifferentiated mass' (see Figure 11.1). This represents a reduction in the *illusion of outgroup homogeneity* ('they all look the same').

Mrs M has had to face the reality of Rasheed as her anaesthetist. If he (or I) can gain her confidence, it may begin to challenge her attitude to all black people.

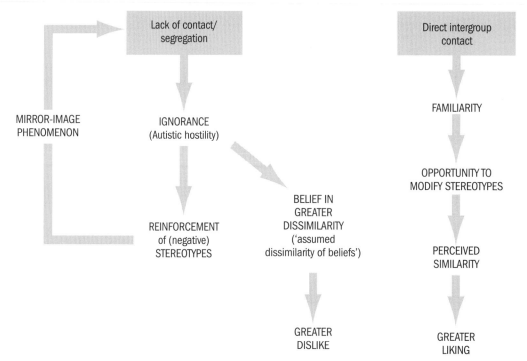

Figure 11.1 Summary of how the negative cycle of lack of contact/segregation between racial/ethnic groups and reinforcement of negative stereotypes can be broken by direct contact (as advocated by Allport's contact hypothesis)

How effective is equal status contact?

It's generally agreed that increased contact alone won't reduce prejudice. Despite evidence that we prefer people who are familiar, if this contact is between people who are consistently of *unequal status*, then 'familiarity may breed contempt'. Aronson (1980) points out that many whites (in the USA) have always had a great deal of contact with blacks – as dishwashers, toilet attendants, domestic servants, and so on. Such contacts may simply reinforce the stereotypes held by whites of blacks as being inferior. Similarly, Amir (1994) argues that we need to ask, 'Under what conditions does intergroup contact have an impact, for whom, and regarding what outcomes?'

A case in point are the findings of Stouffer *et al.* (1949) and Amir (1969) that interracial attitudes improved markedly when blacks and whites served together as soldiers in battle and on ships, but relationships weren't so good at base camp.

This introduces complications. Mrs M will see many black people in lower-status jobs in the hospital. However, there are also many Asian and Afro-Caribbean nurses and doctors.

Pursuit of common (superordinate) goals

In a *cooperative* situation, the attainment of one person's goal enhances the chances of attainment of the goals of other group members; this is the reverse of a competitive situation (Brown, 1986).

One influential attempt to realise both mutual cooperation and equal status contact is Aronson *et al.*'s (1978) *jigsaw method*. This is a highly structured method of interdependent learning, in which children are assigned to six-person, interracial learning groups (see Gross, 2005). According to Aronson (1992, 2000), the jigsaw method consistently enhances students' self-esteem, improves academic performance, increases liking for classmates and improves some interracial perceptions, compared with children in traditional classrooms.

However, although the children of different racial/ethnic groups who'd actually worked together came to like each other better as individuals, their reduced prejudice didn't *generalise* to those ethnic groups as a whole. This may be partly accounted for by the fact that most experiments of this type are small-scale and relatively short-term interventions. The jigsaw method also works best with young children, before prejudiced attitudes have an opportunity to become deeply ingrained (Aronson, 1992).

If it reduces some prejudice towards others it's a start, isn't it? Health care provides a natural programme to promote harmony; the whole health care team is interdependent. Mrs M can see black and white 'groups' working with equal status and collaborating to achieve a common goal: her successful recovery. But will it help change her attitude?

Do common goals always work?

The imposition of superordinate goals may sometimes even *increase* antagonism towards the outgroup – if the cooperation fails to achieve its aims. Groups need distinctive and complementary roles to play, so that each group's contributions are clearly defined. When this doesn't happen, liking for the other group may actually *decrease*, perhaps because group members are concerned with the integrity of the ingroup (Brown, R.J., 1988).

Maintaining group boundaries – *mutual differentiation* (Fiske, 2004) – is essential for promoting generalisation from the particular outgroup members to the whole outgroup (Hewstone, 2003). For example, Harwood *et al.* (2003, in Hewstone, 2003) found that contact with grandparents was a much better predictor of more positive attitudes towards the elderly in general, when young people reported being aware of age groups during contact (see Chapter 19).

But isn't there the danger that emphasising group/category boundaries during contact will *reinforce* perceptions of group differences and increase intergroup anxiety (Islam and Hewstone, 1993, in Hewstone, 2003; see below)? It certainly shouldn't be done in the initial stages of contact, especially when intergroup relationships are very negative. According to Hewstone (2003), the best approach is 'to promote contact that is simultaneously both "interpersonal" (e.g. involving personal exchange within a close relationship) and "intergroup" (i.e. both members are still aware that they belong to different groups) …'.

If something went wrong with Mrs M's recovery, she might look for her scapegoat among the black staff, I suppose. Alternatively, if she sees me as an Asian nurse who cares well for her and likes me, she is more likely to have a favourable impression of all Asian nurses.

An evaluation of the contact hypothesis (CH)

◎ Contact can 'work' via more subtle processes than generalisation (Hewstone, 2003). For example, it can help reduce the 'almost automatic fear' caused by interacting with members of outgroups – 'intergroup awe' (Stephan and Stephan, 1985). Contact has been shown to play a crucial mediating role in reducing anxiety between Hindus and Muslims in Bangladesh, and between Catholics and Protestants in Northern Ireland (Hewstone, 2003). Pettigrew and Tropp (2003, in Hewstone, 2003) have calculated that anxiety reduction accounts for over 20 per cent of the overall effectiveness of contact in reducing prejudice.

◎ According to Pettigrew (1998), generating affective (emotional) ties (including anxiety reduction) is the key mechanism involved in contact. Forming close friendships with outgroup members appears to be the most effective in reducing prejudice, and is certainly more effective than the rather superficial contact that occurs in the neighbourhood or at work.

◎ Pettigrew and Tropp (2003, in Hewstone, 2003) carried out a meta-analysis ('study of studies') of 561 studies, and found a highly significant inverse relationship between contact and prejudice. In other words, the more contact, the less the prejudice. They concluded, emphatically, that 'contact works'.

◎ The CH doesn't apply only to relationships between members of different ethnic/racial groups. The positive effects of contact have also been shown with attitudes towards psychiatric patients, gay men and disabled children (Hewstone, 2003).

And presumably working closely together as a team is the best way to break down barriers between different health care groups, however categorised?

CONCLUSIONS: WHAT TO DO WITH STEREOTYPES?

According to Brislin (1993), 'In many cultures, stereotypes of certain groups are so negative, so pervasive, and have existed for so many generations that they can be considered part of the culture into which children are socialised ...'

As we saw in Chapter 8, stereotypes represent a way of simplifying the extraordinarily complex social world we inhabit by placing people into categories. This alone would explain why they're so resistant to change. But they also influence selective attention and selective remembering, processes that are to a large extent outside conscious control. However, these automatic stereotyped reactions (one of the authors of this book is still 'guilty' of inferring that 'doctor' denotes 'he') can be seen simply as habits that can be broken. Prejudice reduction is a *process*, which involves learning to inhibit these automatic reactions and deciding that prejudice is an inappropriate way of relating to others (Devine and Zuwerink, 1994). But trying to suppress your stereotypes may actually *strengthen* their automaticity. Hogg and Abrams (2000) argue that, 'The knack would seem to be to get people to have insight into their stereotypes – to understand them and see through them rather than merely to suppress them.'

Relying on stereotypes to form impressions of strangers (*category-driven processing*) represents the cognitively easiest, least strenuous route, while relying on their unique characteristics (*attribute-driven processing*) represents the most strenuous route (Fiske and Neuberg, 1990). While people are very skilled at preserving their stereotypes ('You're OK, it's the others'), the more often they come into contact with members of a particular group who don't fit the stereotype, the more likely it is to lose its credibility.

I'm relieved I'm not alone in finding it difficult to change my thinking. My experience with Mrs M showed me some subtle aspects of prejudice and discrimination I may not have acknowledged before. It's also made me think about my own prejudices and lack of awareness of other cultures. I'll try to take much more interest in the socio-cultural factor of assessment, be more aware, and respectful, of other ethnic groups. I also need to be more aware of the political aspects of the NHS. Meanwhile, I've noted that developing a warm, trusting relationship with others is a powerful way to reduce prejudice; I shall make it my goal to achieve this with Mrs M!

CHAPTER SUMMARY

◎ As an extreme attitude, **prejudice** comprises **cognitive (stereotype)**, **affective (hostility)** and **behavioural components**. **Discrimination** usually refers to any kind of prejudiced behaviour.

◎ Most definitions of prejudice identify it as the characteristic of an individual, but it's often associated with **intergroup conflict**. Racism, sexism, heterosexism, ageism, sizeism and 'HIV/AIDS-ism' can all be regarded as **ideologies**, which are characteristics of society, not individuals.

◎ The most influential 'individual' theory of prejudice is the **authoritarian personality**. Adorno *et al.* argued that the authoritarian personality is prejudiced in a **generalised** way.

◎ Rokeach's theory of **ideological dogmatism** identifies authoritarianism as an extreme way of thinking (the 'closed mind'), rather than a particular political persuasion.

◎ According to the **frustration–aggression hypothesis**, frustration-induced aggression is often displaced onto minority groups, which act as **scapegoats**.

◎ According to **realistic group conflict theory** (RGCT), **competition** between groups for scarce resources is a sufficient condition for intergroup hostility.

◎ **Minimal group experiments** demonstrate that intergroup conflict can occur without competition, and that the **mere categorisation** of oneself as belonging to one group rather than another is sufficient for intergroup discrimination.

◎ The minimal group effect is explained in terms of **social identity theory** (SIT), according to which we try to increase self-esteem by accentuating the desirability of our ingroup(s). Prejudice can be seen as part of the attempt to boost self-image.

◎ An important framework for attempts to reduce prejudice is Allport's **contact hypothesis** (CH), which stresses the need for **equal status contact** and the **pursuit of common (superordinate) goals** between members of different ethnic groups.

◎ Group segregation can produce **autistic hostility** and the related **mirror-image phenomenon**, with the likely reinforcement of negative stereotypes. Unequal status contact can also reinforce stereotypes.

◎ In **equal status** situations, there needs to be a balance between **mutual group differentiation** (which maintains **intergroup contact**) and **interpersonal contact**.

- ◎ There's considerable support for the CH, including the **jigsaw method** of learning. The key mechanism involved seems to be creating **affective ties**, including the reduction of **intergroup awe**.
- ◎ Stereotypes (**category-driven processing**) are very resistant to change, because they often form part of the culture. They can be activated automatically/ unconsciously, but may be broken if people are encouraged to focus on the unique characteristics of individuals (**attribute–driven processing**).

CONFORMITY AND GROUP INFLUENCE

12

INTRODUCTION AND OVERVIEW

It's impossible to live among other people and not be influenced by them in some way. According to Allport (1968), social psychology as a discipline can be defined as 'an attempt to understand and explain how the thoughts, feelings and behaviours of individuals are influenced by the actual, imagined, or implied presence of others'.

Sometimes, other people's attempts to change our thoughts or behaviour are very obvious, as when, for example, a ward sister tells a junior nurse to attend to a particular patient. If we do as we're told, we're demonstrating *obedience*, which implies that one person (in this example, the ward sister, an authority figure) has more social power than others (junior nurses). Obedience is discussed in Chapter 13. In common with obedience, other forms of *active social influence* involve deliberate attempts by one person to change another's thoughts or behaviour.

However, on other occasions social influence is less direct and deliberate, and may not involve any explicit requests or demands at all. For example, sometimes the mere presence of other people can influence our behaviour, either inhibiting or enhancing it (see Gross, 2005).

Another form of indirect or passive social influence occurs when your choice of clothes or taste in music is affected by what your friends wear or listen to. This is *conformity*. Your peers (equals) exert pressure on you to behave (and think) in particular ways, a case of the majority influencing the individual (*majority influence*). But majorities can also be influenced by minorities (*minority influence*).

Is there anything that these different forms of social influence have in common? According to Turner (1991):

> The key idea in understanding what researchers mean by social influence is the concept of a social norm. Influence relates to the processes whereby people agree or disagree about appropriate behaviour, form, maintain or change social norms, and the social conditions that give rise to, and the effects of such norms ...

Turner defines a social norm as 'a rule, value or standard shared by the members of a social group that prescribes appropriate, expected or desirable attitudes and conduct in matters relevant to the group ...'.

From my diary (20): Year 2/Surgical Ward

This afternoon I was working with Susan, the preceptee, admitting a patient for hemicolectomy when I noticed the HCA, on her own, changing an IVI at the other end of

ASK YOURSELF ...
- Try to identify some of the social norms that operate in the different nursing situations you have experienced.

the ward. When we left the patient, I said to Susan I thought HCAs weren't supposed to change IVIs. She said that officially they weren't, but the ward was always so busy Sister and the two senior Staff Nurses seemed to allow it. She sounded non-committal, changed the subject and began checking Mr Reardon's assessment with me. I didn't like to question a qualified nurse, but after work I felt uncomfortable and wondered if I should ask Sister about it. I've not been very good at challenging practice, but after my experience with a doctor telling me to mark an operation site (see my diary entry in Chapter 13, page 237) I am more aware of the issue of accountability. I think I should ask about it – and I've decided I won't change an IVI unsupervised, however busy we are.

ASK YOURSELF ...
- What do these definitions have in common?

CONFORMITY

WHAT IS CONFORMITY?

Conformity has been defined in a number of ways. For Crutchfield (1954), it is 'yielding to group pressure'. Mann (1969) agrees with Crutchfield, but argues that it may take different forms and be based on motives other than group pressure. Zimbardo and Leippe (1991) define conformity as 'a change in belief or behaviour in response to real or imagined group pressure when there is no direct request to comply with the group nor any reason to justify the behaviour change'.

Group pressure is the common denominator in definitions of conformity, although none of them specifies particular groups with particular beliefs or practices. Pressure is exerted by those groups that are important to the individual at a given time. Such groups may consist of 'significant others', such as family or peers (*membership groups*), or groups whose values a person admires or aspires to, but to which s/he doesn't actually belong (*reference groups*).

Conformity, then, doesn't imply adhering to any particular set of attitudes or values. Instead, it involves yielding to the real or imagined pressures of any group, whether it has majority or minority status (van Avermaet, 1996).

For Susan the trained ward staff represent a membership group; for me they are still a reference group.

EXPERIMENTAL STUDIES OF CONFORMITY

A study by Jenness (1932) is sometimes cited as the very first experimental study of conformity. Jenness asked individual students to estimate the number of beans in a bottle, and then had them discuss it to arrive at a group estimate. When they were asked individually to make a second estimate, there was a distinct shift towards the group's estimate. Sherif (1935) used a similar procedure in one of the classic conformity experiments.

> **KEY STUDY 12.1 If the light appears to move, it must be the Sherif (Sherif, 1935)**
>
> - Sherif used a visual illusion called the *autokinetic effect*: a stationary spot of light seen in an otherwise dark room appears to move.

- He told participants he was going to move the light, and their task was to say how far they thought the light moved.
- They were tested individually at first, being asked to estimate the extent of movement several times. The estimates fluctuated to begin with, but then 'settled down' and became quite consistent. However, there were wide differences between participants.
- They then heard the estimates of two other participants (the group condition). Under these conditions, the estimates of different participants *converged* (they became more *similar*). Thus, a *group norm* developed, which represented the average of the individual estimates.
- Just as different individuals produced different estimates, so did different groups. This happened both under the conditions already described and when participants were tested in small groups right from the start.

According to Sherif, participants used others' estimates as a frame of reference in what was an ambiguous situation. Note that:
◎ participants weren't in any way instructed to agree with the others in the group (unlike the Jenness study), despite initially wide differences between individuals
◎ when participants were tested again individually, their estimates closely resembled the group norm (rather than their original, individual estimates).

Susan was using the other staff as a 'frame of reference' in this situation, although she did indicate that she knew the behaviour of the HCA wasn't officially correct.

An evaluation of Sherif's experiment

According to Brown (1996), Sherif's study is one of the classics of social psychology. But it seems to raise questions rather than provide answers:
◎ In what sense can Sherif's participants be described as a group?
◎ Can we speak of group norms without any direct interaction taking place or participants seeing themselves as engaged in some kind of joint activity?
In post-experimental interviews, participants all denied being influenced by others' judgements. They also claimed that they struggled to arrive at the 'correct' answers on their own. In other words, they didn't consider themselves part of a group.

While Sherif believed he'd demonstrated conformity, others, notably Asch, disagreed. According to Asch, the fact that the task used by Sherif was *ambiguous* (there was no right or wrong answer) made it difficult to draw any definite conclusions about conformity. Conformity should be measured in terms of the individual's tendency to agree with other group members who unanimously give the *wrong answer* on a task where the solution is obvious or unambiguous. This is a much stricter test of conformity than where there's no correct or incorrect answer to begin with. Asch devised a simple perceptual task that involved participants deciding which of three comparison lines of different lengths matched a standard line.

From a research point of view this is important – we need to be sure we're measuring what we think we are measuring! But what were Sherif's participants demonstrating if not conformity?

In a pilot study, Asch tested 36 participants individually on 20 slightly different versions of the task shown in Figure 12.1. They made a total of only 3 mistakes in the 720 trials (an error rate of 0.42 per cent).

ASK YOURSELF ...
- What was the purpose of the pilot study?

- What conclusions do you think Asch drew from its results?

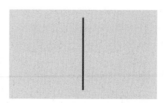

Standard line

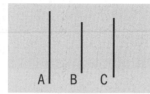

Comparison lines

Figure 12.1 Stimulus cards used in Asch's conformity experiments (1951, 1952, 1956)

The purpose of the pilot study (which involved participants who weren't to take part in the actual experiment) was to establish that the task really was simple, and the answers obvious and unambiguous. Asch concluded that they were. Because his procedure for studying conformity can be adapted to investigate the effects of different variables on conformity, it's known as the *Asch paradigm*.

> **Box 12.1 The Asch paradigm**
>
> - Some of the participants who'd taken part in the pilot study were asked to act as 'stooges' (or 'confederates' – accomplices of the experimenter). The stooges were told they'd be doing the task again, but this time in a group. They were also told that the group would contain one person (a naïve participant) who was completely ignorant that they were stooges.
>
> - On certain *critical* trials, which Asch would indicate by means of a secret signal, all the stooges were required to say out loud the same *wrong answer*. In Asch's original experiment, the stooges (usually seven to nine of them) and the naïve participant were seated either in a straight line or round a table. The situation was rigged so that the naïve participant was always the last or last but one to say the answer out loud (see photo opposite).
>
> - On the first two trials (*neutral* trials), all the stooges gave the correct answers. But the next trial was a critical one (the stooges unanimously gave a wrong answer). This happened a further 11 times (making 12 critical trials in total), with 4 additional neutral trials (making 6 in total) between the critical trials.

The important measure in the Asch paradigm is whether the naïve participant conforms and gives the same wrong answer as the unanimous stooges on the critical trials, or remains independent and gives the obviously correct answer. Asch found a mean conformity rate of 32 per cent – that is, participants agreed with the incorrect majority answer in about one-third of the critical trials.

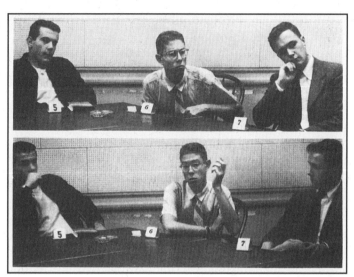

A minority of one faces a unanimous majority (Courtesy William Vandivert and *Scientific American*, November 1955)

Given that the task was simple and unambiguous, such findings indicate a high level of conformity. As van Avermaet (1996) has remarked, 'The results reveal the tremendous impact of an "obviously" incorrect but unanimous majority on the judgements of a lone individual.'

By admitting she knew the HCA's behaviour was wrong and going along with it, Susan conformed to the norms of her membership group.

How did the naïve participants explain their behaviour?

When interviewed at length following the experiment, participants gave a number of specific reasons for conforming:

◎ Some wanted to act in accordance with the experimenter's wishes and convey a favourable impression of themselves by not 'upsetting the experiment' (which they believed they would have done by disagreeing with the majority); they thought some obscure 'mistake' had been made.

◎ A few, who had no reason to believe that there was anything wrong with their eyesight, genuinely doubted the validity of their own judgements by wondering whether they were suffering from eye strain, or whether their chairs had been moved so that they couldn't see the cards properly.

◎ Some denied being aware of having given incorrect answers – they'd unwittingly used the confederates as 'marker posts' (Smith, 1995).

◎ Others said they wanted to be like everyone else, didn't want to 'appear different', 'be made to look a fool', a 'social outcast' or 'inferior'. So, for these participants, there was a discrepancy between the answer they gave in the group and what they *privately believed*: they *knew* the 'wrong' answer was wrong, but went along with it nonetheless. Contrast this with Sherif's participants, for whom there was no conflict between the group's estimate and their own, individual estimates.

This last reason was probably Susan's; she had only recently qualified, there was a Sister, a senior Staff Nurse and another Staff Nurse allowing this behaviour.

Factors affecting conformity

So far, we've described the original, basic experiment. Asch (1952, 1955) subsequently manipulated different variables in order to identify the crucial influences on conformity.

Size of the majority and unanimity

With one naïve participant and just one stooge, conformity was very low (about 3 per cent), ('it's my word against yours'). Where there were two stooges and one participant, conformity increased to 14 per cent and, with three stooges, it reached the 32 per cent that Asch originally reported. But beyond three, conformity didn't continue to rise. This suggests that it's the *unanimity* of the majority that is important (the stooges all agree with each other), rather than the actual size of the majority (the number of stooges).

This was demonstrated when one of the stooges (a *dissenter*) agreed with the naïve participant. With one 'supporter', conformity dropped from 32 to 5.5 per cent. Significantly, a dissenter who disagrees with *both* the naïve participant and the majority has almost as much effect on reducing conformity as one who gives the correct answer (that is, agrees with the naïve participant). In both cases, the majority is no longer unanimous. Thus, just breaking the unanimity of the majority is sufficient to reduce conformity (Allen and Levine, 1971). According to Asch (1951), 'a unanimous majority of three is, under the given conditions, far more effective than a majority of eight containing one dissenter …'

However, this reduction in conformity seems only to apply to unambiguous stimulus situations (like Asch's perceptual task) and not where opinions are being asked for (Allen and Levine, 1968).

Also, Gerard *et al.* (1968) and Latané and Wolf (1981) claim that adding more stooges *will* increase conformity, although the *rate of increase* falls with each extra majority member. According to Hogg and Vaughan (1995), the most robust finding is that conformity reaches its full extent with a three- to five-person majority, with additional members having little effect.

Variables that are changed/manipulated (e.g. the number of trained staff condoning the HCA's action) are the Independent Variables. The degree to which the participants conform (e.g. Susan accepting ward practice) is the Dependent Variable.

Fear of ridicule

In the original experiment, it seems that participants were justified in fearing they'd be ridiculed by the rest of the group if they gave the answer they believed to be correct. When a group of 16 naïve participants and a single stooge were tested, the stooge's wrong answers on the critical trials were greeted with sarcasm, exclamations of disbelief and mocking laughter!

Task difficulty

When Asch made the comparison lines more similar in length (making the task more difficult), participants were more likely to yield to the incorrect majority answer. This was especially true when they felt confident that there was a right answer. When tasks are more ambiguous, in the sense that they involve expressing opinions or stating preferences (there's no objectively correct answer), conformity actually decreases.

Giving answers in private

Critics of Asch's experiment have pointed out that participants may conform because they're reluctant or too embarrassed to expose their private views in face-to-face situations (as many of them indicated in post-experimental interviews). If so, the level of conformity should decrease if they're allowed to write down their answers, or where they remain anonymous in some other way. For example, Deutsch and Gerard (1955) used partitions that shielded participants from each other, with responses showing up on a light panel in front of them – the naïve participant had to press one of three buttons. Under these conditions, conformity was lower than in Asch's face-to-face situation. Indeed, when Asch himself allowed the naïve participant to answer in writing (while the stooges still gave their answers publicly), conformity dropped to 12.5 per cent.

Crutchfield (1954) also used a non-face-to-face procedure. He criticised Asch's experiments for being time-consuming and uneconomical, since only one participant could be tested at a time. He changed the experimental situation so that several (usually five) naïve participants could be tested at the same time. Altogether, he tested over 600 (see Gross, 2005).

The ability to analyse research evidence is part of our study skills and reflective practice. I can see that manipulating the independent variables allowed Asch to find out how different group conditions affected conformity; he found a majority of three (as in Susan's case) is enough to maximise conformity. Using interviews as well allowed him to find out why people conformed.

I intuitively accept the 'fear of ridicule' explanation – that's exactly what happened when I blurted out the wrong answer to a research question in class; I felt so stupid.

Replications of Asch's research

Were Asch's findings a reflection of the times?

The Asch studies have stimulated a great deal of research. Larsen (1974) found significantly lower conformity rates than Asch had found among groups of American students, and suggested that this was because of a changed climate of opinion in America in the 1970s towards independence and criticism, and away from conformity. However, in a later (1979) study, Larsen *et al.* found results very similar to those of Asch. Perhaps the pendulum had begun to swing back again. Why might this have happened?

The early 1950s was the era of 'McCarthyism' in America. This is named after the US Senator Joseph McCarthy, who claimed to have unearthed an anti-American

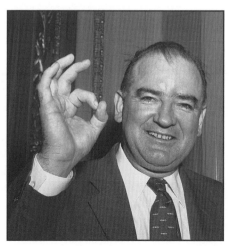

Senator Joseph McCarthy (1908–1957)

Communist plot. This resulted in a witch-hunt of alleged Communist sympathisers, which included academics and Hollywood stars. Under these social and political conditions, high conformity is to be expected (Spencer and Perrin, 1998). By the early 1970s, there was a more liberal climate, but this may have changed again by the late 1970s.

In Britain, Perrin and Spencer (1981) found very low rates of conformity among university students during a period of self-expression and tolerance. As Spencer and Perrin (1998) say, 'The Asch findings are clearly an indicator of the prevailing culture.'

I've learned that good research stimulates more research. Larsen's findings that the degree of conformity (the DV) changed over time within the same culture suggests an IV must have changed – in this case the social conditions.

> **ASK YOURSELF …**
> • Perrin and Spencer (1981) tested young offenders on probation, with probation officers as stooges.
> • How do you think conformity rates with these participants compared with those of Asch?
> • Explain your answer.

We might expect the general social and political climate in Britain in the early 1980s to have had a different impact on university students than on young offenders. Additionally, the stooges were adult authority figures, which means that the group wasn't composed of peers (or equals). Not surprisingly, conformity rates were much higher than for the undergraduates and were similar to those reported by Asch.

It's also possible that experimenters exert an influence. As Brown (1985) has noted, experimenters may also have changed over time. Perhaps their expectations of the amount of conformity that will occur in an experiment are unwittingly conveyed to the participants, who respond accordingly (see Chapter 3, page 16).

I checked this; it is a 'demand characteristic' – responding as you think the experimenter wants, or expects (see Chapter 1). In higher education, students (including nurses since Project 2000 took training into higher education) are encouraged to challenge accepted norms. However, Susan is a newcomer to the qualified team; the three others obviously agree on policy and I can see it would be difficult for her to challenge their authority.

Cross-cultural studies of conformity

As shown in Table 12.1, the vast majority of conformity studies using the Asch paradigm have been carried out in Britain and America. However, using meta-analysis (a 'study of studies'), Bond and Smith (1996) were able to compare the British and American studies with the small number carried out in other parts of the world. After all relevant factors have been taken into account, the studies can be compared in terms of an *averaged effect size* – in this case, the conformity rate.

According to Smith and Bond (1998), the countries represented in Table 12.1 can be described as *individualist* (such as the USA, the UK and other western European countries) or *collectivist* (such as Japan, Fiji and the African countries). In individualist cultures, one's identity is defined by personal choices and achievements, while in collectivist cultures it's defined in terms of the collective group one belongs to (such as the family or religious group). As might be expected, the tendency is for more conformity in collectivist cultures (see Gross, 2005).

> **ASK YOURSELF …**
> • Are there any patterns in the conformity rates (averaged effect size) in Table 12.1?
> • For example, are those countries with the highest and lowest conformity geographically and/or culturally related?

Table 12.1 Asch conformity studies by national culture (based on Bond and Smith, 1996; taken from Smith and Bond, 1998)

Nation	Number of studies	Averaged effect size
Asch's own US studies	18	1.16
Other US studies	79	0.90
Canada	1	1.37
UK	10	0.81
Belgium	4	0.91
France	2	0.56
Netherlands	1	0.74
Germany	1	0.92
Portugal	1	0.58
Japan	5	1.42
Brazil	3	1.60
Fiji	2	2.48
Hong Kong	1	1.93
Arab samples (Kuwait, Lebanon)	2	1.31
Africa (Zimbabwe, Republic of the Congo [Zaire], Ghana)	3	1.84

So being Asian and still influenced by my culture, I might be expected to be more conforming than Susan. But I think we should challenge the behaviour of the HCA while Susan doesn't seem to want to. What are the other IVs that might explain her decision? Personality, class, education – the nature of the group?

An evaluation of the Asch paradigm

◎ According to Fiske (2004), 'Asch's groups weren't very groupy.' In other words, he focused on participants as individuals within a group as distinct from a group process as such.

◎ He concentrated on individual naïve participants' *independence*, rather than group members' *interdependence* (Leyens and Corneille, 1999).

◎ This mirrors Brown's criticism of Sherif's experiments (see above).

Although every health professional is individually accountable, Susan and the other trained staff are a team and interdependent.

Majority or minority influence in Asch-type experiments?

Typically, the findings from experiments using the Asch paradigm have been interpreted as showing the impact of a (powerful) majority on the (vulnerable) individual (who's usually in a minority of one). While the stooges are, numerically, the majority, Asch himself was interested in the social and personal conditions that induce individuals to *resist* group pressure. (In 1950s' America, this group pressure took the form of McCarthyism – see above.)

Spencer and Perrin (1998) ask if reports of Asch's experiments have overstated the power of the majority to force minority individuals to agree with obviously mistaken judgements. Indeed, Moscovici and Faucheux (1972) argued that it's more useful to think of the naïve participant as the majority (s/he embodies the 'conventional', self-evident 'truth') and the stooges as the minority (they reflect an unorthodox, unconventional, eccentric and even outrageous viewpoint). This corresponds to the distinction between the ingroup and outgroup respectively: Moscovici wanted to demonstrate the conditions under which people actually conform to the outgroup. In Asch's experiments, this minority/outgroup influenced the majority 32 per cent of the time, and it's those participants remaining independent who are actually the conformists!

From Moscovici and Faucheux's (1972) point of view, because the three ward managers are breaking the rules regarding the role of the HCA, they are innovators/a minority outgroup, rebelling against accepted practice. If Susan agrees with them, she is joining the outgroup; if she disagrees then she is identifying with the ingroup – the established majority. So although Susan is a conformer, she's identifying with the non-conformers – and, oh dear, I am, after all, the conforming one!

Is the majority always right?

Looked at from Moscovici and Faucheux's perspective, Asch-type experiments suggest how new ideas may come to be accepted (they explain *innovation*), rather than provide evidence about maintenance of the status quo. If groups always followed a majority decision rule ('the majority is always or probably right, so best go along with it'), or if social influence were about the inevitable conforming to the group, where would innovation come from? (Spencer and Perrin, 1998; see Box 12.2.)

According to Moscovici (1976), there's a *conformity bias* in this area of research, such that all social influence is seen as serving the need to adapt to the status quo for the sake of uniformity and stability – the 'tyranny of the majority' (Martin and Hewstone, 2001; Wood, 2000). However, change is sometimes needed to adapt to changing circumstances, and this is very difficult to explain given the conformity bias. Without *active minorities*, social and scientific innovations would simply never happen (van Avermaet, 1996).

If the tendency to conform to the status quo had persisted, none of the recent changes in nursing would have happened. In this case, the ward staff were responding to the demands of a situation – they were problem solving.

How do minorities exert an influence?

Moscovici (1976) re-analysed the data from one of Asch's (1955) experiments, in which he varied the proportion of neutral to critical trials (where stooges gave the right or wrong answers respectively). In the original experiment this proportion was 1:2 (see Box 12.1). When the proportion was 1:6, the conformity rate was 50 per cent, but when it was 4:1 it dropped to 26.2 per cent.

Moscovici interpreted these findings in terms of *consistency*. When there were more critical than neutral trials (the ratio *decreases*), the stooges (who embody the *minority* viewpoint) appear *more consistent* as a group, and this produces a higher conformity rate. They're more often agreeing with each other about something unconventional or novel, which makes it more likely that they'll change the views of the majority (as represented by the naïve participant).

Moscovici *et al.* (1969) showed that a consistent minority can affect the judgements made by the majority even when this involved the (supposedly objective) colour of

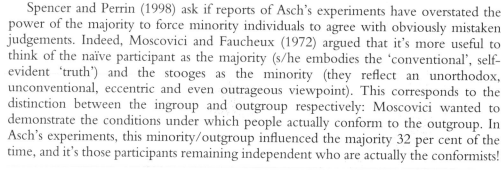

> **ASK YOURSELF ...**
> • Try to account for these findings.
>
> • Why should conformity rates *increase* as the ratio of neutral to critical trials *decreases*, but *decrease* when it *increases*?

slides (see Gross, 2005). Although the minority doesn't have a numerical advantage, their consistent behavioural style makes them influential. In conformity experiments, the influence of the (numerical) majority is evident from the start. But minority influence begins to show only after a while.

However, consistency doesn't necessarily have to involve repeating the same response. Nemeth *et al.* (1974) replicated the Moscovici *et al.* experiment and showed that there's more to minority influence than just consistency: it also matters how the majority interprets the minority's answers. They must relate to the stimulus in some predictable way. In Nemeth *et al.*'s study, the minority's wrong answers (the colour of the slide) depended on another attribute of the stimulus – in this case, the brightness of the slide. So it was the brightness of the slide that counted.

Minority influence is achieved not so much by a particular style of behaviour in the group, but more by a combination of attributes and behaviour (Smith, 1995). Moscovici (1980) proposes that while majorities impose their views through directly requiring compliance (which often requires 'surveillance'), minorities use more *indirect* means to achieve a more lasting conversion.

Susan (and I) could see the reason for her colleagues' attitude to the HCAs; we interpreted it as a response to the problem of chronic shortage of staff on the ward.

> ## Box 12.2 The importance of consistency and other factors in minority influence
>
> According to Hogg and Vaughan (1998), consistency has five main effects.
>
> 1. It disrupts the majority norm, producing uncertainty and doubt.
> 2. It draws attention to itself as an entity.
> 3. It conveys the existence of an alternative, coherent point of view.
> 4. It demonstrates certainty and an unshakeable commitment to a particular point of view.
> 5. It shows that the only solution to the current conflict is the minority viewpoint.
>
> Minorities are more efficient if they:
>
> - are seen to have made significant personal/material sacrifices (*investment*)
> - are perceived as acting out of principle rather than ulterior motives (*autonomy*)
> - display a balance between being 'dogmatic' (*rigid*) and 'inconsistent' (*flexible*)
> - are seen as being *similar* to the majority in terms of age, gender and social category, particularly if they're categorised as part of the ingroup.

Nurse Managers, in consultation with Ward Sisters/Charge Nurses, define the official parameters of the HCA role (the majority group). The ward-trained staff (the minority group) are demonstrating a different point of view, which they see as the only way to solve the 'current conflict': staff shortage.

As the three Registered Nurses are equally accountable for the actions of the HCA, they could be seen as investing personally in the principle of providing adequate care for their patients. This consistent response to a consistent problem may lead to further restructuring of the HCA's role.

When minority group members *consistently* adopt a unique (non-majority, unconventional) response (that is, there's *low consensus*), this is likely to lead majority members to make an *internal/dispositional* attribution (they sincerely believe in what they say).

According to Wood *et al.* (1994), minority influence most often occurs *privately* – that is, on measures that protect the converted majority individuals from appearing publicly to abandon their majority position. For the same reason, influence is often *indirect*, emerging on issues merely *related* to the controversial issues or *delayed* beyond the immediate context (Crano, 2000). 'Thus, majorities can be converted by minorities, but majority individuals do not admit it to others, and perhaps not to themselves, thereby avoiding public identification with the unpopular minority position ...' (Fiske, 2004).

Susan appeared to be complying with her colleagues' policy decision, which is a kind of conformity. However, if privately her attitude conflicts with theirs, when she is registered and in a more senior position, she may challenge it.

WHY DO PEOPLE CONFORM?

Different types of social influence

One very influential and widely accepted account of group influence is Deutsch and Gerard's (1955) distinction between *informational social influence* (ISI) and *normative social influence* (NSI).

Informational social influence (ISI)

Underlying ISI is the need to be right, to have an accurate perception of reality. So when we're uncertain or face an ambiguous situation, we look to others to help us perceive the stimulus situation accurately (or define the situation – see Gross, 2005). This involves a *social comparison* with other group members in order to reduce the uncertainty.

As we saw earlier, Sherif's experiment involves an inherently ambiguous situation: there's no actual movement of the light and so there cannot be any right or wrong answers. Under these conditions, participants were only too willing to validate their own estimates by comparing them with those of others. The results were consistent with Sherif's *social reality hypothesis*, which states that, 'The less one can rely on one's own direct perception and behavioural contact with the physical world, the more susceptible one should be to influence from others ...' (Turner, 1991).

According to Festinger's (1954) *social comparison theory*, people have a basic need to evaluate their ideas and attitudes and, in turn, to confirm that they're correct. This can provide a reassuring sense of control over one's world, and a satisfying sense of competence. In novel or ambiguous situations, social reality is defined by what others think and do. Significantly, Sherif's participants were relatively unaware of being influenced by the other judges (see above).

As a student, I look to others all the time for reassurance that I'm doing the right thing, although reading this chapter is making me more wary of doing so!

Normative social influence (NSI)

Underlying NSI is the need to be accepted by other people, and to make a favourable impression on them. We conform in order to gain social approval and avoid rejection – we agree with others because of their power to reward, punish, accept or reject us.

In Asch's experiment, most participants weren't unsure about the correct answer. Rather, they were faced with a *conflict* between two sources of information, which in unambiguous situations normally coincide – namely their own judgement and that of others. If they chose their own judgement, they risked rejection and ridicule by the majority. Recall, though, that some participants were unaware of any conflict or of having given an incorrect response.

Susan was faced with two conflicting sources of information: the official protocols and their interpretation 'in the real world' by senior staff. This conflict in the knowledge, or cognitive, element of her attitude could lead to cognitive dissonance.

Internalisation and compliance

Related to ISI and NSI are two kinds of conformity.

1. *Internalisation* occurs when a private belief or opinion becomes consistent with a public belief or opinion. In other words, we say what we believe and believe what we say. Mann (1969) calls this *true conformity*, and it can be thought of as a *conversion* to other people's points of view, especially in ambiguous situations.

2. *Compliance* occurs when the answers given publicly aren't those that are privately believed (we say what we don't believe and what we believe we don't say). Compliance represents a compromise in situations where people face a conflict between what they privately believe and what others publicly say they believe.

So if Susan believes her colleagues' behaviour is right and publicly supports them, it will be true conformity; if she just goes along with it, believing it's wrong, she's complying.

> ### ASK YOURSELF ...
> • Which kind of conformity was most common in Sherif's and Asch's experiments?
>
> • How are internalisation and compliance related to NSI and ISI?

In Sherif's experiment, participants were *internalising* others' judgements and making them their own. Faced with an ambiguous situation, participants were guided by what others believed to reduce their uncertainty. So, internalisation is related to ISI.

By contrast, most of Asch's participants knew that the majority answers on the critical trials were wrong, but often agreed with them publicly. They were *complying* with the majority to avoid ridicule or rejection. So, compliance is related to NSI.

I couldn't tell if Susan was internalising the 'minority' ward attitude – she was complying with it, for whatever reason.

Do we have to choose between ISI and NSI?

Remember that when Asch made the three comparison lines much more similar – and hence the task more difficult – conformity increased. Clearly, ISI was involved here. If we believe there's a correct answer and are uncertain what it is, it seems quite logical to expect that we'd be more influenced by a unanimous majority. This is why having a supporter, or the presence of a dissenter, has the effect of reducing conformity. By breaking the group consensus, the participant is shown both that disagreement is possible and that the group is fallible. As Turner (1991) puts it:

> ... the more consensual the group and the more isolated the individual (i.e. the less others agree with the deviant), the greater the power of the group to define reality,

induce self-doubt in the deviant as to both her competence and social position, and threaten her with ridicule and rejection for being different.

In other words, both ISI and NSI can operate in conjunction with each other and shouldn't be seen as opposed processes of influence.

As well as deferring to the unanimous judgement of the group, Susan was no doubt anxious to be accepted by them as well. Both could influence her.

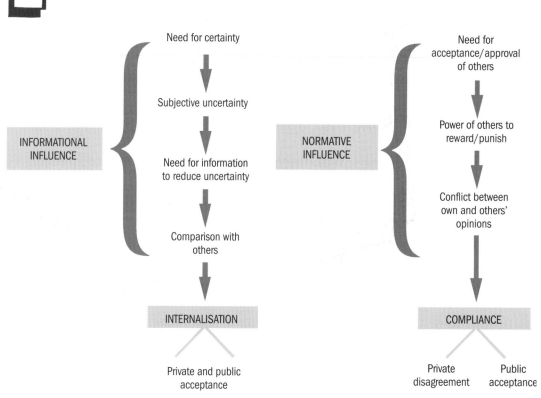

Figure 12.2 The relationship between different kinds of influence and different kinds of conformity

Conformity and group belongingness

The distinction between NSI and ISI has been called the *dual process dependency model* of social influence (e.g. Turner, 1991). But this model underestimates the role of group 'belongingness'. One important feature of conformity is that we're influenced by a group because, psychologically, we feel we belong to it. This is why a group's norms are relevant standards for our own attitudes and behaviour. The dual process dependency model emphasises the *interpersonal* aspects of conformity experiments, which could just as easily occur between individuals as group members.

The *self-categorisation approach* suggests that – in Sherif's experiment, for example – participants assumed that the autokinetic effect was real and expected to agree with each other. In support of this, it's been shown that when participants discover that the autokinetic effect is an illusion, mutual influence and convergence cease – the need to agree at all is removed (Sperling, 1946). If, however, we believe that there *is* a correct answer, and we're uncertain what it is, then those whom we categorise as belonging to 'our' group will influence our judgements. As Brown (1988) has remarked, 'There is more to conformity than simply "defining social reality": it all depends on who is doing the defining.'

KEY STUDY 12.2 Knowing what to think by knowing who you are (Abrams *et al.*, 1990)

- Abrams *et al*. replicated Sherif's experiment with psychology students, but manipulated categorisation: stooges were introduced as students at a nearby university, but were either fellow psychology students or students of ancient history.

- Convergence occurred only when others were categorised as being equivalent to self – that is, a member of the ingroup (fellow psychology students). So self-categorisation may set limits on ISI.

- It should also set limits on NSI, since individuals will presumably have a stronger desire to receive rewards, approval and acceptance from those categorised in the same way as themselves than from those categorised differently.

- Using the Asch paradigm but again manipulating categorisation, Abrams *et al*. found that conformity exceeded the usual level of 32 per cent in the ingroup condition, but was greatly below this level in the outgroup condition.

---

*So Susan would value the point of view **and** the good opinion of her new membership group (the ward staff) more than that of another group (e.g. Nurse Managers)?*

Abrams *et al*. (1990) argue that we experience uncertainty only when we disagree with those with whom we expect to agree. This is especially likely when we regard those others as members of the same category or group as ourselves with respect to judgements made in a shared stimulus situation. Social influence occurs, then, when we see ourselves as belonging to a group and possessing the same characteristics and reactions as other group members.

Turner (1991) calls this kind of self-categorisation, in which group membership is relevant, *referent social influence* (RSI). What's important isn't the validation of physical reality or the avoidance of social disapproval, but the upholding of a *group norm*: people are the source of information about the appropriate ingroup norm.

According to Fiske (2004), a social categorisation approach sees the NSI/ISI distinction as (another) false dichotomy (see above), since 'Information is intrinsically social …'.

Conformity: good or bad?

Sometimes, dissent is just an expression of disagreement, a refusal to 'go along with the crowd' (Maslach *et al.*, 1985). On other occasions, it's more creative or constructive, as when someone suggests a better solution to a problem. A refusal to 'go along with the crowd' may be an attempt to remain independent *as a matter of principle* (what Willis, 1963, calls *anticonformity*), and may betray a basic fear of a loss of personal identity.

According to Zimbardo and Leippe (1991), in most circumstances conformity serves a valuable social purpose in that it '… lubricates the machinery of social interaction [and] enables us to structure our social behaviour and predict the reactions of others'.

For most people, though, the word 'conformity' has a negative connotation. As a result, it's implicitly assumed that independence is 'good' and conformity is 'bad', a value judgement made explicit by Asch (1952). However, conformity can be highly functional, helping us to satisfy social and non-social needs, as well as being necessary (at least to a degree) for social life to proceed at all.

Since each of us has a limited (and often biased) store of information on which to make decisions, other people can often provide valuable additional information and expertise. Conforming with others under these circumstances may be a rational judgement. However, while conformity can help preserve harmony, 'There are obvious dangers to conformity. Failure to speak our minds against dangerous trends or attitudes (for example, racism) can easily be interpreted as support' (Krebs and Blackman, 1988).

The term conformity is often used to convey undesirable behaviour. In laboratory research, it has most often been studied in terms of the 'conspiratorial group … [being] shown to limit, constrain, and distort the individual's response …' (Milgram, 1965). However, in the context of his famous studies of obedience, Milgram showed that the presence of two defiant peers significantly reduced the obedience rate among naïve participants, and he wrote an article (1965) called 'Liberating effects of group pressure' (see Chapter 13).

Also, whether conformity is considered good or bad is a matter of *culture*. In *individualist* cultures, people are often distressed by the possibility that others can influence their behaviour against their will: they prefer to believe they're in control of their destiny. So 'conformity', 'compliance', 'obedience' and other similar terms have negative connotations. But in *collectivist* cultures, adjusting one's behaviour to fit the requests and expectations of others is highly valued, and sometimes even a moral imperative (Fiske *et al.*, 1998). In these cultures, conformity is seen as necessary for social functioning, rather than a sign of weakness (Nagayama Hall and Barongan, 2002).

Whether conformity is good or bad surely depends on the situation? If HCAs acting outside their role compromise standards of care, Susan's silence would be dangerous and unethical.

Individual differences in conformity

Another way of trying to understand why people conform is to consider whether some people are more likely to conform than others and, if so, why.

Crutchfield (1954) found that people who conform tend to be intellectually less effective, have less ego strength, less leadership ability, less mature social relationships, and feelings of inferiority. They also tend to be authoritarian, more submissive, narrow-minded and inhibited, and have relatively little insight into their own personalities compared with those who tend not to conform. However, *consistency across situations* isn't high (McGuire, 1969), and the authoritarian personality (Adorno *et al.*, 1950 – see Chapter 11) is perhaps as close to a 'conforming personality type' as can be found.

In general, men conform less than women. This is at least partly because men are traditionally more likely to see dissent or independence as a way of expressing their competence, while women tend to see cooperation and agreement with others as expressing competence (Zimbardo and Leippe, 1991). However, men with personal qualities and interests that are stereotypically 'feminine' conform as much as women with these same qualities and interests. Conversely, women and men with stereotypically 'masculine' qualities and interests conform less.

The incident with the HCA has made me aware that conformity is about accepting the status quo. I can recognise the difference between conformity, compliance and obedience. I recognise that the danger of conformity lies in the subtle way it operates and is based on a desire to belong and to 'fit in'.

Asch's classic experiments (1952, 1955) showed why the small number of staff agreeing a policy was enough to induce Susan's conformity. As a new and inexperienced member of staff, she would rely on her senior colleagues as a source of information about the appropriate 'ingroup norm' (Turner, 1991).

Moscovici and Faucheux's (1972) view of Asch's experiment showed how the three ward managers can be seen as an innovative minority. If Susan does conform to this 'minority group' and they challenge accepted practice, the role of the HCA might further change and could result in an improvement in the delivery of care.

However, conformists (as high self-monitors) may have a desire to cooperate, and may be willing to compromise in solving problems, which at times can be positive qualities. Deciding whether conformity is a good or bad thing must, I think, be judged in each different situation.

CHAPTER SUMMARY

◎ **Social influence** can be **active** or **deliberate**, as in persuasive communication and obedience, or **passive** or **non-deliberate**, as in social facilitation and conformity. A common feature of all social influence is the concept of a **social norm**.

◎ Definitions of **conformity** commonly refer to **group pressure**, whether the group is a **membership** or a **reference** group.

◎ In Sherif's experiment using the **autokinetic effect**, individual estimates **converged** to form a group norm. Asch criticised Sherif's use of an ambiguous task, and in his own experiments used a 'comparison of lines' task for which there was a correct answer.

◎ Asch found that the **unanimity/consensus of the majority** is crucial, not its size. The presence of a **supporter** or **dissenter** reduces conformity, because the majority is no longer unanimous.

◎ Conformity is increased when the task is made **more difficult** (more **ambiguous**) and reduced when participants give their answer **anonymously**.

◎ Replications of Asch's experiment have produced higher or lower rates of conformity according to when and where they were conducted. Both **socio-historical** and **cultural factors** seem to play a part.

◎ Asch's findings are usually interpreted as showing the impact of **majority influence**. But Moscovici believes that the stooge majority should be thought of as embodying unconventional, minority beliefs, and that conformity experiments show how new ideas come to be accepted (**innovation**).

◎ One way in which **minority influence** works is by displaying **consistency**, together with **investment**, **autonomy** and a balance between **rigidity** and **flexibility**.

◎ Two major **motives for conformity** are the need to be right (**informational social influence**/ISI) and the need to be accepted by others (**normative social influence**/NSI).

◎ ISI is related to Sherif's **social reality hypothesis** and Festinger's **social comparison theory**, and is demonstrated through **internalisation/true conformity**. NSI is linked to **compliance**.

OBEDIENCE

13

INTRODUCTION AND OVERVIEW

Obedience is an active or deliberate form of social influence, which involves someone in authority requiring us to behave in a particular way in a particular situation. If we obey, we are said to be *complying* with the authority figure's request or instruction. Compliance is a major kind of conformity, namely one in which overt behaviour doesn't reflect private beliefs.

Compliance also occurs whenever we do what someone else 'asks' us to do – that is, whenever people make direct requests, such as when a friend asks us for a 'favour' or a salesperson 'invites' us to try a product or service. Many researchers believe that attempts to gain compliance through direct requests is the most common form of social influence (Hogg and Vaughan, 1995).

In the context of nursing, obedience can be seen to operate both *within* the profession (as when junior nurses comply with the wishes/requests of the Charge Nurse or Ward Sister) and *between* nursing staff and doctors. While Florence Nightingale may well have been offended by doctors' definition of nurses as 'devoted and obedient', she must take the blame for starting the militaristic hierarchy that still survives (Heenan, 1990).

In the context of health psychology, compliance refers to 'the extent to which the patient's behaviour (in terms of taking medications, following diets or other lifestyle changes) coincides with medical or health advice' (Haynes *et al.*, 1979).

Damrosch (1995) prefers the term *adherence*, since this implies a more mutual relationship between the patient and the practitioner. 'Compliance' implies that the practitioner is an authority figure, while the patient is a fairly passive recipient.

From my diary (10): Year 1/Orthopaedic Ward

Not the best of days – I managed to trigger a power struggle between a doctor and Staff Nurse. I'd got Mr Price, in for a hip replacement, ready for theatre but the operation site hadn't been marked. Staff asked me to ring the house surgeon. He said he was in ITU and couldn't come. I told him Mr Price was next on the list and he said, 'You do it, then.' I started to say I wasn't allowed to but he interrupted with, 'You'll have to – for heaven's sake, it's quite obvious which hip it is.' He sounded agitated, so I just said, 'All right', and put the phone down. When I told Staff, she went marching off to the phone and five minutes later the doctor came flying into the ward; he looked furious. He stopped and spoke to her and they were obviously arguing. I kept out of his way!

ASK YOURSELF ...
• Try to identify some of the basic *similarities and differences* between conformity and obedience. (See Chapter 12.)

DISTINGUISHING BETWEEN CONFORMITY AND OBEDIENCE

According to Milgram (1992), both conformity and obedience involve the 'abdication of individual judgement in the face of some external social pressure'. However, there are three major *differences* between them.

1. In conformity, there's no explicit requirement to act in a certain way, whereas in obedience we're being ordered or instructed to do something.
2. In conformity, those who influence us are our *peers* (*equals*) and people's behaviour becomes more *alike* (*homogenisation of behaviour*). In obedience, there's a *difference in status* from the outset, with the authority figure influencing another person who has inferior power or status: there's no mutual influence.
3. Conformity has to do with the psychological 'need' for acceptance by others and entails going along with one's peers in a group situation. Obedience has to do with the social power and status of an authority figure in a hierarchical situation. Although we typically deny that we conform (because it seems to detract from our sense of *individuality*), we usually *deny responsibility* for our behaviour in the case of obedience ('He made me do it', or 'I was only doing what I was told').
4. In addition, Brown (1986) says that conformity behaviour is affected by *example* (from peers or equals), while obedience is affected by *direction* (from somebody in higher authority).

Although staff asked me politely to phone and the doctor ordered me to mark the operation site, I perceived them both as directions from authority figures who should be obeyed.

EXPERIMENTAL STUDIES OF OBEDIENCE

In the experiments of Sherif and Asch (see Chapter 12), participants showed conformity by giving a verbal response of some kind, or pressing buttons representing answers on various tasks. In the most famous and controversial of all obedience experiments, Milgram's participants were required to 'kill' another human being.

Well, I know I wouldn't do that! Marking an operation site isn't comparable.

MILGRAM'S RESEARCH

Milgram was attempting to test 'the "Germans are different" hypothesis'. This has been used by historians to explain the systematic destruction of millions of Jews, Poles and others by the Nazis during the 1930s and 1940s. It maintains that the Germans have a basic character defect, namely a readiness to obey authority without question, regardless of the acts demanded by the authority figure. It's this readiness to obey that provided Hitler with the cooperation he needed. After piloting his research in America, Milgram planned to continue it in Germany, but his results showed this was unnecessary.

The participants

The participants in the original (1963) experiment were 20–50-year-old men, from all walks of life. They answered advertisements that came by post or appeared in local newspapers, which asked for volunteers for a study of learning to be conducted at Yale University. It would take about one hour and there would be a payment of $4.50.

The basic procedure

Box 13.1 The basic procedure used in Milgram's obedience experiment

- When participants arrived at Yale University psychology department, they were met by a young man in a grey laboratory coat, who introduced himself as Jack Williams, the experimenter. Also present was a Mr Wallace, introduced as another participant, in his late fifties, an accountant, a little overweight and generally a very mild and harmless-looking man.

- In fact, Mr Wallace was a stooge, and everything that happened after this was preplanned, staged and scripted: everything, that is, except the degree to which the real participant obeyed the experimenter's instructions.

- The participant and Mr Wallace were told that the experiment was concerned with the effects of punishment on learning. One of them was to be the teacher and the other the learner. Their roles were determined by each drawing a piece of paper from a hat: both, in fact, had 'teacher' written on them. Mr Wallace drew first and called out 'learner', so, of course, the real participant was always the teacher.

- They all went into an adjoining room, where Mr Wallace was strapped into a chair with his arms attached to electrodes, which would deliver a shock from the shock generator situated in an adjacent room.

- The teacher and experimenter then moved next door, where the generator was situated. The teacher was given a 45-volt shock to convince him/her that it was real, for s/he was to operate the generator during the experiment. However, that was the only real shock that either the teacher or the learner was to receive throughout the entire experiment.

- The generator had a number of switches, each clearly marked with voltage levels and verbal descriptions, starting at 15 volts and going up to 450 in intervals of 15:

15–60	Slight shock
75–120	Moderate shock
135–180	Strong shock
195–240	Very strong shock
255–300	Intense shock
315–360	Intense to extreme shock
375–420	Danger: severe shock
435–450	XXX

- The teacher had to read out a series of word pairs (e.g. 'blue–girl', 'nice–day', 'fat–neck'), and then the first of one pair (the stimulus word) followed by five words, of which one was the original paired response. The learner had to choose the correct response to the stimulus word by pressing one of four switches, which turned on a light on a panel in the generator room. Each time he made a mistake, the teacher had to deliver a shock, and each successive mistake was punished by a shock 15 volts higher than the one before.

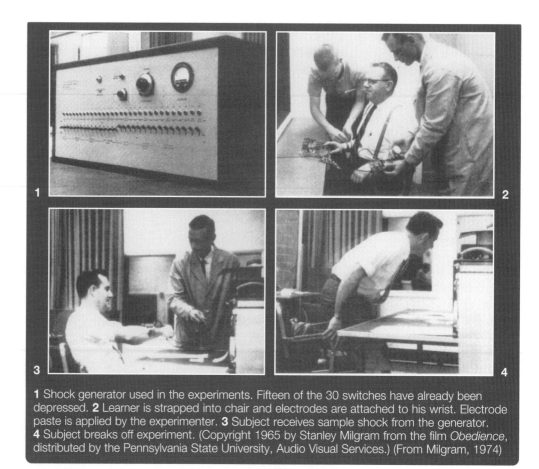

1 Shock generator used in the experiments. Fifteen of the 30 switches have already been depressed. **2** Learner is strapped into chair and electrodes are attached to his wrist. Electrode paste is applied by the experimenter. **3** Subject receives sample shock from the generator. **4** Subject breaks off experiment. (Copyright 1965 by Stanley Milgram from the film *Obedience*, distributed by the Pennsylvania State University, Audio Visual Services.) (From Milgram, 1974)

Milgram had asked 14 psychology students to predict what would happen for 100 participants in this situation. They thought that a few would break off early on, most would stop somewhere in the middle, and a few would continue right up to 450 volts. He also asked 40 psychiatrists, who predicted that, on average, less than 1 per cent would administer the highest voltage.

I can't imagine that anybody in a caring situation would progress very far on such a scale, and certainly not to the point of causing a patient harm or danger.

These estimates were based on what Milgram called the *remote-victim condition*, which was the first of a series of 18 different experiments, all variations on the same basic theme. In this particular experiment, Mr Wallace was scripted to pound loudly on the wall at 300 volts and, after 315 volts, to stop pounding and give no further answers. In the second experiment (*voice feedback*), teachers heard a tape-recorded series of verbal responses, which they believed were the spontaneous reactions of Mr Wallace to the increasing shock levels. For example:

◎ at 75, 90 and 105 volts, he made a little grunt
◎ at 120 volts, he shouted to the experimenter that the shocks were becoming painful
◎ at 150 volts, he cried out, 'Experimenter, get me out of here! I won't be in the experiment any more! I refuse to go on!'; this continued with rising intensity until at 180 volts, he shouted, 'I can't stand the pain!'

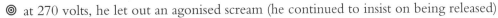

ASK YOURSELF ...

- If you'd been one of Milgram's teacher-participants, how far up the voltage scale would you have continued to punish 'wrong answers'?

◎ at 270 volts, he let out an agonised scream (he continued to insist on being released)
◎ after 330 volts, ominous silence!

The teacher was instructed to treat no response as if it were an incorrect response, so the shocks could continue beyond 300 volts. In addition, the experimenter had a script prepared for whenever the teacher refused to continue or showed any resistance or reluctance to do so:

◎ 'Please continue' or 'Please go on'
◎ 'The experiment requires that you continue'
◎ 'It's absolutely essential that you continue'
◎ 'You have no other choice, you must go on.'

There were also 'special prods' to reassure the participant that s/he wasn't doing the learner any permanent harm: 'Although the shocks may be painful there is no permanent tissue damage, so please go on.'

The results

In the first (remote-victim) experiment, every teacher shocked up to at least 300 volts, and 65 per cent went all the way up to 450 volts. In the voice-feedback condition, 62.5 per cent of participants went on giving shocks up to 450 volts.

Many displayed great anguish, attacked the experimenter verbally, twitched nervously, or broke out into nervous laughter. Many were observed to 'sweat, stutter, tremble, groan, bite their lips and dig their nails into their flesh. Full-blown, uncontrollable seizures were observed for three subjects' (Milgram, 1974). Indeed, one experiment had to be stopped because the participant had a violently convulsive seizure.

I find it difficult to believe these results; two-thirds of the 'teachers' (in spite of their mental conflict) were prepared to risk killing the 'learner'!

To determine why the obedience levels were so high, Milgram conducted several variations using the voice-feedback condition as his baseline measure. In all, a further 16 variations were performed.

ASK YOURSELF ...

- For each of the variations described in Key Study 13.1, estimate the rates of total obedience (those participants going all the way up to 450 volts).

- Try to explain why it might have been higher or lower than the 62.5 per cent in the voice-feedback condition.

KEY STUDY 13.1 Some variations on Milgram's basic procedure

Institutional context (variation 10): in interviews following the first experiment, many participants said they continued delivering shocks because the research was being conducted at Yale University, a highly prestigious institution. So, Milgram transferred the experiment to a run-down office in downtown Bridgeport.

Proximity and touch proximity (variations 3 and 4): in the original procedure, the teacher and learner were in adjacent rooms and couldn't see one another. But in variation 3, they were in the same room (about 46 cm apart), and in variation 4 the teacher was required to force the learner's hand down on to the shock plate.

Remote authority (variation 7): the experimenter left the room (having first given the essential instructions) and gave subsequent instructions by telephone.

Two peers rebel (variation 17): the teacher was paired with two other (stooge) teachers. The stooge teachers read out the list of word-pairs and informed the learner whether the response was correct. The naïve participant delivered the shocks. At 150 volts, the first stooge refused to continue and moved to another part of the room. At 210 volts, the second stooge did the same. The experimenter ordered the real teacher to continue.

A peer administers the shocks (variation 18): the teacher was paired with another (stooge) teacher and had only to read out the word-pairs (the shock being delivered by the stooge).

- In variation 10, the obedience rate was 47.5 per cent. This still very high figure suggests that the institutional context played some part, but wasn't a crucial factor.
- In variation 3, the obedience rate dropped to 40 per cent, and in variation 4 it dropped further to 30 per cent. While it became much more uncomfortable for participants to see – as well as hear – the effects of their obedience, the figures are still very high.
- In variation 7, obedience dropped to 20.5 per cent. Indeed, participants often pretended to deliver a shock or delivered one lower than they were asked to. This suggests that they were trying to compromise between their conscience and the experimenter's instructions. In his absence, it was easier to follow their conscience.

If the doctor had stood in front of me and ordered me to mark the leg, it would have been more difficult to refuse/avoid.

- In variation 17, there was only 10 per cent obedience. Most stopped obeying when the first or second stooge refused to continue. According to Milgram (1965), 'The effects of peer rebellion are most impressive in undercutting the experimenter's authority.' In other words, seeing other participants (our peers) disobey shows that it's *possible* to disobey, as well as *how* to disobey. Indeed, some participants said they didn't realise they *could*. This is a demonstration of the effects of *conformity*.
- In variation 18, obedience rose to 92.5 per cent. This shows that it's easier for participants to shift responsibility from themselves to the person who actually 'throws the switch'.

All these are external influences on behaviour. Why did so many people behave as though they had no choice until shown? But (like those in variation 7 in Milgram) I pretended to comply with the doctor, didn't I? Why didn't I simply say 'no'? And by reporting it to Staff Nurse wasn't I shifting the responsibility to her? I'm no longer so sure I wouldn't have obeyed the experimenter.

WHY DO PEOPLE OBEY?

According to Milgram (1974):

> The most fundamental lesson of our study is that ordinary people simply doing their jobs, and without any particular hostility on their part, can become agents in a terrible destructive process.

Unless there's reason to believe that people who go all the way up to 450 volts are especially sadistic and cruel, or are unusually obedient (which 'the "Germans are different" hypothesis' claimed about a whole nation), explanations of obedience must look 'outside' the individual participant. In this way, the emphasis is shifted away from personal characteristics to the characteristics of the social situation: most people facing that situation would probably act in a similar (obedient) way. What might some of these situational factors be?

Personal responsibility

Many participants raised the issue of responsibility for any harm to the learner. Although the experimenter didn't always discuss this, when he did say 'I'm responsible for what goes on here', participants showed visible relief. Indeed, when participants are told they're responsible for what happens, obedience is sharply reduced (Hamilton, 1978).

Milgram saw this *diffusion of responsibility* as crucial to understanding the atrocities committed by the Nazis, and Eichmann's defence that he was 'just carrying out orders'. (Eichmann was in charge of the transportation of Jews and others to extermination camps, and was eventually tried in Jerusalem, in 1960.)

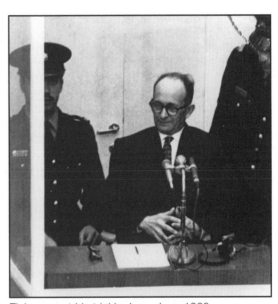

Eichmann at his trial in Jerusalem, 1960

This is about accountability. When we discussed this afterwards, Staff Nurse asked if I would have marked the site knowing I'd be held personally responsible if the surgeon operated on Mr Price's good hip. That made me realise the potential for harm to the patient.

The perception of legitimate authority

As mentioned earlier, many participants showed signs of distress and conflict, and so diffusion of responsibility cannot tell the whole story. The conflict seems to be between two opposing sets of demands – the external authority of the experimenter who says 'Shock' and the internal authority of the conscience which says 'Don't shock'. The point at which conscience triumphs is, of course, where the participant (finally) stops obeying the experimenter, who, in a sense, ceases to be a legitimate authority in the eyes of the participant. In the original experiment 35 per cent reached that point somewhere before 450 volts, and for many, the crucial 'prod' was when the experimenter said, 'You have no other choice, you *must* go on.' They were able to exercise the choice which, of course, they had from the start.

The most common mental adjustment in the obedient participant is to see him/herself as an agent of external authority (the *agentic state*). This represents the opposite of an *autonomous state* and is what makes it possible for us to function in a *hierarchical* social system. For a group to function as a whole, individuals must give up responsibility and defer to others of higher status in the social hierarchy. Legitimate authority thus replaces a person's own self-regulation (Turner, 1991). In Milgram's (1974) words:

> The essence of obedience consists in the fact that a person comes to view himself as the instrument for carrying out another person's wishes, and he, therefore, no longer regards himself as responsible for his actions. Once this critical shift of viewpoint has occurred in the person, all the essential features of obedience follow.

I'm aware the nursing profession is fighting to establish its autonomy, yet I still perceived the doctor's status as higher than ours and felt I should carry out his orders. Staff Nurse certainly had no problem with refusing to be a 'handmaiden'!

Authority figures often possess highly visible symbols of their power or status that make it difficult to refuse their commands. In Milgram's experiments, the experimenter always wore a grey laboratory coat to indicate his position as an authority figure. The impact of such 'visible symbols' was demonstrated by Bushman (1984), who found that a stooge wearing a firefighting uniform was obeyed more often than a stooge dressed as a civilian, even though the request (to give someone a dime) had nothing to do with the authority role in question. For Milgram (1974), 'A substantial proportion of people do what they are told to do, irrespective of the content of the act and without limitations of conscience, so long as they perceive that the command comes from a legitimate authority.'

Another major study that demonstrates the impact of uniforms and other symbols of authority is Zimbardo *et al.*'s (1973) 'prison simulation experiment' (see Gross, 2005).

Most of us wear uniforms, or some indicator of our 'rank', which is significant. (The doctors' symbol of authority – their stethoscopes round their necks – is now being adopted by some nurses too.)

> **ASK YOURSELF ...**
> * What was it about Jack Williams, the experimenter, that conveyed to participants that he was 'in charge' in the experimental situation?

> **ASK YOURSELF ...**
> * If the original advertisement had mentioned electric shocks (which it didn't), do you think there would have been many volunteers?
>
> * In what ways might such volunteers have constituted a more biased sample than those who participated in the actual experiments?

The 'foot in the door' and not knowing how to disobey

According to Gilbert (1981), Milgram's participants may have been 'sucked in' by the series of graduated demands. These began with the 'harmless' advertisement for volunteers for a study of learning and memory, and ended with the instruction to deliver what appeared to be potentially lethal electric shocks to another person. Having begun the experiment, participants may have found it difficult to remove themselves from it.

Much of our work is carrying out doctors' instructions, which makes it more difficult to distinguish what is, and isn't, legitimate.

Presumably, fewer volunteers would have come forward. Those who did may well have been more sadistic than Milgram's sample (assuming that they believed they'd be giving the electric shocks).

Socialisation

Despite our expressed ideal of independence, obedience is something we're socialised into from a very early age by significant others (including our parents and teachers). Obedience may be an ingrained habit that's difficult to resist (Brown, 1986).

An evaluation of Milgram's research

In evaluating Milgram's experiments, *ethical issues* are usually more prominent than scientific ones (see Gross, 2005). However, Milgram asks whether the ethical criticisms are based as much on the nature of the (unexpected) results as on the procedure itself. Aronson (1988) asks whether we would question the ethics if none of the participants had gone beyond the 150-volt level, which is the point at which most people were expected to stop (according to Milgram's students and the 40 psychiatrists he consulted). Aronson manipulated the results experimentally and found that the higher the percentage going right up to 450 volts, the more harmful the effects of the experiment are judged to be.

Methodological issues

◎ Orne and Holland (1968) criticised Milgram's experiments for their lack of *mundane realism* – that is, the results don't extend beyond the particular laboratory setting in which they were collected. They base this claim on the further claim that cues in the experimental setting influenced the participants' perceptions of what was required of them. Obedience, then, might simply have been a response to the *demand characteristics* of the highly unusual experimental setting (see Chapter 1). However, naturalistic studies of obedience dispute this.

KEY STUDY 13.2 A naturalistic study of nurses (Hofling *et al.*, 1966)

- Twenty-two nurses working in various American hospitals received telephone calls from a stooge 'Dr Smith of the psychiatric department', instructing them to give Mr Jones (Dr Smith's patient) 20 mg of a drug called Astrofen.
- Dr Smith said that he was in a desperate hurry and would sign the drug authorisation form when he came to see the patient in ten minutes' time.
- The label on the box containing the Astrofen (which was actually a harmless sugar pill) clearly stated that the maximum daily dose was 10 mg.
- So, if the nurse obeyed Dr Smith's instructions she'd be exceeding the maximum daily dose. Also, she'd be breaking the rules requiring written authorisation before any drug is given and that a nurse be absolutely sure that 'Dr Smith' is a genuine doctor.

ASK YOURSELF ...
- What do you think you'd have done if you'd been one of the nurses?

◎ In interviews, 22 graduate nurses who hadn't participated in the actual experiment were presented with the same situation as an issue to discuss; 21 said they wouldn't have given the drug without written authorisation, especially as it exceeded the maximum daily dose.

◎ A real doctor was posted nearby, unseen by the nurse, and observed what the nurse did following the telephone call; 21 out of the 22 nurses complied without hesitation, and 11 later said they hadn't noticed the dosage discrepancy!

But could the unfamiliarity of Astrofen (a dummy drug, invented for the purposes of the experiment) have influenced the nurses' responses? Also, Hofling *et al.* failed to report what proportion of nurses actually tried to check the instruction with fellow nurses or superiors – they reported only the number of those who (eventually) complied. Rank and Jacobson (1977) repeated the experiment, but with two important changes:

1. they recorded any checking that nurses did
2. they changed the prescription to 30 mg of Valium, with which they were familiar. Under these conditions, only 2 out of 18 nurses were prepared to administer the drug without any checking; 10 prepared the drug but then tried to recontact the doctor, pharmacy, or a supervisor; and 6 tried to check the order before preparing the drug. The limitations of Hofling *et al.*'s experiment, therefore, offer only modest support to Milgram.

Tschudin (2003) states: 'Nurses are always being asked to perform duties for which they may not have been trained.' She also points out that the NMC Code (2002) is specific about such situations: 'You must possess the knowledge, skills and abilities required for lawful, safe and effective practice without direct supervision' (Tschudin, 2003: 99).

As it was, the nurses in the study above were being asked to act against a well-known protocol. What it shows (frighteningly) is that 2 out of 18 (approximately 11 per cent) would have obeyed a doctor and given an overdose of medicine.

ASK YOURSELF ...

• How do you see the relationship between nursing and medical staff?

• Who has more power/authority, and who perceives themselves as having greater power/authority?

• What forms does this greater power/authority take?

• How do these power/authority differences affect patient care?

CRITICAL DISCUSSION 13.1 The nurse–doctor relationship

• Thirty years ago, at least, the stereotypical roles associated with doctors and nurses were very much in place (Robotham, 1999). Stein (1967, in Robotham, 1999) described a definite doctor/nurse 'game' being played out in wards across US hospitals where power was weighted in favour of the medical staff. Nurses were able to suggest courses of action to doctors in such a way as to enable doctors to restate these as their own, so maintaining their superior public image. The system was undeniably hierarchical. This appears to have been replicated in UK hospitals.

• According to Stein *et al.* (1990, in Robotham, 1999), 'The game is dead … one of the players (the nurse) has unilaterally decided to stop playing the game and instead is consciously and actively attempting to change both nursing and how nurses relate to other health professionals.' However, Tellis-Nyak and Tellis-Nyak (1984) and Porter (1995) (both in Rowe, 1999) believe the model still applies.

• While doctors have a lot of respect for nurses, it's often subverted by problems and the issue of *responsibility*. Quite often a task is transferred to the nurse but the responsibility stays with the doctor. According to Hobart (in Robotham, 1999), nursing is a 'culture that acts against taking responsibility'.

• In an interview study of GPs and district nurses, Rowe (1999) found that nurses were keen to expand their roles and it was acknowledged by all participants that district nurses had become experts in certain areas, such as wound care and palliative care. But both groups agreed that the doctors had a continuing responsibility for their registered patients, which made the GPs cautious when delegating care to nursing colleagues. This, in turn, made nurses feel they needed to earn the GPs' trust in order to be able to expand their areas of work. But this sits rather uneasily with the claim that nursing is controlling its own agenda and with the UKCC's *Code of Professional Conduct*, which states that: 'As a registered nurse, midwife or health visitor you are personally accountable for your practice' (Rowe, 1999). GPs felt threatened by nurses taking over areas of work traditionally seen as theirs, making it difficult for them to share responsibility with nurses.

- However, nurses as a whole might look towards midwifery to see which path the nurse–doctor relationship could take. Midwives have been used to working officially with professional accountability and responsibility for some time now (Rowe, 1999).

- According to Brooking (1991), while nurses are no longer subservient to the more powerful medical profession, medicine retains much of its power in relation to nursing for reasons such as:

  (a) doctors usually have legal responsibility for admission, discharge, diagnosis and prescription

  (b) nurses are required (in part of their role at least) to carry out medically prescribed treatment, while the converse isn't true

  (c) doctors see themselves as having overall responsibility for all aspects of care and treatment, so nurses may feel accountable to doctors even for nursing treatments; nurses, in contrast, see very clear role boundaries for themselves and are unlikely to comment to doctors on matters of diagnosis and prescription

  (d) doctors have greater knowledge of disease and its treatment as a result of their longer and more intense education

  (e) nursing is still a predominantly female profession, whereas most senior doctors are male.

- None of these differences would matter if nurses weren't clearly dissatisfied with their relationships with doctors (and vice versa) (Brooking, 1991). But why should this matter? Brooking argues that:

  > ... Sick people need different types of care, best provided by members of different health care professions ... If we can agree that teamwork in health care is essential, it should also be self-evident that teams will function most effectively when their various members understand and respect each other's roles and perspectives ...

Having responsibility means 'to know the boundaries clearly and to be accountable, especially if any limits are overstepped' (Tschudin (2003: 99)). This makes it clear to me that I should have refused immediately to mark Mr Price's leg. By asking a nurse to do it, the doctor was also overstepping boundary limits.

Issues of generalisation

As we noted earlier, Orne and Holland (1968) argued that Milgram's experiments lack mundane realism (or *external* or *ecological validity*). But Milgram (1974) maintains that the process of complying with the demands of an authority figure is essentially the same, whether the setting is the artificial one of the psychological laboratory or a naturally occurring one in the outside world. While there are, of course, differences between laboratory studies of obedience and the obedience observed in Nazi Germany, 'differences in scale, numbers and political context may turn out to be relatively unimportant as long as certain essential features are retained'. The 'essential features' that Milgram refers to is the *agentic state* – seeing yourself as the instrument of someone else's will (see above).

What do Milgram's studies tell us about ourselves?

Perhaps one of the reasons Milgram's research has been so heavily criticised is that it paints an unacceptable picture of human beings. Thus, it's far easier for us to believe that a war criminal like Eichmann was an inhuman monster than that 'ordinary people' can be destructively obedient (what Arendt, 1965, called the *banality of evil*).

THE POWER OF SOCIAL SITUATIONS

Social roles provide models of power and powerlessness, as in parent–child, teacher–student and employer–employee relationships. Rather than asking what makes some people more obedient than others, or how we'd have reacted if we'd been one of Milgram's participants, we could instead ask how we would behave if put into a position of authority ourselves. How easily could we assume the role and use the power that goes with it?

ZIMBARDO'S RESEARCH

Almost as famous – and controversial – as Milgram's obedience studies is the *prison simulation experiment* (Zimbardo *et al.*, 1973). We mentioned earlier that this experiment illustrates the impact of uniforms and other visible symbols of authority, and for this reason it's usually discussed in relation to obedience. However, it's also relevant to certain aspects of *conformity* and, like Milgram's obedience studies, it demonstrates the *power of social situations* to make people act in uncharacteristic ways. A brutalising atmosphere (like a prison) can induce brutality in people who aren't usually brutal (see Gross, 2005).

PATIENT COMPLIANCE: DOING WHAT YOU'RE TOLD

THE CONCEPT OF COMPLIANCE

ASK YOURSELF ...
• Have you ever been non-compliant? For example, have you ever failed to complete a course of antibiotics?

• Why didn't you comply?

• Why do you think it's important to understand non-compliance?

As we noted in the 'Introduction and Overview', the term 'compliance' implies that the patient is passively obeying the requests of the more powerful health professional. Not surprisingly, the traditional concept of compliance is becoming increasingly unsuitable in modern patient-centred nursing. As Marland (1998) puts it, 'The value judgements inherent in the label of non-compliance serve only to scupper any attempts to involve patients as partners in care.'

The traditional definition implies a paternalistic view of the nurse–patient relationship, where the nurse is expert and the patient is in a dependent, childlike role. (This mirrors the view of the doctor/nurse/patient triad, as father/mother/child respectively.) If the patient is not yielding and acquiescent, the label 'non-compliant' may cause the patient to be viewed as troublesome (Holm, 1993, in Marland, 1998). The non-compliant patient may be seen as failing in a moral duty towards the nurse ('letting me down').

Are nurses to patients as doctors are to nurses? The role of both the 'passive nurse' and the role of the 'passive patient' are changing, and patient empowerment is described by the RCN (2003, in Christensen and Hewitt-Taylor, 2006) as a central function in nursing. But Hewitt (2002, in Christensen and Hewitt-Taylor, 2006) suggests that nurses' deference to medical staff leaves the patients with the perception that nurses are powerless, so they're not likely to be seen as facilitators of patients' empowerment. Staff Nurse was!

THE PROBLEM OF NON-COMPLIANCE

As more and more people are being treated with medicines to manage the effects of chronic disease, the issue of compliance is of pressing importance to nursing. It's an important area of research primarily because following health professionals' recommendations is considered essential to patient recovery.

According to Damrosch (1995), poor adherence is almost epidemic. Patients with chronic conditions (such as hypertension and diabetes) are less adherent than those with short-term problems. According to Ekerling and Kohrs (1984, in Marland, 1998), about 50 per cent of patients with enduring health problems don't comply with medical regimes, regardless of diagnosis. This suggests that their non-compliance isn't simply explained in terms of particular symptoms.

But, even with acute conditions, adherence is problematic. Patients are notorious for prematurely discontinuing antibiotics, even if prescribed for just a few days. Remarkably, patients who've undergone renal, liver and heart transplants often fail to comply, despite good adherence prior to the transplant. Despite being informed that this can result in organ rejection and death, 34 per cent of renal patients still non-adhere. About 20 per cent of rejections and deaths in heart recipients are due to non-adherence (Damrosch, 1995). However, patients tend to overestimate their degree of compliance/adherence, because they wish to convey a socially desirable impression. Practitioners also tend to overestimate their patients' compliance. More *objective* methods of assessing compliance include pill counts, records of appointment keeping, physical testing, measures of cholesterol (to check on diet), and electronically monitored bottle caps, which record the date/time of every bottle opening (Damrosch, 1995).

*The findings stated above won't tell us **why** patients aren't adhering. And doesn't wanting to present an **impression** of compliance suggest an 'obedient' attitude? That doesn't seem to fit the idea of autonomous patients.*

Box 13.2 What makes patients comply?

According to Damrosch (1995), there's theoretical agreement regarding the importance of five factors that make patients most likely to comply:

1. They perceive the high severity of the disorder (*serious consequences*). For example, Brewer *et al.* (2002, in Ogden, 2004) examined the relationship between illness cognitions (see Chapter 4) and adherence to medication and cholesterol control in patients with hypercholesterolaemia (very high cholesterol). A belief that the illness has serious consequences was related to medication adherence.

2. They believe the probability of getting the disorder is also high (*personal susceptibility*).

> 3. They have confidence in their ability to perform the behaviour prescribed to reduce the threat (*self-efficacy*).
>
> 4. They're also confident the prescribed regimen will overcome the threat (*response-efficacy*).
>
> 5. They have the intention to perform the behaviour (*behavioural intention*).
>
> Damrosch refers to these five points as the 'double high/double efficacy/behavioural intention model'.

It seems to me that these have little to do with obedience, but are more to do with patients' perception of their illness and their role in controlling it.

According to Marland (1998), chronic illness often involves a close nurse–patient relationship. The nurse may learn why the patient chooses not to follow the advice of health professionals, which may help the nurse gain a deeper understanding of the patient's decision-making processes. This may, in turn, result in interventions that ensure a match between the patient's wishes and therapeutic effectiveness. When patients fail to discuss their medication-taking behaviour openly, they may decide their own level of dose, which may be sub-therapeutic. The prescriber may then decide to increase the dose, as the patient seems not to be responding. If the patient then decides to take the prescribed dose, there may be side-effects or even toxicity (Marland, 1998). As Marland says, 'It is essential … to find ways to establish an open and honest therapeutic alliance. The traditional concept of compliance is a barrier to such a relationship.'

Cheesman (2006) says the term 'compliance' has been replaced by the term 'concordance' – where prescribing and medicine taking are based on partnership – but it hasn't been matched by a shift in ethos. However, I recall Sally (my community mentor) telling me that community matrons will do medicine reviews to ensure greater understanding and effectiveness in prescribing.

PRACTITIONER VARIABLES

Doctors' sensitivity to patients' non-verbal expression of feelings (such as tone of voice) is a good predictor of adherence. For example, Dimatteo *et al.* (1993) conducted a two-year longitudinal study of over 1800 patients with diabetes, heart disease or hypertension, and 186 doctors. The doctors' job satisfaction, willingness to answer questions and practice of scheduling follow-up appointments were all powerful predictors of adherence.

The way practitioners communicate their beliefs to patients also influences compliance. According to Ogden (2000), '… not only do health professionals hold their own subjective views, but … these views may be communicated to the patient in a way that may then influence the patient's choice of treatment.'

Arranging a follow-up appointment, which shows continuing interest, would be likely to encourage compliance.

Doctor–patient communication

According to the traditional model of doctor–patient communication (the 'education' model), the doctor is an expert who communicates his/her knowledge to a naïve

ASK YOURSELF …
- Which models of health behaviour do these five factors derive from (see Chapter 4)?

patient. The doctor is an authority figure, who instructs or directs the patient. Research has suggested that the communication process may be improved if a sharing, more interactive (two-way), patient-centred consulting style is used. This may produce greater patient commitment to any advice given, potentially higher levels of compliance and greater patient satisfaction (implied by the use of 'adherence' – see above).

However, a field experimental study by Savage and Armstrong (1990) of patients attending a group practice in an inner-city area of London found a preference for the education model. Patients (aged 16–75, without serious illnesses) seemed to prefer an authority figure, who offered a formal diagnosis, to a 'sharing' doctor who asked for their views.

People are different! Giving patients more control also means giving them more responsibility and not all of them can cope with that. While on my community placement I went with a diabetic patient to the diabetes clinic. I met one young patient who'd researched her condition on the Internet and knew all about the cause and complications. She was eager to discuss ways to prevent them, asked lots of questions and was very much in control of her diet and regime. My patient was the opposite. She just answered the doctor's questions and kept emphasising she'd stuck faithfully to her diet as if she was trying to please the doctor.

PATIENT AND REGIMEN VARIABLES

Compliance is likely to decrease over time. It's also more problematic for conditions with no obvious symptoms, especially if treatment produces unpleasant side-effects, such as reduced sex drive. Also, the more complex the regimen, the lower the adherence. For example, home monitoring of blood sugar up to ten times per day and multiple insulin injections have been shown to greatly reduce or eliminate adherence. But this is a life-long practice, which is probably daunting to many patients (Damrosch, 1995).

According to Ley's (1981, 1989) *cognitive hypothesis model*, compliance can be predicted by a combination of:
◎ satisfaction with the process of consultation (see above)
◎ understanding of the information given
◎ recall of this information.
Ley's model has been influential in promoting research into communication between health professionals and patients. But it is consistent with the education model of doctor–patient communication and so is subject to the same criticisms (see Ogden, 2004).

Preferring a more interactive approach, Ogden *et al.* (1999, in Ogden, 2000) investigated (a) the level of agreement between patient and health professional, and (b) the impact of this agreement on patient outcome. It's important to understand the extent to which the two individuals 'speak the same language', share the same beliefs, and agree about the desired content and outcome of any consultation. This is especially relevant to general practice, where patient and health professional perspectives are most likely to coincide (see Gross, 2005).

Once a treatment is prescribed, the patient is often left to his/her own devices. Adherence then depends on his/her interpretation of the illness, treatment and symptoms. Siegel *et al.* (1999) studied middle-aged and older HIV-positive people and their drug adherence. Once taking the drugs, they'd question their efficacy and safety if they noticed any unusual symptoms. If they perceived these as side-effects of the drugs, or if the drugs seemed to be having no effect, the conditions were ripe for non-adherence. But according to Forshaw (2002):

◎ because a drug *seems* to be doing nothing that doesn't mean it is, and unpleasant symptoms that appear after taking the drug aren't necessarily caused by the drug

◎ drugs can sometimes take a while to start working, but people often expect immediate results. Also, we often think that if a problem seems to have cleared up, then it has. People commonly stop taking their antibiotics when the symptoms have eased – but these often recur because they're just the final stage of unseen bodily processes. Forshaw recommends that

> Careful education of patients as to exactly what to expect from a treatment can improve adherence, especially in cases where non-adherence stems from lack of knowledge rather than rebelliousness … (Forshaw, 2002).

COMPLIANCE AND THE PLACEBO EFFECT

Evidence suggests that simply adhering to medical recommendations to take pills may benefit patients recovering from a heart attack, *regardless* of whether the pills taken are active drugs or inert placebos (see Gross, 2005). This has implications for understanding the mind–body relationship ('I believe I've taken my medication' is related to actually getting better), and the central role of beliefs and expectations in health and illness (Ogden, 2000).

Ogden cites data suggesting that the best predictor of mortality in men who'd survived a heart attack *wasn't* taking the lipid-lowering drug compared with a placebo, but adherence to taking *any drug at all* (active or placebo). Adherers had lower mortality after five years than non-adherers in both experimental and placebo groups. Ogden concludes by saying, '… "doing as the doctor suggests" appears to be beneficial to health, but not for the traditional reasons ("the drugs are good for you") but perhaps because by taking medication, the patient expects to get better …'

Reflecting on this experience has made me aware of how power affects our relationships. Being professional means being accountable (i.e. accepting responsibility for what we do). Recognising obedience as an abdication of responsibility, rather than a virtue, and seeing the 'agentic state' as the opposite of autonomy, will give me confidence in future to question instructions that worry me. Marking an operation site, knowing I shouldn't, would have been irresponsible, even as a student. I need to be aware of what students are allowed to do.

It's also made me realise that as health professionals we're equally responsible, although our roles are very different; only nurses provide care, psychological support and advocacy on a continuous basis. It's a role that should be subservient to none. Sorting out these ideas has helped me understand why 'concordance', where autonomous patients see themselves as partners in their own care, is more likely to produce adherence to therapeutic behaviour.

CHAPTER SUMMARY

◎ **Compliance** is a factor in different kinds of social influence, including conformity, obedience and our responses to other people's direct requests.

◎ While both conformity and obedience involve the **abdication of personal responsibility**, **obedience** involves orders from someone in **higher authority**, with influence being in one direction only.

◎ Milgram's series of 18 obedience experiments involves a basic procedure (**remote victim/voice feedback**) and variations on this, involving the manipulation of critical variables.

◎ Increasing the proximity to the victim, reducing the proximity of the experimenter and having the social support of 'rebel' fellow teachers all reduced obedience, while having someone else actually deliver the shock increased it.

◎ Two related variables that are crucial for understanding obedience are **acceptance/denial of responsibility** and the '**agentic state**'. The wearing of uniform and other such symbols of authority are also important.

◎ Milgram's experiments have caused great ethical controversy, but have also been criticised on scientific grounds.

◎ The **mundane realism** of the procedure is supported by Hofling *et al.*'s naturalistic experiment involving nurses, and Milgram believes that obedience is essentially the same process regardless of the particular context.

◎ Research indicates that **patient non-compliance/non-adherence** is very common, although this varies depending on the particular disorder. It applies to both chronic and acute conditions, and to organ transplant patients. The **double high/double efficacy/behavioural intention model** identifies the five factors that make compliance most likely.

◎ Compliance is affected by both **practitioner** and **patient/regimen variables**. The former include how doctors **communicate** their beliefs to patients, and the latter include patients' **satisfaction** with the consultation, and their **understanding/recall** of the information given.

EARLY EXPERIENCE AND SOCIAL DEVELOPMENT

14

INTRODUCTION AND OVERVIEW

The study of attachments and their loss or disruption represents an important way of trying to understand how early experience can affect later development. Although it was a central tenet of Freud's psychoanalytic theory that experience during the first five years of life largely determines the kind of adults we become, it's really only since the 1950s that developmental psychologists have systematically studied the nature and importance of the child's tie to its mother.

This began with the English psychiatrist John Bowlby. He was commissioned by the World Health Organization to investigate the effects on children's development of being raised in institutions (in the aftermath of the Second World War). The central concept discussed in his report (*Maternal Care and Mental Health*, 1951) was *maternal deprivation*, which has become almost synonymous with the harmful effects of not growing up within a family.

However, Bowlby has been criticised for exaggerating the importance of the mother–child relationship. There's much more to attachment than attachment to the mother. Fathers are attachment figures in their own right, as are siblings. Children's social development involves the expansion of the network of relationships to include teachers, neighbours and classmates, some of whom will become their friends.

There's now a considerable body of research into attachments beyond infancy and childhood, especially between adult sexual partners, and many psychologists have questioned the deterministic nature of the early years (see Gross, 2005).

According to Schaffer (2004), 'relationships provide the context in which all of a child's psychological functions develop ... Understanding relationship formation is thus an essential part of understanding child development.'

From my diary (3): Year 1/Community (Health Visitor)

During my Primary Care experience, I made a home visit with a Health Visitor (Chris) to a family on the Child Protection Register. Nicky is 21 and has 2 children – Ben (22 months), from a previous relationship, and Julie (10 weeks), from her present one. We heard the baby crying before Nicky answered the door, carrying Ben. When she put him down, he hid behind her and clung to her legs until she sat him in front of the TV, where, thumb in mouth, he watched Bob the Builder. The baby's nappy was soaked when we undressed her to weigh her; she also had a 'sticky eye', which Nicky hadn't noticed. Julie's weight was under the lowest percentile for her age and Nicky said she 'didn't seem to want' all her feeds. Chris suggested Nicky dress the baby while she 'had a chat' with Ben, but I saw she was also observing Nicky. The baby was smiling but Nicky hardly responded at all and didn't talk to her. Afterwards Chris checked how Nicky made up the feeds (she wasn't measuring the food properly) and showed her how to bathe the baby's eyes with cool, boiled water. She also encouraged her to talk to the baby more.

THE DEVELOPMENT AND VARIETY OF ATTACHMENTS

WHAT IS ATTACHMENT?

According to Kagan *et al.* (1978), an attachment is:

> … an intense emotional relationship that is specific to two people, that endures over time, and in which prolonged separation from the partner is accompanied by stress and sorrow.

While this definition applies to attachment formation at any point in the life cycle, our first attachment acts as a *prototype* (or model) for all later relationships. Similarly, although the definition applies to any attachment, the crucial first attachment is usually taken to be with the mother.

PHASES IN THE DEVELOPMENT OF ATTACHMENTS

The attachment process can be divided into several phases (Schaffer, 1996a), as follows:

1. The *pre-attachment phase* lasts until about three months of age. From about six weeks, babies develop an attraction to other human beings in preference to physical aspects of the environment. This is shown through behaviours such as nestling, gurgling and smiling (the *social smile*), which are directed to just about anyone.
2. At about three months, infants begin to discriminate between familiar and unfamiliar people, smiling much more at the former (the social smile has now disappeared). However, they'll allow strangers to handle and look after them without becoming noticeably distressed, provided they're cared for adequately. This *indiscriminate attachment phase* lasts until around seven months.
3. From about seven or eight months, infants begin to develop specific attachments. This is demonstrated through actively trying to stay close to certain people (particularly the mother) and becoming distressed when separated from them (*separation anxiety*). This *discriminate attachment phase* occurs when an infant can consistently tell the difference between its mother and other people, and has developed *object permanence* (the awareness that things – in this case, the mother – continue to exist even when they cannot be seen; see Chapter 15).

   Also at this time, infants avoid closeness with unfamiliar people and some display the *fear-of-strangers response*. This includes crying and/or trying to move away, which are usually triggered only when a stranger tries to make direct contact with the baby (rather than when the stranger is just 'there').
4. In the *multiple attachment phase* (from about nine months onwards), strong additional ties are formed with other major caregivers (such as the father, grandparents and siblings) and with non-caregivers (such as other children). Although the fear-of-strangers response typically weakens, the strongest attachment continues to be with the mother.

Baby Julie is in the pre-attachment phase; when I took her from Nicky and began to talk to her, she responded with smiles and little excited movements. By hiding from us, Ben showed he didn't trust strangers.

THEORIES OF THE ATTACHMENT PROCESS

'CUPBOARD LOVE' THEORIES

According to *psychoanalytic* accounts, the infant becomes attached to its caregiver (usually the mother) because of his/her ability to satisfy its instinctual needs. For Freud (1926):

> The reason why the infant in arms wants to perceive the presence of its mother is only because it already knows that she satisfies all its needs without delay.

Freud believed that healthy attachments are formed when feeding practices satisfy the infant's needs for food, security and oral sexual gratification (see Chapters 2 and 6). Unhealthy attachments occur when infants are *deprived* of food and oral pleasure, or are *overindulged*. Thus, psychoanalytic accounts stress the importance of feeding, especially breastfeeding, and of the maternal figure.

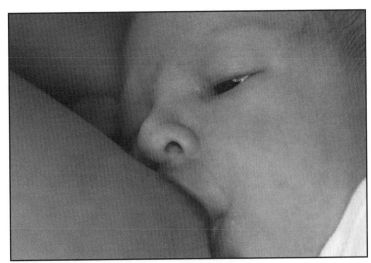

Is this really all there is to attachment formation?

ASK YOURSELF ...
• What do you think the *behaviourist* account of attachment might be (see Chapter 2)?

Chris said Nicky had breastfed Ben for a few weeks, but didn't succeed with Julie and wasn't responding well to the baby's physical or psychological needs.

The *behaviourist* view of attachment also sees infants as becoming attached to those who satisfy their physiological needs. Infants associate their caregivers (who act as *conditioned* or *secondary reinforcers*) with gratification/satisfaction (food being an *unconditioned* or *primary reinforcer*), and they learn to approach them to have their needs met. This eventually generalises into a feeling of security whenever the caregiver is present.

In that case, the baby should attach to Nicky as she is the only one feeding her. The father appears periodically but doesn't stay for more than a day or two at a time.

An evaluation of 'cupboard love' theories

◎ Both behaviourist and psychoanalytic accounts of attachment as 'cupboard love' were challenged by Harlow's studies involving rhesus monkeys (e.g. Harlow, 1959; Harlow and Zimmerman, 1959; see Gross, 2005). In the course of studying learning, Harlow separated new-born monkeys from their mothers and raised them in individual cages. Each cage contained a 'baby blanket', to which the monkey became intensely attached, showing great distress when it was removed for any reason. This apparent attachment to its blanket, and the display of behaviour comparable to that of an infant monkey actually separated from its mother, seemed to contradict the view that attachment comes from an association with nourishment. (For an account of Harlow's research using wire and cloth (terry-towelling) surrogate monkey mothers see Gross, 2005.)

◎ Although attachment clearly doesn't depend on feeding alone, the rhesus monkeys reared exclusively with their cloth 'mothers' failed to develop normally. They became extremely aggressive adults, rarely interacted with other monkeys, made inappropriate sexual responses and were difficult (if not impossible) to breed. So, in monkeys at least, normal development seems to depend on factors other than having something soft and cuddly to provide comfort. Harlow's research indicates that one of these is *interaction with other members of the species* during the first six months of life.

Many young children have an 'attachment' article – a soft blanket or cuddly toy that presumably provides a feeling of warmth and security. As well as food, breastfeeding provides warmth and softness naturally for the baby; bottle feeding can be less intimate. During our visit I saw little interaction between Nicky and the baby – or with Ben.

◎ Research on attachment in humans also casts doubt on 'cupboard love' theories.

KEY STUDY 14.1 Feeding isn't everything for Scottish infants (Schaffer and Emerson, 1964)

- Sixty infants were followed up at four-weekly intervals throughout their first year, and then again at eighteen months.

- Mothers reported on their infants' behaviour in seven everyday situations involving separations, such as being left alone in a room, with a babysitter, and put to bed at night. For each situation, information was obtained regarding whether the infant protested or not, how much and how regularly it protested, and whose departure elicited this reaction.

- Infants were clearly attached to people who didn't perform caretaking activities (notably the father). Also, in 39 per cent of cases, the person who usually fed, bathed and changed the infant (typically the mother) wasn't the infant's primary attachment figure.

Schaffer and Emerson (1964) concluded that the two features of a person's behaviour that best predicted whether s/he would become an attachment figure for the infant are:

1. *responsiveness* to the infant's behaviour
2. the *total amount of stimulation* s/he provided (such as talking, touching and playing).

For Schaffer (1971), 'cupboard love' theories of attachment put things the wrong way round. Instead of infants being passive recipients of nutrition (they 'live to eat'), he prefers to see them as *active seekers of stimulation* (they 'eat to live').

Schaffer and Emerson's (1964) research indicates the reason Chris intends to bring a video on massage to encourage Nicky to have more tactile contact with the baby. The baby needs to be talked to and cuddled as well as fed.

ETHOLOGICAL THEORIES

The term 'attachment' was actually introduced to psychology by *ethologists* (zoologists who study the evolutionary functions of the 'natural' behaviour of non-human animals). Lorenz (1935) showed that some non-humans (including geese) form strong bonds with the first moving objects they encounter (usually, but not always, the mother). Since this *imprinting* occurs simply through perceiving the caregiver without any feeding taking place, it too makes a 'cupboard love' account of attachment seem less valid, at least in goslings (see Gross, 2005).

Most psychologists would agree that the only way to be sure about a particular species is to study that species. To generalise the findings from rhesus monkeys and goslings to human infants is dangerous (although less so in the case of rhesus monkeys). However, Harlow's and Lorenz's findings can suggest how attachments might be formed in humans. Indeed, Bowlby was greatly influenced by ethological theory, especially by Lorenz's concept of imprinting.

Normally, the baby is given to the mother immediately after birth for skin-to-skin contact to encourage attachment. I discovered Julie went to intensive care for 24 hours on delivery; Nicky didn't see her baby until the next day, which might be significant.

BOWLBY'S THEORY

This represents the most comprehensive theory of human attachment formation. Bowlby (1969, 1973) argued that because new-born human infants are entirely helpless, they're *genetically programmed* to behave towards their mothers in ways that ensure their survival.

> ### Box 14.1 Species-specific behaviours used by infants to shape and control their caregivers' behaviour
>
> **Sucking:** While sucking is important for nourishment, not all sucking is nutritive. *Non-nutritive sucking*, also seen in non-humans, seems to be an innate tendency which inhibits a new-born's distress. In western societies, babies are often given 'dummies' (or 'pacifiers') to calm them when they're upset.

> **Cuddling:** Human infants adjust their postures to mould themselves to the contours of the parent's body. The reflexive response that encourages front-to-front contact with the mother plays an important part in reinforcing the caregiver's behaviour.
>
> **Looking:** When parents don't respond to an infant's eye contact, the infant usually shows signs of distress. An infant's looking behaviour, therefore, acts as an invitation to its mother to respond. If she fails to do so, the infant becomes upset and avoids further visual contact. By contrast, mutual gazing is rewarding for an infant.
>
> **Smiling:** This seems to be an innate behaviour, since babies can produce smiles shortly after birth. Although the first 'social smile' doesn't usually occur before six weeks (see page 256), adults view the smiling infant as a 'real person', which they find very rewarding.
>
> **Crying:** Young infants usually cry only when hungry, cold or in pain, and crying is most effectively ended by picking up and cuddling them. Caregivers who respond quickly during the first three months tend to have babies that cry *less* during the last four months of their first year than infants with unresponsive caregivers (Bell and Ainsworth, 1972).

Baby Julie demonstrated all these behaviours. Ben wrapped himself around Nicky's legs so his whole body was in contact with her and, when he was removed, comforted himself by non-nutritive sucking. Freud would say it was satisfying an oral sexual need; a behaviourist would say it was a conditioned response eliciting the security experienced during feeding.

The mother also inherits a genetic blueprint which programmes her to respond to the baby. There's a critical period during which the *synchrony of action* between mother and infant produces an attachment. In Bowlby's (1951) view, mothering is useless for all children if delayed until after two-and-a-half to three years, and for most children if delayed until after twelve months.

Bowlby believed that infants display a strong innate tendency to become attached to one particular adult female (not necessarily the natural mother), a tendency he called *monotropy*. This attachment to the mother figure is *qualitatively* different (different in kind) from any later attachments. For Bowlby (1951), 'Mother love in infancy is as important for mental health as are vitamins and proteins for physical health.'

Chris is worried as this doesn't seem to be happening with Julie, who for some reason isn't a 'thriving' baby. Also, Ben isn't getting enough stimulation.

ASK YOURSELF ...

• Do you agree with Bowlby that the infant's relationship with its mother is unique, or are men just as capable as women of providing adequate parenting and becoming attachment figures for their young children?

An evaluation of Bowlby's theory

◎ Bowlby's views on monotropy have been criticised. For example, infants and young children display a whole range of attachment behaviours towards a variety of attachment figures other than their mothers. In other words, the mother isn't special in the way the infant shows its attachment to her (Rutter, 1981).

◎ Although Bowlby didn't deny that children form multiple attachments, he saw attachment to the mother as being unique: it's the first to develop and is the strongest of all. However, Schaffer and Emerson's (1964) study (see Key Study 14.1) showed that multiple attachments seem to be the rule rather than the exception. For example: at about seven months, 29 per cent of infants had already formed several attachments simultaneously (10 per cent had formed five or more), and by 10 months, 59 per cent had developed more than one attachment.

Although there was usually one particularly strong attachment, most infants showed multiple attachments of varying intensity:

(a) only half of the 18 month olds were most strongly attached to their mothers
(b) almost one-third were most strongly attached to their fathers
(c) about 17 per cent were equally attached to both parents.

Ben seems to be lacking attachment figures; his father left when Ben was six months old, there are no grandparents locally, and he doesn't go to a playgroup. Nicky said when her new partner is around he's 'good with Ben'.

What about fathers?

For Bowlby, the father is of no direct emotional significance to the young infant, but only of indirect value as an emotional and economic support for the mother. *Evolutionary psychologists* (see Gross, 2005) see mothers as having a greater *parental investment* in their offspring and hence are better prepared for child-rearing and attachment (Kenrick, 1994). However, Bowlby's views on fathers as attachment figures are disputed by findings such as those of Schaffer and Emerson (1964).

CRITICAL DISCUSSION 14.1 How good are fathers at being mothers?

- Framing the question this way, of course, rests on the implicit assumption that women are 'natural' parents. This view of women is reflected in Bowlby's theory of monotropy and the complementary responsiveness of mothers to their babies (the 'maternal instinct').

- Based on this view of women-as-mothers, any departure from the traditional division of labour in child care has been greeted with suspicion: men inevitably will provide inferior parenting (Schaffer, 2004).

- Although *men as principal parents* is still a minority phenomenon, it's by no means as unusual as it used to be. Fathers' participation in child-rearing has certainly become much more common and an increasing number of children now live in father-headed families.

- There's considerable cultural variation in the extent of fathers' involvement in child care. This suggests that whatever sex differences exist in this respect are a matter of *social convention* and not an 'immutably fixed part of being male or female' (Schaffer, 2004) or *biology*.

- Although the evidence is sparse, there's no indication that the development of children brought up by a man differs in any way from others. Direct observation of men in their fathering role has shown them to be as capable of as much warmth and sensitivity as women (Schaffer, 2004).

- Rather than being poor substitutes for mothers, fathers make their own unique contribution to the care and development of infants and young children (at least in two-parent families). Children's developmental outcome is affected not by the parents' gender but by the kind of relationship that exists within each individual parent–child couple (Parke, 2002).

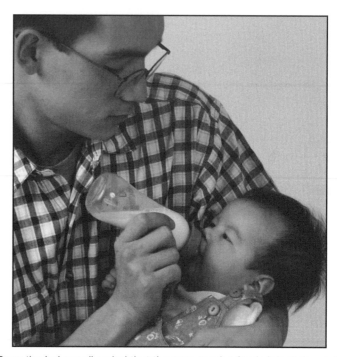

Does the baby really mind that the person who feeds it isn't female?

This is an example of the need to evaluate research findings in historical context; Bowlby was writing when mothers were considered the natural carers – whatever their inclination. Nicky said her partner was 'good with Ben'; did she mean he just plays with him, or assumes a 'mothering' role? In this situation, shouldn't we assess Julie's father's relationship with both children?

INDIVIDUAL VARIATIONS IN ATTACHMENT

Ainsworth *et al.*'s (1971, 1978) famous Baltimore, USA, study involved both interviews and naturalistic observation and was also *longitudinal*: 26 mother–infant pairs were visited at home every 3–4 weeks, each visit lasting 3–4 hours, for the first year of the baby's life. In order to make sense of the enormous amount of data collected for each pair (72 hours' worth), there needed to be an *external criterion measure* (some standard against which to compare the observations). The criterion chosen was the *Strange Situation* (SS) (see Figure 14.1 and Table 14.1).

Group data confirmed that babies explored the playroom and toys more vigorously in the mothers' presence than after the stranger entered or while the mother was absent. However, Ainsworth was particularly fascinated by the unexpected variety of infants' reactions to the mothers' return (*reunion behaviours* – see Table 14.2).

In the strange situation technique, although every aspect of the participants' reactions is observed and videotaped, it's the child's response to the mother's return that's given the most attention. This provides a clearer picture of the state of attachment than even the response to separation itself (Marrone, 1998).

Table 14.1 The eight episodes of the 'Strange Situation'

Episode	Persons present	Duration	Brief description
1	Mother, baby, observer	30 seconds	Observer introduces mother and baby to experimental room, then leaves
2	Mother, baby	3 minutes	Mother is non-participant while baby explores; if necessary, play is stimulated after two minutes
3	Stranger, mother, baby	3 minutes	Stranger enters. First minute: stranger silent. Second minute: stranger converses with mother. Third minute: stranger approaches baby. After three minutes, mother leaves unobtrusively
4	Stranger, baby	3 minutes or less★	First separation episode. Stranger's behaviour is geared to the baby's
5	Mother, baby	3 minutes or more★★	First reunion episode. Stranger leaves. Mother greets and/or comforts baby, then tries to settle baby again in play. Mother then leaves, saying 'bye-bye'
6	Baby	3 minutes or less★	Second separation episode
7	Stranger, baby	3 minutes or less★	Continuation of second separation. Stranger enters and gears her behaviour to baby's
8	Mother, baby	3 minutes	Second reunion episode. Mother enters, greets baby, then picks up baby. Meanwhile, stranger leaves unobtrusively

★ Episode is ended early if baby is unduly distressed.
★★ Episode is prolonged if more time is required for baby to become reinvolved in play.
(Based on Ainsworth *et al.*, 1978; Krebs and Blackman, 1988)

The dynamics of the attachment relationship can be seen in terms of a balance between (a) exploratory behaviour directed towards the environment, and (b) attachment behaviour directed towards the caregiver. Looked at in this light, securely attached babies have got the balance right (Meins, 2003). But in both patterns of insecure attachment, the balance is tipped to one or other extreme: the anxious-avoidant baby shows high levels of environment-directed behaviour to the detriment of

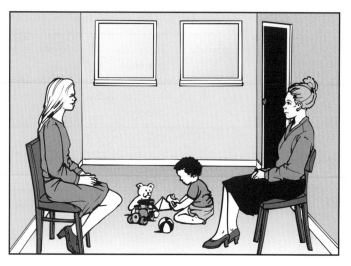

Figure 14.1 One of the eight episodes in the 'Strange Situation'

Table 14.2 Behaviour associated with three types of attachment in one year olds using the 'Strange Situation'

Category	Name	Sample (%)
Type A	**Anxious–avoidant**	**15**

Typical behaviour: Baby largely ignores mother, because of *indifference* towards her. Play is little affected by whether she's present or absent. No or few signs of distress when mother leaves, and actively ignores or avoids her on her return. *Distress is caused by being alone*, rather than being left by the mother. Can be comforted as easily by the stranger as by the mother. In fact, *both adults are treated in a very similar way.*

Category	Name	Sample (%)
Type B	**Securely attached**	**70**

Typical behaviour: Baby plays happily while the mother is present, whether the stranger is present or not. Mother is largely 'ignored', because she can be trusted to be there if needed. Clearly distressed when the mother leaves, and play is considerably reduced. Seeks immediate contact with mother on her return, quickly calms down in her arms and resumes play. The *distress is caused by the mother's absence*, not by being alone. Although the stranger can provide some comfort, *she and the mother are treated very differently.*

Category	Name	Sample (%)
Type C	**Anxious–resistant**	**15**

Typical behaviour: Baby is fussy and wary while the mother is present. Cries a lot more than types A and B, and *has difficulty using mother as a safe base*. Very distressed when she leaves, seeks contact with her on her return, but simultaneously shows anger and resists contact (may approach her and reach out to be picked up, then struggles to get down again). This demonstrates the baby's *ambivalence* towards her. Doesn't return to play readily. *Actively resists stranger's efforts to make contact.*

attachment behaviour, while the anxious–resistant baby is preoccupied with the caregiver to the detriment of exploration and play.

Although not in a 'strange situation', Ben's behaviour was more like the anxious-resistant group; he kept checking his mother was in sight.

THE ROLE OF MATERNAL SENSITIVITY

The crucial feature determining the quality of attachment is the mother's *sensitivity*. The sensitive mother sees things from her baby's perspective, correctly interprets its signals, responds to its needs, and is accepting, cooperative and accessible. By contrast, the insensitive mother interacts almost exclusively in terms of her own wishes, moods and activities. According to Ainsworth *et al.*, sensitive mothers tend to have babies who are *securely attached*, whereas insensitive mothers have *insecurely attached* babies (either *anxious–avoidant/detached* or *anxious–resistant/ambivalent*).

During the past 20 years or so, several studies with larger samples have tested, and supported, the original claim that parental sensitivity actually *causes* attachment security (van Ijzendoorn and Schuengel, 1999). However, sensitivity isn't an *exclusive* condition for attachment security – other parenting qualities play a part (e.g. DeWolff and van Ijzendoorn, 1997). Conversely, even abusive parents don't necessarily produce deviant forms of attachment. According to Schaffer (2004), although maltreated children are clearly at risk:

◎ they usually show some signs of attachment to their abusing parents, although this may be confused and disorganised (see below); the attachment system seems to be so powerful that even in the absence of consistent love and emotional warmth, children persist in trying to form attachments
◎ there are always some children (although a small minority – about 15 per cent) who form secure attachments; they enjoy good relationships with peers and others, and by no means all abused children become abusing adults.

(For an evaluation of the SS and a discussion of cultural differences in attachment, see Gross, 2005.)

*Schaffer's (2004) conclusions and reference to the attachment system as 'powerful' suggest an infant's instinctive need to attach. But the **development** of attachment seems to depend on the sensitivity and responsiveness of the carer, whoever it is.*

DEPRIVATION AND PRIVATION

BOWLBY'S MATERNAL-DEPRIVATION HYPOTHESIS (MDH)

As noted earlier, Bowlby argued for the existence of a critical period in attachment formation. This, along with his theory of monotropy (see page 260), led him to claim that the mother–infant attachment couldn't be broken in the first few years of life without serious and permanent damage to social, emotional and intellectual development. For Bowlby (1951), 'An infant and young child should experience a warm, intimate and continuous relationship with his mother (or permanent mother figure) in which both find satisfaction and enjoyment.'

Bowlby's *maternal-deprivation hypothesis* (MDH) was based largely on studies conducted in the 1930s and 1940s of children brought up in residential nurseries and other large institutions (such as orphanages).

KEY STUDY 14.2 Some early research findings on the effects of institutionalisation

Goldfarb (1943): 15 children raised in institutions from about six months until three and a half years of age were matched with 15 children who'd gone straight from their mothers to foster homes. The institutionalised children lived in almost complete social isolation during their first year. The matching was based on genetic factors and natural mothers' education and occupational status.

At age three, the institutionalised group was behind the fostered group on measures of abstract thinking, social maturity, rule-following and sociability. Between 10 and 14, the institutionalised group continued to perform more poorly on the various tests, and their average IQs (intelligence quotients) were 72 and 95 respectively.

This is similar to what Chris described as a 'failure to thrive' baby. I can see why Chris is worried Nicky isn't responding adequately to her children.

Those who appeared to be brighter or more easy-going, more sociable and healthy were more likely to have been fostered. In this case, the differences in development of the two groups might have been due to these initial characteristics. However, Goldfarb concluded that all the institutionalised children's poorer abilities were due to the time spent in the institutions.

Spitz (1945, 1946); Spitz and Wolf (1946): Spitz found that in some very poor South American orphanages, overworked and untrained staff rarely talked to the infants, hardly ever picked them up even for feeding, gave them no affection and provided no toys. The orphans displayed *anaclitic depression* (a reaction to the loss of a love object). This involves symptoms such as apprehension, sadness, weepiness, withdrawal, loss of appetite, refusal to eat, loss of weight, inability to sleep, and developmental retardation. It's similar to *hospitalism*.

After three months of unbroken deprivation, recovery was rarely, if ever, complete. In their study of 91 orphanage infants in the USA and Canada, Spitz and Wolf found that over one-third died before their first birthdays, despite good nutrition and medical care.

Interpreting the findings from studies of institutions

Bowlby, Goldfarb, Spitz and Wolf explained the harmful effects of growing up in an institution in terms of what Bowlby called maternal deprivation. In doing so, they failed:

◎ to recognise that poor, unstimulating environments are generally associated with learning difficulties and retarded language development (vital for overall intellectual development); hence, a crucial variable in intellectual development is the amount of *intellectual stimulation* a child receives, *not* the amount of mothering (Rutter, 1981)

◎ to distinguish between the effects of deprivation and privation. Strictly, *deprivation* ('de-privation') refers to the loss, through separation, of the maternal attachment figure (which assumes that an attachment has already developed); *privation* refers to

---

ASK YOURSELF ...

• What characteristics of the children might have determined whether they were fostered or kept in the institution?

• How might this have accounted for the results?

---

the absence of an attachment figure – there's been no opportunity to form an attachment in the first place (Rutter, 1981).

The studies described in Key Study 14.2 (on which Bowlby originally based his MDH) are most accurately thought of as demonstrating the effects of *privation*. However, Bowlby's own theory and research were mainly concerned with *deprivation*. By using only the one term (deprivation), he confused two very different types of early experience, which have very different types of effect (both short- and long-term).

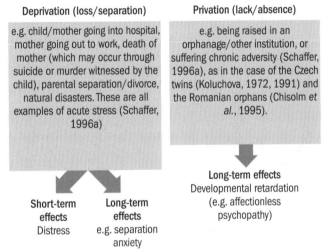

Figure 14.2 Examples of the difference between deprivation and privation, including their effects

I can see there is a distinct difference between maternal deprivation and privation. Nicky's children are not suffering from either, but from poor quality of care.

DEPRIVATION (SEPARATION OR LOSS)

Short-term deprivation and its effects

One example of short-term deprivation (days or weeks, rather than months or years) is that of a child going into a nursery while its mother goes into hospital. Another is that of the child itself going into hospital (see Critical Discussion 14.2). Bowlby and Robertson showed that when young children go into hospital, they display *distress*, which typically involves three components or stages.

Box 14.2 The components or stages of distress

- **Protest:** The initial, immediate reaction takes the form of crying, screaming, kicking and generally struggling to escape, or clinging to the mother to prevent her from leaving. This is an outward and direct expression of the child's anger, fear, bitterness and bewilderment.

- **Despair:** The struggling and protest eventually give way to calmer behaviour. The child may appear apathetic, but internally still feels all the anger and fear previously displayed. It keeps such feelings 'locked up' and wants nothing to do with other people. The child may no longer anticipate the mother's return, and barely reacts to others' offers of comfort, preferring to comfort itself by rocking, thumb-sucking, and so on.

- **Detachment:** If the separation continues, the child begins to respond to people again, but tends to treat everyone alike and rather superficially. However, if reunited with the mother at this stage, the child may well have to 'relearn' its relationship with her and may even 'reject' her (as she 'rejected' her child).

ASK YOURSELF ...

- Distress (especially protest and despair) can be thought of as an extreme display of attachment behaviours. Looked at this way, what factors do you think are likely to make separation most distressing for the child?

Factors influencing distress

Evidence suggests that not all children go through the stages of distress, and that they differ in how much distress they experience. Separation is likely to be most distressing:

◎ when there is no mother substitute to take the mother's place
◎ between the ages of 7 and 8 months (when attachments are just beginning to develop – see above) and 3 years, with a peak at 12–18 months (Maccoby, 1980). This is related to the child's inability to retain a mental image of the absent mother, and its limited understanding of language
◎ for boys (although there are also wide differences within each gender)
◎ if there have been any behaviour problems, such as aggression, that existed before the separation; such problems are likely to be accentuated if separation occurs
◎ if the mother and child have an extremely close and protective relationship, in which they're rarely apart, and the child is unused to meeting new people; children appear to cope best if their relationship with their mother is stable and relaxed, but not too close, and if they have other attachment figures (such as their fathers) who can provide love and care.

Many institutions used to be run in a way that made the development of substitute attachments very difficult (see page 271). One *long-term* effect of short-term separation is *separation anxiety*. This is also associated with long-term deprivation and is discussed below.

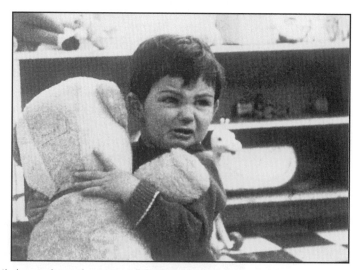

John (17 months) experienced extreme distress while spending 9 days in a residential nursery when his mother was in hospital having a second baby. According to Bowlby, he was grieving for the absent mother. Robertson and Robertson (1969) (who made a series of films called *Young Children in Brief Separation*) found that the extreme distress was caused by a combination of factors: multiple caretakers, lack of a mother substitute, loss of the mother and strange environment and routines

CRITICAL DISCUSSION 14.2 Children in hospital (Devlin, 1989)

- In many children's wards in the mid-1950s, visiting was restricted to a couple of hours at the weekend.

- James Robertson, a psychoanalyst who worked with Anna Freud and Dorothy Burlingham in the 1940s, made films of children before, during and after hospital admission – including *A Two-year-old Goes to Hospital* (1952) and *Going to Hospital with Mother* (1958). These are still used to train paediatric staff.

- The films captured the stages of distress and helped sow the seeds of a revolution which ensured that children have a better experience of hospital. Robertson argued that parents should be allowed to be with their children throughout their stay.

- However, the struggle even to begin to change attitudes wasn't an easy one. The two films were used in evidence to the committee that produced the Platt Report (1959). This was the first of several government circulars and reports during the 1960s and 1970s, all recommending that:

  (a) there should be unrestricted visiting

  (b) there should be overnight accommodation for parents

  (c) children shouldn't be nursed on adult wards.

- Robertson encouraged parents to form pressure groups. The National Association for the Welfare of Children in Hospital (NAWCH) first reported (in 1962) that most hospitals still allowed afternoon visiting only. Even by 1982, parents were still regarded as visitors in half of all acute children's wards in England, overnight accommodation for parents was far from satisfactory, and at least half the wards nursing children weren't part of comprehensive paediatric units.

- In 1986, NAWCH reported a huge improvement in the proportion of wards with entirely unrestricted access for parents. But conditions are still far from ideal.

Why, in spite of such compelling evidence and recommendations, did it take such a long time (30 years!)? Was this an example of entrenched attitudes preventing change, or was it about money? Thankfully, it's no longer the case. When my own daughter was in hospital, I stayed with her, including overnight.

Long-term deprivation and its effects

Long-term deprivation includes the permanent separation resulting from *parental death* and the increasingly common separation caused by *divorce*. Perhaps the most common effect of long-term deprivation is what Bowlby called *separation anxiety* – the fear that separation will occur again in the future (see Gross, 2005).

Day care is also regarded by some as another form of long-term deprivation (again, see Gross, 2005).

As so many nurses (including me) are now working parents, I found this worrying. So it was a relief to find that Schaffer (2004, in Gross, 2005) concludes, 'where conditions are optimal, children of employed mothers may actually benefit compared to those of unemployed mothers ...' Clarke Stewart (1989, in Gross, 2005) argues, 'The issue today is not whether infants should be in day care but how to make their experiences there and at home supportive of their development and of their parents' peace of mind.'

Being divorced, I find it reassuring to know Schaffer (2004) also finds the generalisation that children are damaged for life by divorce unjustified.

Privation

As we noted earlier, privation is the failure to develop an attachment to any individual. Given the importance of the child's first relationship as a model or prototype of relationships in general, failure to develop an attachment of any kind is likely to adversely affect all subsequent relationships.

Affectionless psychopathy

According to Bowlby, maternal deprivation in early childhood causes *affectionless psychopathy*. This is the inability to care and have deep feelings for other people and the consequent lack of meaningful interpersonal relationships, together with the inability to experience guilt.

KEY STUDY 14.3 Growing up with TB (Bowlby *et al.*, 1956)

- Bowlby *et al.* studied 60 children aged 7–13, who'd spent between 5 months and 2 years in a tuberculosis (TB) sanatorium (which provided no substitute mothering) at various ages up to 4.
- About half had been separated from their parents before they were two years old.
- When compared with a group of non-separated 'control' children from the same school classes, the overall picture was that the two groups were more similar than different.
- The separated children were more prone to 'daydreaming', showed less initiative, were more overexcited, rougher in play, concentrated less well and were less competitive. But they weren't more likely to show affectionless psychopathy, regardless of when their separation had occurred (before or after the age of two).

Bowlby *et al.* admitted that 'part of the emotional disturbance can be attributed to factors other than separation', such as the common occurrence of illness and death in the sanatorium children's families. So, there was very little evidence for the link between affectionless psychopathy and *separation* (or *bond disruption*). However, Bowlby may have provided evidence for an association with privation instead (a failure to form bonds in early life). According to Rutter (1981), privation is likely to lead to:
- an initial phase of clinging, dependent behaviour
- attention-seeking, and uninhibited, indiscriminate friendliness
- a personality characterised by lack of guilt, an inability to keep rules, and an inability to form lasting relationships.

Julie is obviously not suffering maternal deprivation but unless Nicky responds more to her, they may not bond satisfactorily.

Are the effects of privation reversible?

There are (at least) three kinds of study which demonstrate that it's possible to undo the effects of early privation.

1. *Case studies* of children who've endured extreme early privation, often in near complete isolation. Examples include the Czech twins studied by Koluchova (1972, 1991) and concentration camp survivors (Freud and Dann, 1951; see Gross, 2005).

2. Studies of *late adoption*: children raised in institutions are adopted after Bowlby's critical period for attachment development (twelve months for most children, up to two and a half/three years for the rest). Studies include those of Tizard and her colleagues (e.g. Hodges and Tizard, 1989; see Key Study 14.4) and Chisolm *et al.* (1995; see Gross, 2005).

3. Studies of *developmental pathways* (see page 272).

Studies of late adoption

Tizard (1977) and Hodges and Tizard (1989) studied children who, on leaving care between the ages of two and seven, were either adopted or returned to their own families. The institutions they grew up in provided good physical care and appeared to provide adequate intellectual stimulation, but the children had little opportunity to form close, continuous relationships with adults. For example, by age two, they'd been looked after for at least a week by an average of 24 different caregivers. The children's attachment behaviour was very unusual and, in general, the first opportunity to form long-term attachments came when they left the institutions and were placed in families.

By age eight, most of the adopted children had formed close attachments to their adoptive parents (who very much wanted a child), despite the lack of early attachments in the institutions (Tizard and Hodges, 1978). But only some of those children returned to their own families had formed close attachments. As reported by their teachers, the ex-institutional children as a whole displayed attention-seeking behaviour, restlessness, disobedience and poor peer relationships.

> ### KEY STUDY 14.4 Ex-institution children at age 16 (Hodges and Tizard, 1989)
>
> - At age 16, the family relationships of most of the adopted children seemed satisfactory, for both them and their parents. They differed little from a non-adopted comparison group who'd never been in care. Hence, early institutional care hadn't necessarily led to a later inability to form a close attachment to parents (contrary to Bowlby's predictions).
>
> - By contrast, those children returned to their families still suffered difficulties and poor family relationships. These included mutual difficulty in showing affection, and the parents reported feeling closer to the children's siblings than to the returned children.
>
> - *Outside* the family, however, *both* the adopted and returned children showed similar relationships with peers and adults. Compared with a control group, they were:
>
>   (a) still more likely to seek adult affection and approval
>
>   (b) still more likely to have difficulties in their relationships with peers

(c) less likely to have a special friend or to see peers as sources of emotional support

(d) more likely to be friendly to any peer rather than choosing their friends.

These findings *are* consistent with Bowlby's MDH.

Hodges and Tizard's research indicates that children who fail to enjoy close and lasting relationships with adults in the first years of life can make such attachments later on. But these depend on the adults concerned and how they nurture such attachments.

These ex-institution children have now been followed up into adulthood (average age 31 years). There were very few significant differences between the ex-institution group and the comparison group. While acknowledging the small sample size (22 ex-institution, 23 comparisons), Hodges (personal communication, 2000) states that, 'the evidence seems to support both the view that the effects of earlier adversity fade given the right later circumstances, and the view that there are some enduring effects producing continuities in personal characteristics.'

Developmental pathways

Quinton and Rutter (1988) wanted to find out whether children deprived of parental care become depriving parents themselves. They observed one group of women, brought up in care, interacting with their own children, and compared them with a second group of non-institutionalised mothers. The women brought up in care were, as a whole, less sensitive, supportive and warm towards their children.

However, there was also considerable variability *within* the group brought up in care, with some women displaying good parenting skills. This could be explained in terms of *developmental pathways* (what Schaffer, 2004, calls *developmental trajectories*). For example, some of the women had more positive school experiences than others. This made them three times more likely as adolescents or young adults to make proper career and marriage partner choices (Rutter, 1989). Such positive experience represents an escape route from the early hardships associated with being brought up in care.

Similar adverse childhood experiences can have multiple outcomes (Schaffer, 1996b, 2004). *Starting off* at a disadvantage doesn't necessarily mean having to *finish up* at a disadvantage. In other words, early disadvantage doesn't inevitably set off a chain reaction of more and more disadvantage. Periodically, individuals reach *turning points* where choices must be made, and the path that's taken can either reinforce or help to minimise the consequences of previous experience (Schaffer, 2004).

The developmental pathways concept makes me feel more optimistic about Nicky. I discovered that, after being in three different foster homes, at 13 she ended up in a care home. Chris emphasised Nicky's need for careful monitoring and proper support; if she responds well it could be a turning point for her.

CRITICAL DISCUSSION 14.3: The effects of 'reduced' or 'minimal parenting'

- Due to advances in reproductive technologies, it's become possible for children to be conceived and born 'artificially' to parents who'd otherwise remain childless.

  (a) *In vitro fertilisation* (IVF): sperm and egg are provided by the father and mother, but they're combined in the laboratory.

(b) *Egg donation:* the father's sperm fertilises another woman's egg – so the child will be genetically related only to him.

(c) *Donor insemination* (DI)/*artificial insemination by donor* (AID): the mother is impregnated by the sperm of a male other than the husband – so the child will be genetically related only to her.

- Almost 18,000 babies have been born in the UK through donated gametes (sperm and eggs) and embryos since the Human Fertilisation and Embryology Authority (HFEA) was created in 1991. Currently, birth certificates reveal nothing about the genetic father, and the law, as it stands, prevents revelation of the donor's identity. However, that's set to change.

- There are various potential problems that may arise: the often stressful nature of prolonged fertility treatment; the secrecy surrounding the act of conception; the possibility of tension between the parents because one of them is infertile, as well as that parent's feelings of inadequacy or guilt; children's realisation that they're somehow different; and the absence of a genetic link with one or both parents involved in some of the techniques used (Schaffer, 2004).

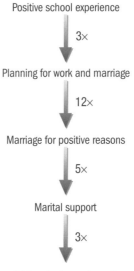

Figure 14.3 A simplified adaptive chain of circumstances in institution-raised women (based on Quinton & Rutter, 1988; Rutter, 1989)

ASK YOURSELF ...
- What do you think the effects on children brought into the world by such 'unnatural' means might be?

◎ Golombok and her colleagues (Golombok *et al.*, 1995, 1999, 2001) have conducted some of the few follow-up studies of children conceived in these various ways. They compared families with a child (aged between 4 and 12) conceived by each of the three methods described above with two control groups: (i) naturally conceived children, and (ii) children adopted at birth.

◎ There was no evidence that these new reproductive technologies have negative consequences – for either child or parent. Neither lack of genetic relationship nor manner of conception had any implications for their well-being.

◎ Together with studies of adopted children (see above), Golombok's research shows that 'a "blood-bond" is not necessary for the development of sound parent–child relationships: this can be found even when the role of parenthood is fragmented between a biological and psychological parent …' (in Schaffer, 2004).

But all these relationships exist from the baby's birth. It may be different for later-adopted babies. Hodges and Tizard's research seems to indicate that children who suffered from early adversity did have relationship difficulties but, optimistically, **can** recover if their later attachments are carefully nurtured. I hope this applies to Nicky.

Discussing the visit afterwards, Chris was pleased I already knew about the local 'Sure Start' group; this will help Nicky develop her parenting skills. It would also provide social interaction for her and play opportunities for Ben.

This experience has shown me that much health care is about problem solving! It reinforced the idea that in some cases it is psychological and social factors that lead to health problems and therefore psychological and social care that will prevent them. Chris was hopeful that, in Julie's case, early intervention may prevent poor attachment becoming a problem. It seems a good example of the 'proactive' approach within the biopsychosocial model of health that is a basic principle of health visiting.

CONCLUSIONS

Schaffer (1998) believes that psychological development is far more flexible than was previously thought. Our personalities aren't fixed once and for all by events in the early years and, given the right circumstances, the effects of even quite severe and prolonged deprivation can be reversed. As Clarke and Clarke (2000) conclude, 'For most children … the effects of such experiences represent no more than a first step in an ongoing lifepath …'

CHAPTER SUMMARY

◎ **Attachments** are intense, enduring emotional ties to specific people. The **mother–child relationship** is usually taken as a model for all later relationships.
◎ The attachment process can be divided into **pre-attachment**, **indiscriminate**, **discriminate** and **multiple attachment phases**.
◎ The development of specific attachments is shown through **separation anxiety**. Some babies also display the **fear-of-strangers response**.
◎ According to **'cupboard love' theories**, attachments are learned through satisfaction of the baby's need for food. However, Schaffer and Emerson found that not only were infants attached to people who didn't perform caretaking activities, but those who did weren't always their primary attachment figures.
◎ According to Bowlby, new-born humans are **genetically programmed** to behave towards their mothers in ways that ensure their survival. There's a **critical period** for attachment development, and attachment to the mother figure is based on **monotropy**.
◎ The **Strange Situation** (SS) is used to classify the baby's basic attachment to the mother into three main types: **anxious–avoidant**, **securely attached** and **anxious–resistant**. The crucial feature determining the quality of attachment is the mother's **sensitivity**.

◎ Bowlby's **maternal–deprivation hypothesis** (MDH) was used to explain the harmful effects of growing up in institutions. But this fails to recognise the understimulating nature of the institutional environment, and to disentangle the different kinds of retardation produced by different types of **privation**.

◎ According to Bowlby's theory, **short–term deprivation** produces **distress**. **Privation** produces long-term **developmental retardation** (such as **affectionless psychopathy**).

◎ Parental death and divorce are examples of **long-term deprivation** and are associated with long-term effects, particularly **separation anxiety**. Another example is day care.

◎ Case studies of children who've endured **extreme privation**, studies of **late adoption**, and Quinton and Rutter's study of **developmental pathways** all indicate that the effects of early privation are **reversible**.

COGNITIVE DEVELOPMENT 15

INTRODUCTION AND OVERVIEW

According to Meadows (1993, 1995), cognitive development is concerned with the study of 'the child as thinker'. However, different theoretical accounts of how the child's thinking develops rest on very different images of what the child is like:

◎ Piaget sees the child as an *organism adapting to its environment*, as well as a *scientist constructing its own understanding of the world*

◎ Vygotsky, in contrast with Piaget, sees the child as a *participant in an interactive process*, by which socially and culturally determined knowledge and understanding gradually become *individualised*

◎ Bruner, like Vygotsky, emphasises the *social* aspects of the child's cognitive development (see Gross, 2005).

Some years ago, Piaget's theory was regarded as the major framework or paradigm within child development. Despite remaining a vital source of influence and inspiration, both in psychology and education, today there are hardly any 'orthodox' Piagetians left (Dasen, 1994). Many fundamental aspects of Piaget's theory have been challenged, and fewer and fewer developmental psychologists now subscribe to his or other 'hard' stage theories (Durkin, 1995). Nonetheless, Piaget's is still the most comprehensive account of how children come to understand the world (Schaffer, 2004). Arguably, however, it was a little too 'cold' – that is, concerned with purely *intellectual* functions that supposedly can be studied separately from socio-emotional functions. Vygotsky tried to redress the balance (Schaffer, 2004).

From my diary (4): Year 1/Community (Health Visitor)

Following my visit with Chris (the HV) to Nicky and her two children (see my diary entry on page 255), Chris expressed her concern about the older child's cognitive development. To help assess his progress, she suggested I read some child development theory and said Piaget was a good place to start.

When we arrived on our next visit, Ben, who is 22 months, was watching TV. When I showed him the toy tractor I'd brought, he agreed to switch off the TV. We could see his reflection in the blank screen and I asked him who it was.

He looked at it for few seconds, then smiled. 'That Ben,' he said, pointing to himself. He grabbed the toy. I asked him who had a tractor like that and he replied, 'Bob builder!' We talked about the programme; he knew the names of all the characters and when I asked, 'Can we fix it?' he laughed and completed the catchphrase by adding, 'Yes, we can!'

Later, I 'hid' under a cup a tiny packet containing a few raisins; he found and ate them. I did it again, using another cup, and he did the same. The third time I put the raisins under one cup and the empty box under a nearer one. He found the box and when he discovered it was empty he looked puzzled, then turned up the other cup and – to his delight – found them.

PIAGET'S THEORY: THE CHILD-AS-SCIENTIST

Rather than trying to explain individual differences (why some children are more intelligent than others – see Gross, 2005), Piaget was interested in how intelligence itself changes as children grow. He called this *genetic epistemology*.

According to Piaget, cognitive development occurs through the interaction of innate capacities with environmental events, and progresses through a series of *hierarchical, qualitatively different stages*:

◎ All children pass through the stages in the *same sequence* without skipping any or (except in the case of brain damage) regressing to earlier ones (they're *invariant*).
◎ The stages are also the *same for everyone* irrespective of culture (they're *universal*).
◎ Underlying the changes are certain *functional invariants*, fundamental aspects of the developmental process which remain the same and work in the same way through the various stages. The most important of these are *assimilation*, *accommodation* and *equilibration*.
◎ The principal *cognitive structure* that changes is the *schema* (plural *schemas* or *schemata*).

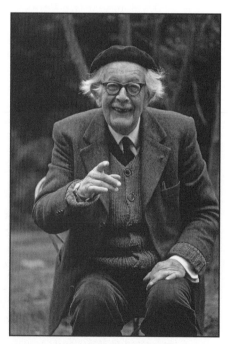

Jean Piaget (1896–1980)

SCHEMAS (OR SCHEMATA)

A *schema* (or *scheme*) is the basic building block or unit of intelligent behaviour. Piaget saw schemas as mental structures which organise past experiences and provide a way of understanding future experiences. Life begins with simple schemas, which are largely confined to inbuilt reflexes (such as sucking and grasping). These operate independently of other reflexes, and are activated only when certain objects are present. As we grow, so our schemas become increasingly complex.

ASSIMILATION, ACCOMMODATION AND EQUILIBRATION

Assimilation is the process by which we incorporate new information into existing schemas. For example, babies will reflexively suck a nipple and other objects, such as a finger. To learn to suck from a bottle or drink from a cup, the initial sucking reflex must be modified through *accommodation*.

When a child can deal with most, if not all, new experiences by assimilating them, it's in a state of *equilibrium*. This is brought about by *equilibration*, the process of seeking 'mental balance'. But if existing schemas are inadequate to cope with new situations, cognitive *disequilibrium* occurs. To restore equilibrium, the existing schema must be 'stretched' in order to take in (or 'accommodate') new information. The necessary and complementary processes of assimilation and accommodation constitute the fundamental process of *adaptation* (see Figure 15.1).

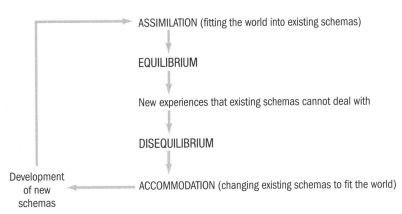

Figure 15.1 Relationship between assimilation, equilibrium, disequilibrium and accommodation in the development of schemas

Ben's ten-week-old baby sister Julie's 'drinking schema' consists only of sucking, whereas Ben's has accommodated drinking from a cup, a bottle and through a straw.

STAGES OF COGNITIVE DEVELOPMENT

Each of Piaget's four stages represents a stage in the development of intelligence (hence *sensorimotor intelligence*, *pre-operational intelligence*, and so on) and is a way of summarising the various schemas a child has at a particular time. The ages shown in Table 15.1 are approximate, because children move through the stages at different rates due to differences in both the environment and their biological maturation. Children also pass through transitional periods, in which their thinking is a mixture of two stages.

Table 15.1 Piaget's four stages of cognitive development

Stage	Approximate age
Sensorimotor	0–2 years
Pre-operational	2–7 years
Concrete operational	7–11 years
Formal operational	11 years onwards

The sensorimotor stage

This lasts for approximately the first two years of life. Infants learn about the world primarily through their senses ('sensori-'), and by doing ('motor'). Based on observations of his own children, Piaget (1952) divided the sensorimotor stage into six sub-stages.

Object permanence

Frequent interaction with objects ultimately leads to the development of *object permanence*. In the second sub-stage (*primary circular reactions*: one to four months), an infant will look where an object disappears for a few moments, but won't search for it. If the object doesn't reappear, the infant apparently loses interest. Piaget called this *passive exploration*, because the infant expects the object to reappear but doesn't actively search for it ('out of sight is out of mind').

In the third sub-stage (*secondary circular reactions*: four to ten months), an infant will reach for a partially hidden object, suggesting that s/he realises that the rest of it is attached to the visible part. But if the object is completely hidden, infants make no attempt to retrieve it. In the fourth sub-stage (*the coordination of secondary circular reactions*: 10–12 months), a hidden object will be searched for ('out of sight' is no longer 'out of mind'), but the infant will persist in looking for it where it was last hidden, even when it's hidden somewhere else.

 This explains why attachment peaks at this age: the older child can retain an image of the attachment figure and will make efforts to 'find' him or her.

While after 12 months infants will look for an object where they last saw it hidden, object permanence isn't yet fully developed. Suppose an infant sees an object placed in a matchbox, which is then put under a pillow. When it's not looking, the object is removed from the matchbox and left under the pillow. If the matchbox is given to the infant, it will open it expecting to find the object. On not finding it, the infant won't look under the pillow. This is because it cannot take into account the possibility that something it's not actually seen might have happened (*failure to infer invisible displacements*). Once the infant can infer invisible displacements (after 18 months), the development of object permanence is complete.

Julie and Ben are at different sub-stages within the sensorimotor stage. Julie 'passively explores'. By continuing his search for the raisins, Ben showed he can infer invisible displacement, so has achieved that particular 'milestone'.

> **Box 15.1 The general symbolic function**
>
> • Other cognitive structures that have developed by the end of the sensorimotor stage include *self-recognition* (see Chapter 16) and *symbolic thought* (such as *language*).
>
> • Two other manifestations of the *general symbolic function* are *deferred imitation* and *representational* (or *make-believe*) *play*.
>
> • Deferred imitation is the ability to imitate or reproduce something that's been perceived but is no longer present (Meltzoff and Moore, 1983).
>
> • Representational play involves using one object as though it were another. Like deferred imitation, this ability depends on the infant's growing ability to form mental images of things and people in their absence (to *remember*).

Ben recognised his reflection as himself. Names and words are symbols representing objects, so he can use symbolic thought; his quoting 'Yes we can!' showed deferred imitation. I was pleased at how much I discovered through play. Chris and I agreed his language skills were underdeveloped – not surprising in view of his lack of social interaction. Happily, Nicky is keen to go to Sure Start.

The pre-operational stage

Probably the main difference between this and the sensorimotor stage is the continued development and use of internal images (or 'interiorised' schemas), symbols and language, especially important for the child's developing sense of self-awareness (see Chapter 16). However, the child tends to be influenced by how things *look*, rather than by logical principles or operations (hence the term 'pre-operational').

Piaget sub-divided the stage into the *pre-conceptual* (ages two to four) and the *intuitive sub-stages* (ages four to seven). The *absolute* nature of the pre-conceptual child's thinking makes relative terms such as 'bigger' or 'stronger' difficult to understand (things tend to be 'biggest' or just 'big'). The intuitive child can use relative terms, but its ability to think logically is still limited.

From my diary (5): Year 1/Children's Ward

To extend my experience to sick children, Chris helped me arrange a week at a local children's ward. Having read about Piaget, I realised it also gave me an opportunity to observe children in different stages of cognitive development.

Today I helped Staff Nurse look after three patients. Peter (two and a half) has severe eczema, Lucy (six) is in for surgery to pin back her ears, and Jacob (twelve and a half) is in traction for a fractured femur. Peter was physically demanding, following me around everywhere; Lucy demanded lots of verbal interaction, and Jacob didn't seem to want any; I later discovered differently. Peter is in the preconceptual sub-stage and Lucy in the intuitive sub-stage of Piaget's pre-operational stage.

Seriation and artificialism

In *seriation*, the pre-conceptual child has difficulty arranging objects on the basis of a particular dimension, such as increasing height (Piaget and Szeminska, 1952). *Artificialism* is the belief that natural features have been designed and constructed by people. For example, the question 'Why is the sky blue?' might produce the answer 'Somebody painted it'.

Transductive reasoning and animism

Transductive reasoning involves drawing an inference about the relationship between two things based on a single shared attribute – for example, if both cats and dogs have four legs, then cats must be dogs. This sort of reasoning can lead to *animism* – the belief that inanimate objects are alive. (This is relevant to the child's understanding of death; see Chapter 20.)

> **Box 15.2 Examples of children's animism during the pre-operational stage (from Piaget, 1973)**
>
> - Cli (three years nine months) speaking of a motor in a garage: 'The motor's gone to bye-byes. It doesn't go out because of the rain …'
>
> - Nel (two years nine months) seeing a hollow chestnut tree: 'Didn't it cry when the hole was made?' To a stone: 'Don't touch my garden! … My garden would cry.' Nel, after throwing a stone on to a sloping bank, watching the stone rolling down, said: 'Look at the stone. It's afraid of the grass.'
>
> - Nel scratched herself against a wall. Looking at her hand: 'Who made that mark? – It hurts where the wall hit me.'
>
> - Dar (one year eight months/two years five months) bringing his toy motor to the window: 'Motor see the snow.' Dar stood up in bed, crying and calling out: 'The mummies (the ladies) all on the ground, hurt!' Dar was watching the grey clouds. He was told that it was going to rain. 'Oh, look at the wind! Naughty wind, smack wind.' On a morning in winter when the sun shone into the room: 'Oh, good! The sun's come to make the radiator warm.'

ASK YOURSELF …
- Can you think of any examples of adults displaying animistic thinking?

- Do you ever think this way yourself?

Centration

Centration involves focusing on only a single perceptual quality at a time. A pre-conceptual child asked to divide apples into 'big and red' ones and 'small and green' ones will either put all the red (or green) apples together irrespective of their size, or all the big (or small) apples together irrespective of their colour. Until the child can *decentre*, it will be unable to classify things logically or systematically. Centration is also associated with the *inability* to conserve (see below).

Staff Nurse explained that young children can deal with complex information only in short, separate sessions. This is why we did Lucy's magic ointment (to stop the needle hurting) preparation in the morning and left the post-operative (bandaging of her ears) preparation until the afternoon.

Egocentrism

According to Piaget, pre-operational children are *egocentric*, that is, they see the world from their own standpoints and cannot appreciate that other people might see things differently. They cannot put themselves 'in other people's shoes' to realise that other people don't know or perceive everything they themselves do. Consider the following example (Phillips, 1969) of a conversation between an experimenter and a four-year-old boy:

Experimenter:	'Do you have a brother?'
Child:	'Yes.'

Experimenter:	'What's his name?'
Child:	'Jim.'
Experimenter:	'Does Jim have a brother?'
Child:	'No.'

KEY STUDY 15.1 The 'Swiss mountain scene' test of egocentrism (Piaget and Inhelder, 1956)

- The three papier-mâché model mountains shown in Figure 15.3 are of different colours. One has snow on the top, one a house and one a red cross.

- The child walks round and explores the model, and then sits on one side while a doll is placed at some different location. The child is shown ten pictures of different views of the model and asked to choose the one that represents how the doll sees it.

- Four-year-olds were completely unaware of perspectives other than their own, and always chose a picture which matched *their* views of the model. Six-year-olds showed some awareness, but often chose the wrong picture. Only seven- and eight-year-olds consistently chose the picture that represented the *doll's* view.

- According to Piaget, children below the age of seven are bound by the *egocentric illusion*. They fail to understand that what they see is *relative to their own* positions, and instead take it to represent 'the world as it really is'.

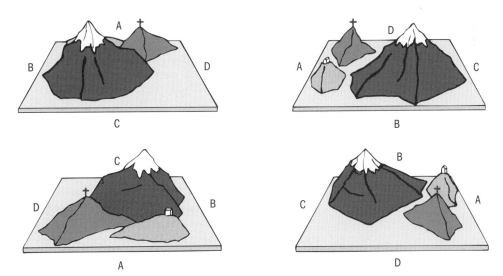

Figure 15.2 Piaget and Inhelder's three-mountain scene, seen from four different sides (from Smith & Cowie, 1988)

Just after the 'pretend' local anaesthetic was applied to her hand, Lucy's father rang. I heard her say, 'See, I have a plaster!' and then, 'No – it's Tigger!' in a surprised tone as if he should have known she had an 'animal' plaster.

283

Conservation

Conservation is the understanding that any quantity (such as number, liquid quantity, length, or substance) remains the same despite physical changes in the arrangement of objects. Piaget believed that pre-operational children cannot conserve because their thinking is dominated by the *perceptual* nature of objects (their 'appearance').

The inability to conserve is another example of centration. With liquid quantity, for example, the child centres on just one dimension of the beaker, usually its height, and fails to take width into account (see Figure 15.3).

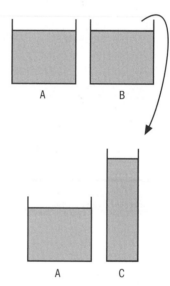

Figure 15.3 The conservation of liquid quantity. Although the child agrees that there's the same amount of liquid in A and B, when the contents of B are poured into C, the appearance of C sways the child's judgement so that C is now judged to contain more liquid than A ('it looks more' or 'it's taller'). Although the child has seen the liquid poured from B into C and agrees that none has been spilled or added in the process (what Piaget calls 'identity'), the appearance of the higher level of liquid in the taller, thinner beaker C is compelling

Only in the concrete operational stage do children understand that 'getting taller' and 'getting narrower' tend to cancel each other out (*compensation*). If the contents of the taller beaker are poured back into the shorter one, the child will again say that the two shorter beakers contain the same amount. But it cannot perform this operation mentally and so lacks *reversibility* (understanding that what can be done can be undone without any gain or loss). These same limitations apply to other forms of conservation, such as number (using two rows of counters) and substance/quantity (using plasticine) (see Gross, 2005).

Box 15.3 Imaginary friends (based on Darbyshire, 1986a)

- Swendsen (1934, in Darbyshire, 1986a) defined an imaginary friend as 'an invisible character named and referred to in conversation with other persons, or played with directly for a period of time ... having an air of reality for the child but no apparent objective basis'. It may be a toy or doll, especially a favourite one, or a creature or animal.

- Most researchers agree that imaginary friends first appear at around two and a half years and disappear around five or six. This corresponds to Piaget's pre-operational stage. Girls are three times more likely to have an imaginary friend (Swendsen, in Darbyshire, 1986a).

- The child tends to attribute adult qualities to the friend, such as knowledge, authority and power. It may be given an ordinary boy's or girl's name or a pet (invented) name.

- Young children will often use their imaginary friend to help them bridge the gap between external controls (usually the parents) and the internal ones represented by the superego (see Chapters 2 and 6). The child may ask the friend what to do in a particular situation and the friend will then 'tell them' what to do.

- The imaginary friend can also become a very convenient scapegoat for the child's naughtiness. She may attribute this to the friend in order to avoid parental disapproval. This isn't simply a case of the young child lying to avoid punishment, but an important stage in the developing process of self-criticism and self-control (Nagera, 1969, in Darbyshire, 1986a).

- Several researchers have claimed that only children, or those who have been neglected or rejected, are more likely to have an imaginary friend. For example, Nagera gives several accounts of children who have created their imaginary friend at a time of stress and conflict, such as shortly after parental divorce or after the birth of a new baby.

- Going into hospital is another stressful situation in which imaginary friends may appear. It's tempting for a nurse to use the friend as a means of reassuring the child. For example, 'You don't have to worry about having a little injection because X is going to have one as well and he's not afraid, is he?' But the child may become confused if the nurse later tries to deny the nature of the friend; for instance, when the child says she's not taking that medicine because X says it's horrible.

The concrete operational stage

The child is now capable of performing logical operations, but only in the presence of actual objects. S/he can conserve, and shows reversibility and more logical classification.

Further examples of the child's ability to decentre include his/her appreciation that objects can belong to more than one class (as in the case of Andrew being Bob's brother *and* Charlie's best friend). There's also a significant *decline* in egocentrism (and the growing *relativism* of the child's viewpoint), plus the onset of seriation and reciprocity of relationships (such as knowing that adding one to three produces the same amount as taking one from five).

KEY STUDY 15.2 What are nurses like? (Price, 1988)

- Price reports the findings from a survey of 203 7–12 year olds (corresponding to the whole of the concrete operational stage and the early part of the formal operational stage). All but seven were aged 7–11.

- For children of this age, their mother might put on a uniform and become a nurse, but this doesn't prevent her from returning that night as mummy once more. Even though she wears a uniform and is a nurse, she's still mummy 'underneath'. This demonstrates conservation (specifically, the idea of reversibility – see above).

- Children were asked to complete a written questionnaire, which included six open-ended questions on nurses and one on doctors.

- 'What nurses do' produced responses that Price classified as: (a) *the expressive/feminine role* (nurses fulfil traditionally expressive roles similar to that of mothers, such as giving cuddles or making a fuss of children when they feel lonely or sore; they read bedtime stories and play); (b) *nurses as clinicians* (nurses use skills such as 'give you stitches and operations', 'operate on you' and 'dus tings lck sowe your stumoc together' [*sic*]. They also give injections, medicines and pills); (c) *nurses as doctors' assistants* (nurses often help the doctor, in the operating theatre, clinic and treatment room). A total of 27 children said that nurses explain what the doctor does, and 9 felt that the doctors help the nurses!

- The 'nice' things that nurses do centred on the expressive communication role, such as explaining, 'chat', tactile comfort, story-telling and being honest.

- Surprisingly, there were few 'nasty' things that nurses do. These centred on giving injections and lying about operations/procedures that 'would not hurt'.

- Doctors were seen to function during short visits and were more technical and less communicative. They look at X-rays, cure disease, treat wounds, do operations, 'put soap in your tummy' and test your heart and ears.

- The most important qualities for nurses to have are patience (76), kindness (63) and bravery (57). They were also thought to be 'brainy', 'clever' and talkative.

- These qualities were to be displayed in a wide range of settings: hospital, surgery, old people's homes, 'around the district', hospices, in aeroplanes and at accidents. They expected to see nurses in their own homes, at school and in the army.

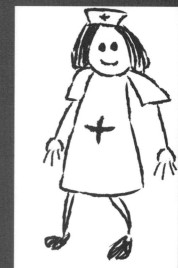

- Drawings of nurses always included a uniform, usually with red crosses on it, a fob watch, and often a belt and hat. Typical accoutrements included syringes, stethoscopes, first-aid boxes and a saw!

- Because children at this stage are reasoning from what they've actually experienced, the role of the nurse as communicator has never been more important. The findings suggest that nurses can expect a degree of trust from children, but that they should act as an 'interpreter' of nursing events. Failure to do so will traumatise the child (Price, 1988).

The Price (1988) survey seems to sum up what should be our role behaviour: patience, kindness and tactile comfort, communication and honesty. Might a survey of adult patients produce a similar result?

Price also says children reason from experience (Piaget's concrete operational stage). So, to prepare Lucy for post-operative bandaging, I suggested she became a nurse; she let me bandage her head to demonstrate how to bandage mine. We pretended we couldn't hear anything at all and used exaggerated gestures to convey meanings, which made her laugh.

The formal operational stage

While the concrete operational child is still concerned with manipulating things (even if this is done mentally), the formal operational thinker can manipulate *ideas* or *propositions*, and can reason solely on the basis of verbal statements ('first order' and 'second order' operations respectively). 'Formal' refers to the ability to follow the form of an argument without reference to its particular content. In *transitivity problems*, for example, 'If A is taller than B, and B is taller than C, then A is taller than C' is a form of argument whose conclusion is logically true, regardless of what A, B and C might refer to.

Formal operational thinkers can also think *hypothetically* – that is, they can think about what *could be* as well as what *actually is*. For example, asked what it would be like if people had tails, they might say, 'Dogs would know when you were happy' or 'Lovers could hold their tails in secret under the table.' Concrete operational thinkers might tell you 'not to be so silly', or say where on the body the tail might be, showing their dependence on what they've actually seen (Dworetzky, 1981). This ability to imagine and discuss things that have never been encountered is evidence of the continued decentration that occurs beyond concrete operations.

As Jacob is in the formal operational stage, he can imagine 'what if' something goes wrong. As he didn't speak much, I watched him play a game on his laptop and asked him how it worked. He explained it so enthusiastically! Afterwards, I asked if he was worried about anything. After a while, he admitted he was 'a bit concerned' his leg might not heal properly and he wouldn't get back into the school football team. He sounded casual, but I sensed that it mattered to him.

An evaluation of Piaget's theory

As we noted in the 'Introduction and Overview' section of this chapter, Piaget's theory has had an enormous impact on our understanding of cognitive development. However, as Flavell (1982) and others (e.g. Siegal, 2003) have remarked:

> Like all theories of great reach and significance … it has problems that gradually come to light as years and years of thinking and research get done on it. Thus, some of us now think that the theory may in varying degrees be unclear, incorrect and incomplete.

Egocentrism

Gelman (1979) has shown that four-year-olds adjust their explanations of things to make them clearer to a blindfold listener. This isn't what we'd expect if, as Piaget claims, children of this age are egocentric. Nor would we expect four-year-olds to use simpler forms of speech when talking to two-year-olds (Gelman, 1979) or choose appropriate birthday presents for their mothers (Marvin, 1975, in Morris, 1988).

Critics of the 'Swiss mountain scene' test (Key Study 15.1) see it as an unusually difficult way of presenting a problem to a young child. Borke (1975) and Hughes (cited in Donaldson, 1978) have shown that when the task is presented in a meaningful context (making what Donaldson calls 'human sense'), even three-and-a-half-year-olds can appreciate the world as another person sees it. These are all examples of perspective-taking. According to Siegal (2003), 'A reasonable conclusion is that young children are not egocentric all of the time, but their perspective-taking skills clearly improve during childhood ...'

Box 15.4 Perspective-taking, false beliefs and theory of mind

- According to Flavell *et al.* (1990), there are two levels of perspective-taking (PT) ability:

  (a) *level 1* (two-to-three-year-olds) – the child knows that some other person experiences something differently (*perceptual* PT)

  (b) *level 2* (four-to-five-year-olds) – the child develops a whole series of complex rules for figuring out precisely what the other person sees or experiences (*affective* and *cognitive* PT).

- In a study of children's ability to distinguish between appearance and reality, Flavell (1986) showed children a sponge painted to look like a rock. They were asked what it looked like and what it 'really' was. Three-year-olds said either that it looked like a sponge and was a sponge, or that it looked like a rock and was a rock. However, four-to-five-year-olds could say that it looked like a rock but was in fact a sponge.

- Gopnik and Astington (1988) allowed children to *feel* the sponge before asking them the questions used in Flavell's study. They were then told: 'Your friend John hasn't touched this, he hasn't squeezed it. If John just sees it over here like this, what will he think it is? Will he think it's a rock or a sponge?'

- How do you think the three year olds answered?

- How do you think the four to five year olds answered?

- Typically, three-year-olds said that John would think it was a sponge (which it is), while four-to-five-year-olds said he'd think it was a rock (because he hadn't had the opportunity of touching/squeezing it). In other words, the older children were attributing John with a *false belief*, which they could only do by taking John's perspective.

- Evidence like this has led several theorists (e.g. Gopnik and Wellman, 1994) to propose that four-to-five-year-olds have developed a quite sophisticated *theory of mind* (Premack and Woodruff, 1978). This refers to the understanding that people (and not objects) have desires, beliefs and other mental states, some of which (such as beliefs) can be false (*cognitive* PT). The older children in Gopnick and Astington's study understood that John wouldn't know something which *they did*.

When Lucy cried because her mother left, Peter also became upset and ran to comfort her. Perceptual perspective-taking explains how Peter could perceive (Level 1 PT) Lucy's distress, but not that he seemed able, at two-and-a-half, to empathise with her.

Conservation

The ability to conserve also seems to occur earlier than Piaget believed. Rose and Blank (1974) showed that when the *pre-transformation question* (the question asked before one row of counters, say, is rearranged) was dropped, six-year-olds often succeeded on the number conservation task. Importantly, they made fewer errors on the standard version of the task when tested a week later. These findings were replicated by Samuel and Bryant (1984) using conservation of number, liquid quantity and substance.

According to Donaldson (1978), the standard version of the task unwittingly 'forces' children to produce the wrong answer against their better judgement, by the mere fact that the same question is asked twice, before and after the transformation. Hence, children believe they're expected to give a different answer on the second question. On this explanation, *contextual cues* may override purely linguistic ones. Children may think the experimenter has rejected their first answer, so they feel they're required to give a *different* answer on the second question in order to please the adult questioner. This is the problem of a *clash of conversational worlds* between child and adult (Siegal, 2003).

Bruner (1966) argues that children's attention is so captured by the transformed state that they disregard the pre-transformed state and fail to attend to it when asked the second question.

Isn't this another indication of centration?

Cross-cultural tests of the stages

According to Schaffer (2004), Piaget's account gives the impression that the stages are an inevitable consequence of being human, and that external influences stemming from the social environment play no part. What evidence is there to support this?

The few cross-cultural studies of the sensorimotor stage have shown the sub-stages to be universal. Overall, it seems that ecological or cultural factors *don't* influence the sequence of stages, but *do* affect the rate at which they're attained (Segall *et al.*, 1999).

Conservation experiments have been conducted with Aborigines in remote parts of the central Australian desert (Dasen, 1994), as well as Eskimo, African (Senegal and Rwande), Hong Kong and Papua New Guinea samples. Consistent with Dasen's findings, children from non-western cultures often show a considerable lag in acquiring operational thought, but this applies mainly to those having minimal contact with white culture. Where Aborigines, for example, live in white communities and attend school there, they perform at a similar level to whites. Even where there is a lag in development compared with whites, the stages still appear in the same order. So (as with the sensorimotor sub-stages), 'Cultural factors … can affect *rate* of attainment; they do not alter developmental *sequence*' (Schaffer, 2004).

As Dasen (1994) puts it:

> The deep structures, the basic cognitive processes, are indeed universal, while at the surface level, the way these basic processes are brought to bear on specific contents, in specific contexts, is influenced by culture. Universality and cultural diversity are not opposites, but are complementary aspects of all human behaviour and development.

Perrin and Perrin (1983, in Taylor et al., 1999) found that clinicians (paediatricians, nurses and child development students) correctly estimated children's ages less than 40 per cent of the time. They concluded that physicians and nurses make little use of the notion of developmental stages, and approach all children as if they were in middle childhood or in the Piagetian stage of concrete operations. Other evidence suggests that even if we get the age right, we shouldn't assume it determines developmental stage.

The role of social factors in cognitive development

Meadows (1995) maintains that Piaget implicitly saw children as largely independent and isolated in their construction of knowledge and understanding of the physical world (children as scientists). This excluded the contribution of other people to children's cognitive development. The social nature of knowledge and thought is a basic proposition of Vygotsky's theory (see below). According to Vygotsky (1987):

> The child [in Piaget's theory] is not seen as part of the social whole, as a subject of social relationships. He is not seen as a being who participates in the societal life of the social whole to which he belongs from the outset. The social is viewed as something standing outside the child.

Despite all these (and other) criticisms, Siegal (2003) believes that:

> ... Piaget's intriguing observations opened up many fruitful lines of enquiry and ... while many of his interpretations have by and large been modified or superseded, he set the agenda for a vast body of productive research in the twentieth and twenty-first centuries.

VYGOTSKY'S THEORY: THE CHILD-AS-APPRENTICE

Vygotsky didn't produce a fully formed theory or coherent body of research, and many of his ideas weren't spelled out in detail. His works were published in the former Soviet Union in the 1920s and 1930s, but weren't translated into English until the early 1960s.

Vygotsky and Piaget agree that development doesn't occur in a vacuum: knowledge is constructed as a result of the child's active interaction with the environment. But, as we've seen, for Piaget that environment is essentially *asocial* (so, his account is described as *constructivist*). But for Vygotsky,

> Human nature cannot be described in the abstract; whatever course children's mental growth takes is to a large extent a function of the cultural tools that are handed down to them by other people ...

(in Schaffer, 2004).

So, for Vygotsky, cognitive development is a thoroughly *social* process (hence, he's a *social constructivist*). His aim was to spell out and explain how the higher mental functions (reasoning, understanding, planning, remembering, and so on) arise out of children's social experiences. He did this by considering human development in terms of three levels: the *cultural*, *interpersonal* and *individual*. He had much more to say about the first two, so we'll concentrate on these here.

Vygotsky believed we understand the world (other people?) through our routine interactive processes, which is a very good reason for taking time to play with the children in the ward. (I think this is similar to the social constructionist theory I read about in Chapter 2.)

THE CULTURAL LEVEL

Children don't need to 'reinvent the world anew' (as Piaget seemed to believe). They can benefit from the accumulated wisdom of previous generations; indeed, they cannot avoid doing so through interactions with caregivers. So, each generation stands on the

ASK YOURSELF ...
- Can you think of examples of *cultural tools* that might be especially important for children's cognitive development?

shoulders of the previous one, taking over the particular culture – including its intellectual, material, scientific and artistic achievements – in order to develop it further before handing it on, in turn, to the next generation (Schaffer, 2004).

*However, Piaget emphasised cognitive **development** – this helps explain, for example, how Lucy perceives the world differently from Peter.*

Cultural tools are what the child 'inherits'. These can be:
◎ *technological* (clocks, bicycles and other physical devices)
◎ *psychological* (concepts and symbols, such as language, literacy, maths and scientific theories)
◎ *values* (such as speed, efficiency and power).
It's through such tools that children learn to conduct their lives in socially effective and acceptable ways, as well as understanding how the world works.

Schaffer (2004) gives the example of *computers* as a major – and relatively recent – cultural tool:

> There are few instances in history where a new technical invention has assumed such a dominant role in virtually all spheres of human activity as the computer… in the space of just a few decades computing expertise is regarded as an essential skill for even quite young children to acquire …

Jacob has his own laptop and there is a computer in the activities room. All the children love it – even Peter!

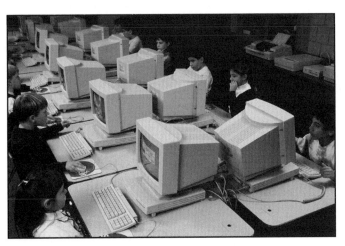

The computer: a powerful and pervasive cultural tool

The most essential cultural tool is *language*.
◎ It's the pre-eminent means of passing on society's accumulated knowledge: how others speak and what they speak about is the main channel of communicating culture from adult to child.
◎ It enables children to regulate their own activities.
◎ At about age seven, speech becomes internalised to form internal thought: an essential *social* function thus becomes the major tool for *cognitive* functioning.

This reminds me why we should be concerned about Ben's lack of language development (see my notes on page 281).

THE INTERPERSONAL LEVEL

It's here that culture and the individual meet, and it's the level at which Vygotsky made his major contribution.

Internalisation and the social nature of thinking

The ability to think and reason by and for ourselves (inner speech or verbal thought) is the result of a fundamentally *social* process. At birth, we're social beings capable of interacting with others, but able to do little either practically or intellectually, by or for ourselves. But gradually, we move towards self-sufficiency and independence, and by participating in social activities, our abilities become transformed. For Vygotsky, cognitive development involves an active *internalisation* of problem-solving processes that takes place as a result of mutual interaction between children and those with whom they have regular social contact (initially the parents, but later friends and classmates and teachers).

This is the reverse of how Piaget (at least initially) saw things. Piaget's idea of 'the child as a scientist' is replaced by the idea of 'the *child as an apprentice*', who acquires the culture's knowledge and skills through graded collaboration with those who already possess them (Rogoff, 1990). According to Vygotsky (1981),

> any function in the child's cultural development appears twice, or on two planes. First it appears on the social plane, and then on the psychological plane.

So, cognitive development progresses from the *intermental* to the *intramental* (from joint regulation to self-regulation).

Scaffolding and the zone of proximal development (ZPD)

The *zone of proximal development* (ZPD) defines those functions that haven't yet matured but are in the process of maturing (Vygotsky, 1978). These could be called the 'buds' or 'flowers' rather than the 'fruits' of development. The actual developmental level characterises mental development *retrospectively*, while the ZPD characterises mental development *prospectively*.

Scaffolding refers to the kind of guidance and support adults provide children in the ZPD by which children acquire their knowledge and skills (Wood *et al.*, 1976; Wood and Wood, 1996). As a task becomes more familiar to the child and more within its competence, those who provide the scaffold leave more and more for the child to do until it can perform the task successfully. In this way, the developing thinker doesn't have to create cognition 'from scratch': there are others available who've already 'served' their own apprenticeship.

The internalised cognitive skills remain social in two senses. First, as mature learners we can 'scaffold' ourselves through difficult tasks (self-instruction), as others once scaffolded our earlier attempts. Second, the only skills practised to a high level of competence for most people are those offered by their culture: cognitive potential may be universal, but cognitive expertise is culturally determined (Meadows, 1995).

'Scaffolding' draws attention to the conditions under which learning usually occurs. It also emphasises the essential *social-interactive* nature of these conditions (Schaffer, 2004). According to Vygotsky, a more knowledgeable child can provide instruction and guidance for another, in order to bring the latter up to a similar level of competence (*peer tutoring* – see Foot and Howe, 1998; Foot *et al.*, 1990).

ASK YOURSELF ...
- How does this distinction between cognitive potential and expertise relate to Dasen's (1994) assessment of Piaget's stages?

ASK YOURSELF ...
• What would you say is the key difference between Vygotsky's and Piaget's theories?

This is why we have mentors! The English National Board (in Downie and Basford, 2003: 228/9) defines a mentor as 'an appropriately qualified and experienced first level nurse/midwife/health visitor who, by example and facilitation, guides, assists and supports the student in learning new skills, adopting new behaviour and acquiring new attitudes'.

An evaluation of Vygotsky's theory

◎ Vygotsky's theory clearly 'compensates' for one of the central limitations of Piaget's theory. As Segall *et al.* (1999) put it, 'Piaget produced a theory of the development of an "epistemic subject", an idealised, non-existent individual, completely divorced from the social environment.' For Vygotsky, culture (and especially language) plays a key role in cognitive development: the development of the individual cannot be understood – and indeed cannot happen – outside the context of social interaction.

◎ While Vygotsky's theory hasn't been tested cross-culturally as Piaget's has, it has influenced cross-cultural psychology through the development of *cultural psychology* (e.g. Cole, 1990; see Chapter 2, page 35) and related approaches, such as 'socially shared cognition' (Resnick *et al.*, 1991) and 'distributed cognition' (Salomon, 1993). According to all these approaches, '... cognitive processes are not seen as exclusively individual central processors, but ... are situation specific ... therefore cognition is not necessarily situated "within the head" but is shared among people and settings ...' (Segall *et al.*, 1999).

◎ In contrast with Piaget's theory, Vygotsky's isn't truly developmental. His ideas are based on a 'prototype' child, who functions in the same way at age two or twelve: nothing is said about changes in the processes underlying learning (such as attention, memory and intellectual capacities) and how these affect social interaction at different ages.

◎ Schaffer (2004) believes that his neglect of *emotional* factors is a serious omission: he makes no reference to struggles, the frustrations of failure, the joys of success, or generally what *motivates* the child to achieve particular goals: 'While cognition was given a social appearance, Vygotsky's treatment of the child is as "cold" as Piaget's ...' (Schaffer, 2004).

My experiences with the HV and in the children's ward have shown me how relevant developmental theory is to the practical care of children – well or sick. I've also learned that, although theories disagree, they all contribute to understanding. For instance, to understand the world of children we need both Piaget's constructivist and Vygotsky's social interactionist perspectives. Schaffer (2004) says we also need to consider emotion and motivation, which is a humanistic perspective. I need to remember that, with children, it's even more important not to make assumptions based on their chronological age nor, in a multicultural society, from our own cultural point of view. Taylor et al. (1999) suggest that the most constructive starting point for any explanation is the child; they quote Jolly's suggestion (1981) that we should watch what children stare at in hospital and then ask them what they think.

CHAPTER SUMMARY

◎ Piaget sees **intelligence** as **adaptation to the environment**, and he was interested in how intelligence changes as children grow (**genetic epistemology**). Younger children's intelligence is **qualitatively different** from that of older children.

◎ **Cognitive development** occurs through the **interaction** between innate capacities and environmental events. It progresses through a series of **hierarchical**, **invariant** and **universal stages**: the **sensorimotor**, **pre-operational**, **concrete operational** and **formal operational** stages.

◎ Underlying cognitive changes are **functional invariants**, the most important being **assimilation**, **accommodation** (which together constitute **adaptation**) and **equilibration**. The major cognitive structures that change are **schemas/schemata**.

◎ During the **sensorimotor stage**, frequent interaction with objects ultimately leads to **object permanence**, which is fully developed when the child can infer **invisible displacements**.

◎ By the end of the sensorimotor stage, schemas have become '**interiorised**'. **Representational/make-believe play**, like **deferred imitation**, reflects the **general symbolic function**.

◎ **Pre-operational children** have difficulty in **seriation tasks** and also display **transductive reasoning** and **animism**. **Centration** is illustrated by the **inability to conserve**. Pre-operational children are also **egocentric**.

◎ During the **concrete operational stage**, logical operations can be performed only in the presence of actual or observable objects.

◎ **Formal operational thinkers** can manipulate **ideas** and **propositions** ('second order' operations) and think **hypothetically**.

◎ Four-and-five-year-olds are capable of **perspective-taking**, enabling them to attribute **false beliefs** to other people. This is a crucial feature of the child's *theory of mind*.

◎ While basic cognitive processes may be **universal**, how these are brought to bear on specific contents is influenced by **culture**.

◎ According to Vygotsky, the initially helpless baby actively **internalises** problem-solving processes through **interaction with parents**. Vygotsky's **child apprentice** acquires cultural knowledge and skills through **graded collaboration** with those who already possess them (**scaffolding**).

◎ Vygotsky's **zone of proximal development** (ZPD) characterises development **prospectively**. It defines those functions that haven't yet matured but are in the process of maturing.

DEVELOPMENT OF THE SELF-CONCEPT

16

INTRODUCTION AND OVERVIEW

According to Hampson (1995), the human capacity for self-awareness permits us to try to see ourselves as others see us. When personality psychologists study personality via self-reports, such as questionnaires (see Chapter 6), they're assessing people's perceptions of themselves. Social psychologists also study people's self-perceptions through their study of the *self-concept*.

The self-concept (or simply 'self') is a *hypothetical construct:* it's a 'theory' each one of us develops about who we are and how we fit into society. It's repeatedly revised during childhood in the light of both cognitive development and social experience. On the one hand, as children get older they become more competent at self-awareness and more realistic; on the other hand, other people's perceptions and responses will come to play a more central role in shaping the nature of that awareness (Schaffer, 2004).

Adolescence is a crucial period for its development. A major account of how the self-concept changes in adolescence is Erikson's *psychosocial theory* (see Chapter 17). But the formation of the self is never complete. At no time does the self function as a closed system, and it is always affected by others' evaluations of us (Schaffer, 2004). This is consistent with the view of the self as 'social to the core' (Fiske, 2004). Even when tracing how self-perception changes in the individual, this is an *inherently social process*, as reflected in the early theories of James, Cooley and Mead. More recent extensions of these see the self as *constructed in language* (e.g. Harré) (see Gross, 2005).

For many patients, the bodily self – or body image – is a crucial aspect of the self that undergoes revision as a result of their illness and the treatment they receive for it. This is especially true for cancer patients (including women with breast cancer who have a mastectomy, and anyone who undergoes facial surgery for their cancer), ostomy patients and those with HIV/AIDS (who will be some of those with cancer), and people who suffer severe burns or disability as a result of an accident.

From my diary (19): Year 2/Surgical Ward

Clare is a 22-year-old with ulcerative colitis, who I knew from last year on the medical ward. She is pale and very thin; she looks almost anorexic. She had an ileostomy two days ago and today the stoma specialist nurse (Eulette) arrived to change her ileostomy bag for the first time. Staff Nurse, who was the link nurse between Eulette and the ward, suggested I accompany her (a) to learn from an expert and (b) to be a familiar presence to Clare, who was very apprehensive about the procedure.

It did prove difficult for Clare. Although she'd had counselling, met other ileostomy patients and had been fully involved in choosing the ileostomy site, she was unable to cope with the first sight of the stoma and became very distressed. Eulette was very calm and matter of fact; she explained the stoma was bruised and swollen from the operation and that it would look much better in a few days. She reminded Clare that it was the means of 'getting her life back', which seemed to calm her down a bit. Afterwards I sat with Clare while she had a cry. 'I know it will make me better, but I hate it, it's disgusting; I don't feel I'm me any more,' she said.

ASK YOURSELF ...
• What do you think is the difference between consciousness and self-consciousness?

CONSCIOUSNESS AND SELF-CONSCIOUSNESS

When you look in the mirror at your face, you're both the person who's looking and that which is looked at. Similarly, when you think about the kind of person you are or something you've done, you're both the person doing the thinking and what's being thought about. In other words, you're both *subject* (the thinker or looker) and *object* (what's being looked at or thought about). We use the personal pronoun 'I' to refer to ourselves as subject, and 'me' to refer to ourselves as object, and this represents a rather special relationship we have with ourselves, namely *self-consciousness/self-awareness*.

While other species possess consciousness (they have sensations of cold, heat, hunger and thirst, and can feel pleasure, pain, fear, sexual arousal, and so on – they're *sentient* creatures), only humans possess self-consciousness. We often use the term 'self-conscious' to describe our response to situations where we're made to feel object-like or exposed in some way (for example, we leave home in the morning to discover our sweater's on back-to-front). But this is a *secondary* meaning: the *primary* meaning refers to this unique relationship in which the same person, the same self, is both subject and object.

Being ill and in hospital is an experience that, unavoidably, tends to objectify the self. It seems the dramatic change in Clare's objective self, her body image, has changed her subjective self, her idea of who she is.

WHAT IS THE SELF?

'*Self*' and '*self-concept*' are used interchangeably to refer to an individual's overall self-awareness. According to Murphy (1947), 'the self is the individual as known to the individual', and Burns (1980) defines it as 'the set of attitudes a person holds towards himself'.

According to Leary (2004), the self is a *cognitive structure* that permits self-reflection and organises information about oneself. It also has *motivational features*, in particular:
◎ *self-consistency* (to maintain, if not verify, one's existing view of oneself)
◎ *self-evaluation* (self-assessment – to see oneself accurately)
◎ *self-enhancement* (to maintain a positive image of oneself).

One's existing view of oneself is one's *self*-image, and our evaluation of ourselves determines our *self*-esteem. Self-enhancement can be both private and public.
◎ *Private* self-enhancement also relates to *self-esteem*. According to Greenwald (1980), the *self-esteem motive* acts like a totalitarian political regime, which suppresses information and rewrites history to preserve a particular desired image of the government. In the same way, the 'totalitarian ego' distorts facts about the self and rewrites one's memory of personal history in order to maintain one's own positive evaluation.

◎ *Public* self-enhancement relates to *self-presentation* (or *impression management*), our deliberate attempts to influence others' impressions of us – usually in a positive way (see Chapter 8).

My previous impression of Clare had been as a fashionably slim, pretty, young woman. Not surprisingly, she'd had lots of boyfriends, none serious. In spite of her illness, I'd have said she had a very positive, self-enhancing view of herself. Since her operation, clearly this isn't so.

PRIVATE VS PUBLIC SELF

Murphy's and Burns' definitions of the self given above are really definitions of the *private* self. According to Leary (2004):

> … at the most fundamental level, the self is the cognitive apparatus that permits self-reflexive thought – the cognitive structures and associated processes that permit people to take themselves as an object of their own thought and to think consciously about themselves …

This describes the 'subject'/'object' relationship that we discussed above (self-consciousness/awareness) and corresponds to the 'I'/'me' distinction. Leary claims that, strictly, there is only a private self. So, what does the *public* self refer to? It's been used to refer to three distinct entities:

1. the image we convey to others (including reputation and roles)
2. our beliefs about our public image (how we think others perceive us)
3. the impressions others actually form about us.

Whichever of these we mean, the term refers to a very different concept from the private, psychological self, which allows us to think about and control these public impressions: '… this so-called public self resides either within the individual's own private sense of self or in others' minds, respectively. In either case, it is not a "self" in the true sense of the term …' (Leary, 2004).

However, according to Goffman's dramaturgical approach (e.g. 1971), personality is simply the sum total of an individual's social roles. Both this, and the social constructionist approach (see Chapter 2), reject the view of the self as a private feature of individuals, seeing it as wholly social/public (see Gross, 2005).

Until now, Clare's public self has coincided with her private self: attractive, well-groomed and sweet smelling. She now thinks of herself (her body anyway) as 'disgusting'.

COMPONENTS OF THE SELF-CONCEPT

The self-concept is a general term that normally refers to three major components: *self-image*, *self-esteem* and the *ideal self*.

SELF-IMAGE

Self-image refers to the way we describe ourselves, what we think we're like. One way of investigating self-image is to ask people the question 'Who are you?' 20 times (Kuhn and McPartland, 1954). This typically produces two main categories of answer.

1. *Social roles* are usually objective aspects of the self-image (e.g. son, daughter, brother, sister, student). They are 'facts' that can be verified by others.

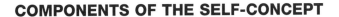

ASK YOURSELF …
• Give 20 different answers to the question 'Who are you?'.

2. *Personality traits* are more a matter of opinion and judgement, and what we think we're like may be different from how others see us. But how others behave towards us has an important influence on our self-perception (see Gross, 2005).

Clare's job is an integral part of her self-concept; she sells a well-known (expensive) brand of make-up in a large store. She is very aware of her physical appearance – she likes to wash her hair every day and is always beautifully made up.

As well as social roles and personality traits, people's answers often refer to their *physical characteristics* (such as tall, short, fat, thin, blue-eyed, brown-haired). These are part of our *body image/bodily self*, the 'bodily me', which also includes bodily sensations, such as pain, cold and hunger. A more permanent feature of our body image relates to what we count as part of our body (and hence belonging to us) and what we don't.

Allport (1955) gives two rather dramatic examples of how intimate our bodily sense is, and just where we draw the boundaries between 'me' and 'not me' (see the 'Ask Yourself' box).

> ### ASK YOURSELF …
> * Imagine swallowing your saliva – or actually do it! Now imagine spitting it into a cup and drinking it! Clearly, once we've spat out our saliva, we've disowned it – it no longer belongs to us.
>
> * Imagine sucking blood from a cut on your finger (something we do quite automatically). Now imagine sucking the blood from a plaster on your finger. Again, once it's soaked into the plaster it has ceased to be part of ourselves.
>
> * Can you think of any exceptions to this 'rule'?

According to Blackmore (1989), the concept of body image has been well defined in nursing literature. For example, Smitherman (1981, in Blackmore, 1989), while acknowledging that body image is only part of our total self-concept, sees it as occupying

> … a very prominent position. Our society is very concerned with physical appearance … the ideal body image … has been said to represent youth, beauty, vigour, intactness and health. There is likely to be a resulting reduced self-esteem, insecurity and anxiety among those who deviate significantly from this ideal.

As a result of her operation, Clare's body is no longer 'intact' and a previously hidden part of her body is now visible. The image she had of herself as having (in spite of her illness) an 'ideal body' is destroyed.

Fawcett and Fry (1980, in Blackmore, 1989) recognise that body image is a complex concept and that 'body perception' (direct mental experience of physical appearance) isn't the whole picture. They identify 'body attitude' as 'the broad spectrum of feelings, attitudes and emotional reactions towards the body'.

Changes in body image as a result of disease and accidents

This complex concept of body image isn't static. Whenever our body changes in some way, so our body image changes (altered body image/ABI – Price, 1986). In extreme cases, we'd expect a correspondingly dramatic change in body image.

According to Price, ABI affects patients in all the usual clinical divisions of the modern hospital, such as dermatology, A&E, surgery, medicine and psychiatry. Some areas, notably oncology, will have a preponderance of ABI problems to deal with.

Clare's private body image has changed drastically but her public one hasn't necessarily done so. She made it clear she wants her altered body to remain secret, that no one should know except her family and her boyfriend.

> ## Box 16.1 Categories of patients with altered body images (ABIs) (based on Price, 1986)
>
> - **Those with congenital/hereditary conditions:** These include a range of paediatric problems, such as cleft lip and palate, spina bifida, Down's syndrome and orthopaedic deformities. Although such altered images affect and persist in adult patients, they have a more acute impact in childhood, when body image hasn't fully developed and is fragile (see text below). It may become increasingly negative through peer criticism and ostracism, especially if the child and its family aren't helped to develop adequate coping strategies.
>
> - **Those who have suffered a traumatic alteration of their body image:** These include those with facial scarring following a road traffic accident or children who have scalded themselves. In these cases, the change in body image is rapid and there's no time to prepare the individual psychologically.
>
> - **Developmental ABIs:** These include psychiatric disorders such as anorexia nervosa (see Gross, 2005). This is developmental to the extent that it's a potentially progressive disorder, and because it affects individuals as they move through the complex changes of body and self-image in puberty (see Chapter 17).
>
> - **Pathological ABIs:** These are legion and include some potentially life-threatening conditions, such as cancers, dermatological conditions and infections. They may develop very slowly, appear to go into remission, or even disappear altogether. There may be time to adapt, but the patient is never certain how the ABI will develop and this causes great insecurity.
>
> - **Sexual body image problems:** These include actual changes in sexual appearance and function, or experience of our sexuality and its appropriateness to our self-image. The surgical amputation of the penis for cancer, or the lack of well-developed masculine characteristics in a young adult male, may both be traumatic in their own ways.

Price believes that *hidden* and *open* ABIs may cross many of these categories. Hidden ABIs aren't necessarily any easier for the patient to deal with. For example, a woman who has undergone a total hysterectomy may not appear to have a body image problem. Other examples include epilepsy, colostomy/ileostomy, and renal failure that requires haemodialysis or continuous ambulatory peritoneal dialysis (CAPD). As far as the outside world is concerned, the problem is hidden (and so appears not to exist), but to the spouse the problem may be open. Equally, if a patient denies having a problem with a new body shape or form, the problem becomes hidden for them too (Price, 1986)!

This is one of Clare's problems. Her ABI is certainly not hidden from her; she is only too aware of all the implications – so much so, that while she was so upset she said she was going to finish with her boyfriend and give up her job. But Eulette persuaded her to postpone any such decisions until she'd recovered from her operation and felt better.

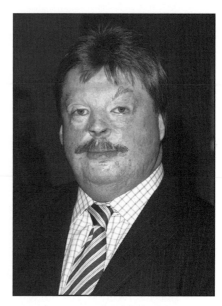

Simon Weston, survivor – and casualty – of the Falklands War in 1982

Price (1990) defines ABI as 'any significant alteration to body image occurring outside the realms of expected human development'. It can arise from either the *external* environment (for example, major surgery, including mastectomy; burns; medical interventions, such as IV lines or naso-gastric tubes) or the *internal* environment (for example, congenital defects such as Down's syndrome; malignant tumours; psychiatric illness such as anorexia nervosa; HIV-related diseases (see below)).

In the context of testicular cancer and its treatment, Blackmore (1989) describes three kinds of loss that occur:

1. *Loss of psychological self* relates to a man's feelings about his masculinity. Many patients who have had a testicle removed (orchidectomy) describe themselves as no longer being a 'real man' or only 'half a man'. The patient may feel he is less virile and less able to perform sexually than before. Related to these feelings about masculinity are feelings about overall self-worth/esteem (see below).

2. *Loss of socio-cultural self* results from the stigma attached not just to the diagnosis of cancer but to disease of the genital organs. Although fears of sexual performance and fertility may be very real or completely unfounded, either way the disease will affect intimate sexual relationships.

3. *Loss of physical self* occurs in many ways after diagnosis and treatment. First, there's the loss of a testicle and a surgical scar from an inguinal incision. If the remaining testicle isn't functioning, testosterone production may be reduced, leading to reduced libido, hot flushes and a slowing of growth of facial hair. There's also likely to be a reduction in fertility. Both radiotherapy and chemotherapy will have similar effects to their use for any other form of cancer.

Patients with breast cancer and mastectomy

According to Willis (1998), a diagnosis of breast cancer is hard to cope with, especially if the recommended treatment is a mastectomy. Dealing with a life-threatening condition is made all the more difficult by the permanent change in body image that

ASK YOURSELF …

• Try to identify similarities and differences between men who've undergone an orchidectomy and women who've had a mastectomy, in terms of the three kinds of loss described above.

breast removal entails. For some women the psychological impact of losing a breast casts a shadow that remains even if the cancer is treated successfully.

Breast reconstruction (BR) can offer solace to some women, but it's not a choice that's automatically extended to everyone who would benefit or is suitable. Women referred to specialist breast care units are most likely to be offered BR, where they have access to plastic surgeons or general surgeons who have sub-specialised in breast cancer surgery and reconstruction. It's often the advocacy of the patient's breast care nurse that ensures women are offered this treatment (Willis, 1998).

Bredin (1999) believes that some women who have had a mastectomy aren't getting enough help in coping with their ABI. Although not all women have problems adjusting, those who do often conceal the fact from health professionals, who may be reluctant to broach the issue. Bredin claims that, 'Conventional management colludes with a sense that their feelings of loss and disfigurement should be kept secret.'

While it's expected that the loss of any part of the body is traumatic, the loss of a part invested with the significance of feminine identity and functioning is even more difficult (Dunn, 1988). In fact, mastectomy has been called one of the most prevalent sexually threatening experiences. Woods (1975, in Dunn) suggests that the loss of a breast has biological, psychological and socio-cultural implications for a woman's sexuality and sexual functioning (see the three kinds of loss involved in orchidectomy, above). For example, if the woman thinks her sexual partner will find the mastectomy mutilating, it can result in avoidance of sexual contact (Dunn, 1988).

This describes Pat's new body image. She was a woman who'd had a mastectomy, and was convinced her partner and family would be revolted by it (see my notes on page 96). At first she refused to let anyone except the Community Nurse and the doctor see it. When I said to Clare that mastectomy patients felt the same as her, she said bitterly, 'Yes, but at least theirs is clean.' I didn't say anything, but of course Pat's wound wasn't – it was discharging – and I realised they were both feeling the same disgust at their inability to control their hygiene.

Patients with HIV/AIDS

In a focused interview study, Firn and Norman (1995) attempted to describe how patients with AIDS and their nurses perceived the emotional and psychological issues faced by people with AIDS and the nurse's role in responding to these issues (see Chapter 3).

Changes in body image were identified by patients as a source of great emotional distress. An instrument designed to identify people at risk of developing a seriously ABI (Price, 1990) identifies three major components:

1. *Body reality* refers to our body as it really is and to the areas of the body that are altered in appearance, with changes in the face, hands and sexual organs potentially causing the greatest distress. These seem to be the areas most affected in HIV disease. For example, Kaposi's sarcoma (KS) is a type of skin cancer that commonly affects the face and is the most common primary tumour found in HIV disease. The lesions are often small, flat, dusky pink or violet areas of skin discolouration that progress, in weeks or months, to raised, painless, hard nodules. Although make-up can disguise many of the lesions and scars, the psychological implications have a massive impact on the patient's mental health (Jamieson, 1996). One of Firn and Norman's participants described it as making her feel 'like a leper'. Others described the very visible effects of weight loss and the distressing effects of repeated infections in the genital area, such as herpes and thrush.

2. *Body presentation* is how we present our body to the world (including how we dress, pose and move). Firn and Norman's participants repeatedly mentioned incontinence as being a particularly distressing loss of bodily control.

I believe the incontinence was Clare's main problem. She is a fastidious young woman; the presence, and more particularly the sight, of her incontinence is revolting to her.

3. *Body ideal* refers to our perceptions of how we expect our body to appear and function. As some people with AIDS are relatively young, it's reasonable to assume that they have high expectations from life and so are less prepared for debilitating illness than people with other potentially life-threatening conditions.

Firn and Norman found that nurses tended to underestimate the extent of the distress experienced by AIDS patients as a result of their ABIs. This is reflected in the AIDS literature (Firn and Norman, 1995).

Patients with a stoma

Stomas are surgically constructed openings made in the wall of the abdomen to eliminate faeces or urine, when obstruction or disease make it necessary to remove part of the normal elimination route (Pullen, 1998). An estimated 100,000 people in the UK have bowel or urinary stomas, with ileostomies, colostomies and urostomies being the most common.

Stomas inevitably change a patient's lifestyle. They must come to terms with altered physical control over their elimination processes, as well as the practicalities of wearing a bag and dealing with problems such as leakage or odour. They often feel frustrated, helpless, embarrassed or disgusted, but the loss of a positive body image can be the most significant difficulty (Pullen, 1998).

When the surgeon recommends an operation, from a strictly medical point of view there may be no good reason for delay – but, from a psychological perspective, delay may be necessary. Patients have to change the way they feel and think about themselves, come to terms with the fact that they're going to have a stoma, probably for the rest of their lives, and that they're going to undergo major surgery. All this has to be accepted and acknowledged as a reality, and involves a fundamental shift in their self-concept; this in itself is threatening (Kelly, 1994). The stoma excretes urine or faeces at will, rendering the patient incontinent. This can have a devastating effect on self-esteem. A bodily function that's usually tucked away out of sight and can be dealt with discreetly is suddenly the focus of attention (Taylor, 1994). Also, a lack of control over elimination can be perceived as returning (regressing) to childhood (Topping, 1990; see also Chapter 6).

Pullen (1998) notes that body image and sexuality are interrelated and both are important factors in the recovery of an ostomy patient. According to Topping (1990), research has consistently found that GPs, surgeons and nurses are unwilling or unable to help them with sexual difficulties.

Eulette's discussions with Clare at the clinic when she was first told she needed an ileostomy, at her home and on the day before her operation had addressed the fact of her permanent 'incontinence'. Eulette told me she'd also tried to discuss how it would affect her relationship with her boyfriend, but Clare had avoided this. I don't find it easy to discuss sexual relationships and told Eulette this. She said we must reassure Clare she could have a healthy sexual relationship and we should be prepared to suggest alternative positions and provide access to attractive coverings to keep the bag in place. It was helpful having positive suggestions to make and afterwards I felt confident enough to encourage Clare to discuss it.

> **Box 16.2 Sexual difficulties faced by stoma patients (based on Topping, 1990)**
>
> - Some male patients become impotent (the inability to have or sustain an erection firm enough for satisfactory intercourse). But there can be a return of erectile function over time and the less a man focuses on having hard erections, the less anxiety will impair what function remains. Treatment options include intercavernosal self-injection of papaverine, penile prostheses and vacuum devices. Careful counselling of both the patient and his partner is essential.
> - Dry orgasm (ejaculation) occurs due to damage to the parasympathetic nerves in the presacral area, or surgical trauma to the prostate, seminal vesicles or the bladder neck. So, some men don't actually ejaculate, while others ejaculate backwards into the bladder. Although the intensity of orgasm may not be disturbed, the experience is different. Any individual affected this way should be offered the opportunity to bank sperm pre-operatively.
> - Dyspareunia (painful intercourse) can result from anatomical changes such as shortening of the vaginal vault, damage to the posterior vaginal wall, or from changes in the volume of vaginal secretions.

Human beings are sexual beings, so sexuality should be an important aspect of nursing care (Taylor, 1994). According to Webb (1985, in Taylor, 1994), 'If nursing is to be truly holistic it must address such a basic part of humanity as sexuality within all care planning.'

However, sex still remains a subject that's avoided when patients are interviewed. Taylor quotes Lion (1982), who claims that, 'Nurses who are comfortable with their own sexuality and the sexuality of others, who have a sexual health knowledge base and who cultivate sensitive and perceptive communication skills, can effectively integrate sex into the nursing process.'

Having been happily married (for a time), I do understand the importance of a good sexual relationship and feel ashamed I have avoided the subject with patients until now. I need to develop the necessary communication skills to talk to patients about it without getting embarrassed. Eulette's matter-of-fact attitude and subsequently talking to Clare has helped; I'll find it easier in future.

Patients with a facial disfigurement

According to Kelly (1990), particular attention has been paid to the effects of breast and bowel cancer and the resultant devastation on the body. But rather less attention (or certainly less publicity) has been given to the effects of a totally *visible* ABI. Surely it's reasonable to assume that a visible change (such as involved in maxillo-facial surgery or facial disfigurement caused by accidents) would cause even more anxiety than one that can be hidden, at least for some of the time, from a partner, and, if one chooses, nearly always from the casual observer.

Clare is able to keep her 'altered body' hidden; if she couldn't do this, I think the task of adjusting to her stoma would be much harder for her.

Surprisingly, oral cancer hasn't been a major focus for psychological research despite the great personal and social significance of the oral cavity and the high mortality rate with more advanced tumours (McEleney, 1992). Surgery for facial cancer results in a permanent, visible alteration of the face that's difficult to disguise. It seems to be only after surgery that facial cancer patients reflect on what mutilation means to them (Barrit, 1982, in McEleney, 1992) – only then do they realise that part of their face is missing (Dropkin, 1979, in McEleney, 1992). If the face is regarded as the outward expression of our inner selves, used to convey all sorts of unspoken messages, what happens to the person whose expression is permanently dictated by external factors, regardless of how s/he might be feeling (Griffiths, 1989)?

Because of its unexpected occurrence, a facial malformation at an advanced age causes a violent mental shock (Barrit, 1977, in McEleney, 1992). Facially disfigured people have more difficulties accepting and adjusting to a new self-image than those who've been deformed since birth and who have regarded this from the beginning as part of themselves (Wellisch *et al.*, 1983, in McEleney, 1992).

Looking in the mirror for the first time and getting used to doing this represents one of the biggest hurdles in the process of recovery (Partridge, 1990, in McEleney, 1992). Patients are confronted with the 'death' of their visual appearance and can be left with a face they may not consider their own (Griffiths, 1989).

Speech, chewing and swallowing are the three main functions commonly affected following treatment to the head and neck, but hearing, vision, taste, smell and sexual expression may also be affected (Kelly, 1990).

Radical surgery is often the treatment of choice for head and neck cancer. The patient, fearing cosmetic disfigurement and functional deficits of speech and swallowing, may be indecisive about the proposed surgery. Nurses are in a unique position to support a patient's decision whether to go ahead with the surgery (Koster and Bergoma, 1990, in McEleney, 1992). They can help the patient to understand the planned surgery, giving further information and discussing the care involved. However, nurses must maintain a positive and supportive attitude if the patient and their family are to be reassured about the surgery being the right course, however radical it may be (McEleney, 1992).

Tschudin (2003) says that full explanations of the details of what, why and how something is being done have to be **offered**, not given only if patients ask for them, and that informed consent can mean saying no as well as yes.

SELF-ESTEEM

While the self-image is essentially *descriptive*, self-esteem (or *self-regard*) is essentially *evaluative*. It refers to how much we like and approve of ourselves, how worthy a person we think we are. Coopersmith (1967) defined it as 'a personal judgement of worthiness, that is expressed in the attitudes the individual holds towards himself'.

How much we like or value ourselves can be an overall judgement, or it can relate to specific areas of our lives. For example, we can have a generally high opinion of ourselves and yet not like certain of our characteristics or attributes (such as our curly hair when we want it straight, or our lack of assertiveness when we want to be more assertive). Conversely, it may be very difficult to have high overall esteem if we're very badly disfigured, or are desperately shy.

Our self-esteem can be regarded as how we evaluate our self-image – that is, how much we like the kind of person we think we are. Clearly, certain characteristics or abilities have a greater value in society generally, and so are likely to influence our self-esteem accordingly – for example, being physically attractive as opposed to unattractive (see Chapter 8). The value attached to particular characteristics will also depend on culture, gender, age and social background (see Gross, 2005).

It was obvious that much of Clare's self-esteem comes from her appearance – her image of herself as an attractive, glamorous young woman – and her job, which is centred around that image.

CRITICAL DISCUSSION 16.1 Is self-esteem all it's cracked up to be?

- According to Fiske (2004), the benefits of high self-esteem are real, but they can be taken too far: 'Nowadays, self-esteem is all the rage, as attested by the self-help section of the nearest bookstore: Self-esteem is the great cure-all, the great panacea for the problems that ail us …'

- But Baumeister (1998) has begun to debunk this myth – in the context of violence and aggression. In a review of the research literature, Baumeister *et al*. (1996) concluded that some of the most aggressive people have incredibly *high* self-esteem. Violence becomes more likely when another person or situation contradicts a person's highly favourable view of themselves.

- Such individuals' self-esteem is also *fragile* and *inflated*. It's this combination that makes them so easily threatened. Violence and aggression may be an attempt at self-protection. Murder, rape, assault and domestic violence are often associated with threats to honour and feelings of male superiority.

Part of Clare's recovery may depend on her ability to derive self-esteem from qualities she has apart from her physical appearance. I know she has a friendly, open and bubbly personality, and takes pleasure from making others feel good about themselves.

THE IDEAL SELF

Self-esteem is also partly determined by how much the self-image differs from the *ideal self*. If our self-image is the kind of person we think we are, then our ideal self (*ego-ideal* or *idealised self-image*) is the kind of person we'd *like to be*. This can vary in extent and degree. We may want to be different in certain aspects, or we may want to be a totally different person. (We may even wish we were someone else!) Generally, the greater the gap between our self-image and our ideal self, the lower our self-esteem (see Rogers' *self theory*, in Gross, 2005).

Most people have a complex self-concept with a relatively large number of *self-schemata* (complex and clear information relating to various aspects of ourselves). These include an array of *possible* selves, *future-orientated* schemata of what we'd like to become (ideal self) (Markus and Nurius, 1986). Visions of future possible selves may influence how we make important life decisions, such as career choice.

The idea of *multiple selves* raises the question of whether there's any one self that's more real or authentic than the others. For example, perhaps we feel most real (most 'ourselves') when with someone we believe sees us as we wish to be seen. Personality theorists tend to assume that the person has a single, unitary self. This is implied by the fact that typical instructions at the top of a personality questionnaire don't specify which self the respondent should describe (Hampson, 1995). By contrast, social psychologists recognise the possibility that the self refers to a complex set of perceptions, composed of a number of schemata relating both to what we're like and how we *could be*.

Before her surgery Clare's self-image and her ideal self were much closer together, in spite of her illness. Now, her body image has been made different, her self-image falls short of her ideal self and threatens at least one future schema – to have a lasting sexual relationship.

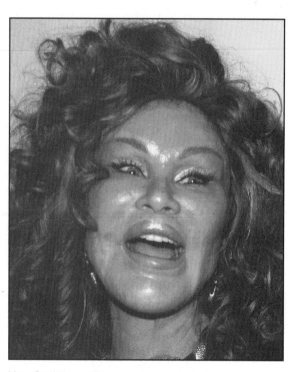

Jocelyne Wildenstein (the 'Cat Woman') has had several plastic surgery procedures to make herself look like a cat

DEVELOPMENTAL CHANGES IN THE SELF-CONCEPT

HOW DO WE GET TO KNOW OURSELVES?

Achieving identity, in the sense of acquiring a set of beliefs about the self (a *self-schema*), is one of the central developmental tasks of a social being (Lewis, 1990). It progresses through several levels of complexity and continues to develop through the lifespan (see Chapters 17–19).

During the first few months, the baby gradually distinguishes itself from its environment and from other people, and develops a sense of *continuity through time* (the *existential self*). But at this stage, the infant's self-knowledge is comparable to that of other species (such as monkeys). What makes human self-knowledge distinctive is becoming aware that we have it – we're conscious of our existence and uniqueness (Buss, 1992).

According to Maccoby (1980), babies are able to distinguish between themselves and others on two counts:

1. their own fingers hurt when bitten (but they don't have any such sensations when they're biting their rattle or their mother's fingers)
2. probably quite early in life, they begin to associate feelings from their own body movements with the sight of their own limbs and the sounds of their own cries. These sense impressions are bound together into a cluster that defines the *bodily self*, so this is probably the first aspect of the self-concept to develop.

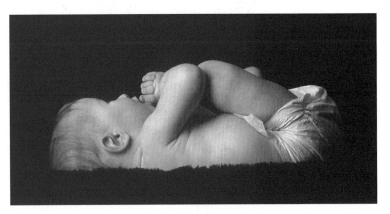

A baby acquiring its bodily self

Other aspects of the self-concept develop by degrees, but there seem to be fairly clearly defined stages of development. Young children may know their own names and understand the limits of their own bodies and yet be unable to think about themselves as coherent entities. So, self-awareness/self-consciousness develops very gradually.

According to Piaget, an awareness of self comes through the gradual process of *adaptation to the environment* (see Chapter 15). As the child explores objects and accommodates to them (thus developing new *sensorimotor schemas*), it simultaneously discovers aspects of its self. For example, trying to put a large block into its mouth and finding that it won't fit is a lesson in selfhood, as well as a lesson about the world of objects.

Self-recognition

One way in which the development of bodily self has been studied is through *self-recognition*; this involves more than just a simple discrimination of bodily features. To determine that the person in a photograph or a film or reflected in a mirror is oneself, certain knowledge seems to be necessary:

◎ at least a rudimentary knowledge of oneself as continuous through time (necessary for recognising ourselves in photographs or movies) and space (necessary for recognising ourselves in mirrors), and
◎ knowledge of particular features (what we look like).

Although other kinds of self-recognition are possible (e.g. one's voice or feelings), only *visual* self-recognition has been studied extensively, both in humans and non-humans.

A number of researchers (e.g. Lewis and Brooks-Gunn, 1979) have used modified forms of Gallup's technique with 6–24-month-old children. The mother applies a dot of rouge (blusher) to the child's nose (while pretending to wipe its face) and the child is observed to see how often it touches its nose. It's then placed in front of a mirror and again the number of times it touches its nose is recorded. At about 18 months, there's a significant change. While touching the dot was never seen before 15 months, between 15 and 18 months, 5–25 per cent of infants touched it and 75 per cent of the 18–20-month-olds did.

In order to use the mirror image to touch the dot on its nose, the baby must also have built up a schema of how its face should look in the mirror before (otherwise, it wouldn't notice the discrepancy created by the dot). This doesn't develop before about 18 months. This is also about the time when, according to Piaget, *object permanence* is completed, so object permanence would seem to be a necessary condition for the development of self-recognition (see Chapter 15).

I've seen photos of Clare when she was younger; in all of them she has pretty clothes and looks attractive, so she has grown up with an image of herself like that.

Self-definition

Piaget, Mead and many others have pointed to the importance of language in consolidating the early development of self-awareness, by providing labels that permit distinctions between self and not-self ('I', 'you', 'me', 'it'). The toddler can then use these labels to communicate notions of selfhood to others. One important kind of label is the child's *name*.

Names aren't usually chosen arbitrarily – either the parents particularly like the name, or they want to name the child after a relative or famous person. Names aren't neutral labels in terms of how people respond to them and what they associate with them. Indeed, they can be used as the basis for *stereotyping* (see Chapter 8 and Gross, 2005).

When children refer to themselves as 'I' (or 'me') and others as 'you', they're having to reverse the labels that are normally used to refer to them by others ('you', 'he', 'she'). Also, of course, they hear others refer to themselves as 'I' and not as 'you', 'he' or 'she'. This is a problem of *shifting reference*. Despite this, most children don't invert 'I' and 'you'. However, two interesting exceptions are autistic and blind children, who often use 'I' for others and 'you' for self (see Gross, 2005).

The psychological self

Maccoby (1980) asks what children mean when they refer to themselves as 'I' or 'me'. Are they referring to anything more than a physical entity enclosed by an envelope of skin?

KEY STUDY 16.1 There's more to children than meets the eye (Flavell *et al.*, 1978)

- Flavell *et al.* (1978) investigated development of the psychological self in two-and-a-half- to five-year-olds.
- In one study, a doll was placed on the table in front of the child, and it was explained that dolls are like people in some ways – they have arms, legs, hands, and so on (which were pointed to). Then the child was asked how dolls are different from people, whether they know their names and think about things, and so on. Most children said a doll doesn't know its name and cannot think about things, but people can.

- They were then asked, 'Where is the part of you that knows your name and thinks about things?' and 'Where do you do your thinking and knowing?' A total of 14 out of 22 children gave fairly clear localisation for the thinking self, namely 'in their heads', while others found it very difficult. The experimenter then looked directly into the child's eyes and asked, 'Can I see you thinking in there?' Most children thought not.

These answers suggest that by three-and-a-half-to-four-years, a child has a rudimentary concept of a private, thinking self that's not visible even to someone looking directly into its eyes. The child can distinguish this from the bodily self, which it knows is visible to others. In other words, by about age four, children begin to develop a *theory of mind*, the awareness that they – and other people – have mental processes (e.g. Leekam, 1993; Shatz, 1994; Wellman, 1990). However, one group failing to develop a theory of mind is that of autistic children (see Gross, 2005).

The categorical self

Age and *gender* are both parts of the central core of the self-image. They represent two of the categories regarding the self that are also used to perceive and interpret the behaviour of others.

Age is probably the first social category to be acquired by the child (and is so even before a concept of number develops). Lewis and Brooks-Gunn (1979) found that 6- to 12-month-olds can distinguish between photographs, slides and papier-mâché heads of adults and babies. By 12 months, they prefer interacting with unfamiliar babies to unfamiliar adults. Also, as soon as they've acquired labels like 'mummy', 'daddy' and 'baby', they almost never make age-related mistakes.

Before age seven, children tend to define the self in *physical* terms: hair colour, height, favourite activities and possessions. Inner, psychological experiences and characteristics aren't described as being distinct from overt behaviour and external, physical characteristics. During middle childhood through to adolescence, self-descriptions now include many more references to internal, psychological characteristics, such as competencies, knowledge, emotions, values and personality traits (Damon and Hart, 1988). However, Damon and Hart also report important cultural differences in how the self-concept develops (see Gross, 2005).

School highlights others' expectations about how the self should develop. It also provides a social context in which new goals are set and comparisons with others (peers) are prompted. This makes evaluation of the self all the more important (Durkin, 1995). This comparison becomes more important still during adolescence (see Chapter 17).

If she is to adapt successfully to her new condition, Clare's attitudes to her self-concept have to change. In our culture, the importance of physical attractiveness is learned at an early age; until now it has been the taken-for-granted source of Clare's self-esteem.

Price's (1990) definition of altered body image from an external source (surgery) applies to Clare. Blackmore's (1989) three dimensions of loss – physical, psychological and socio-cultural – are useful and help me understand the many changes Clare has to adapt to.

I realise the resources of the specialist stoma nurse were invaluable. She provided Clare with practical suggestions, arranged visits from other (successfully adjusted) ileostomy patients of Clare's age, and shared her expertise with ward staff and students.

A positive reaction and support from Clare's family and boyfriend, and the nurses who care for her, should help her regain a positive, if altered, self-concept.

CHAPTER SUMMARY

◎ An important distinction is that between **consciousness** and self-**consciousness/ awareness**. Self-awareness allows us to see ourselves as others see us.

◎ An important distinction is made between the **private** and **public** self.

◎ Our **self-concept** refers to our perception of our personality, and comprises the **self-image** (which includes **body image/bodily self**), **self-esteem** and **ideal self**.

◎ Components of body image include **body reality**, **body presentation** and **body ideal**.

◎ Patients with a wide range of diseases and conditions are likely to experience an **altered body image** (**ABI**), whose effects can be particularly distressing when sexual desire and performance are involved.

◎ The self-concept develops in fairly regular, predictable ways. During the first few months, the **existential self** emerges, but the **bodily self** is probably the first aspect of the self-concept to develop.

◎ The bodily self has been studied through (mainly visual) **self-recognition in mirrors**. Self-recognition appears at about 18 months in children, and is also found in chimps.

◎ **Self-definition** is related to the use of language, including the use of labels, such as names. By three and a half to four, children seem to have a basic understanding of a **psychological self** (or **'theory of mind'**).

◎ **Age** and **gender** are two basic features of the **categorical self**. The categorical self changes from being described in **physical** to more **psychological** terms during middle childhood through to adolescence.

ADOLESCENCE 17

INTRODUCTION AND OVERVIEW

The word 'adolescence' comes from the Latin *adolescere* meaning 'to grow into maturity'. As well as being a time of enormous physiological change, adolescence is marked by changes in behaviour, expectations and relationships with both parents and peers. In western, industrialised societies, there's generally no single initiation rite signalling the passage into adulthood. This makes the transition more difficult than it appears to be in more traditional, non-industrialised societies. Relationships with adults in general, and parents in particular, must be renegotiated in a way that allows the adolescent to achieve greater independence. This process is aided by changing relationships with peers.

Historically, adolescence has been seen as a period of transition between childhood and adulthood. But writers today are more likely to describe it as one of *multiple transitions*, involving education, training, employment and unemployment, as well as transitions from one set of living circumstances to another (Coleman and Roker, 1998).

This change in perspective in many ways reflects changes in the adolescent experience compared with those of previous generations: it starts five years earlier, marriage takes place six to seven years later than it did, and cohabitation, perhaps as a prelude to marriage, is rapidly increasing (Coleman and Hendry, 1990). Passage into

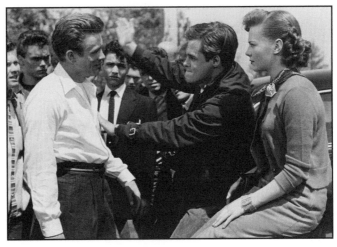

1950s films such as *Rebel Without A Cause*, starring James Dean (left), have been seen as helping to create the concept of the 'rebellious teenager'

adulthood may also be deferred by the delay in acquiring an income: not only has there been an extension in compulsory education, but pressure on the workforce to become more highly skilled places a premium on continuing education (Hendry, 1999).

Coupled with these 'adulthood-postponing' changes, in recent years adolescents have enjoyed greater self-determination at steadily younger ages. Yet this greater freedom carries with it more risks and greater costs when errors of judgement are made. As Hendry (1999) says:

> ... 'dropping out' of school, being out of work, teenage pregnancy, sexually transmitted diseases, being homeless, drug addiction and suicide, are powerful examples of the price that some young people pay for their extended freedom ...

From my diary (16): Year 2/Surgical Ward

One of my allocated patients today was 16-year-old Josh, admitted from A&E at 3 am after being found drunk in a doorway. He had a left temporal contusion, a Glasgow Coma Score (GCS) of 13 and was on hourly neurological observations. The HO had ordered a computed tomogram (CT) scan to exclude neural trauma. Sister suggested I went with Josh. When we arrived in X-ray, the radiographer (Winston) explained to Josh (and me) what was going to happen and kept reassuring him he'd be in the scanner for a very short time. After the initial lateral picture, Winston suggested that, while he set up for the main picture, I should go back in to keep Josh company as he seemed apprehensive – some people found the scanner claustrophobic. I did as he suggested (reproaching myself for not noticing). When we returned to the ward, Josh's mother (Anna) had arrived. I took her to Josh, who burst into tears. I pulled the curtains round the bed while she comforted him, and left them to talk. Later, Sister asked Anna if she minded me sitting in while they discussed Josh.

ASK YOURSELF ...
- What kinds of transition do adolescents in western societies experience?

- Are they necessarily the same for all adolescents?

NORMATIVE AND NON-NORMATIVE SHIFTS

One way of categorising the various transitions involved in adolescence is in terms of *normative* and *non-normative shifts* (Hendry and Kloep, 1999; Kloep and Hendry, 1999).

◎ *Normative, maturational shifts* include the growth spurt (both sexes), menarche (first menstruation), first nocturnal emissions ('wet dreams'), voice breaking (boys), changes in sexual organs, beginning of sexual arousal, changed romantic relationships, gender-role identity, changed relationships with adults, increasing autonomy and responsibility.

◎ *Normative, society-dependent shifts* include the change from primary to secondary school, leaving school, getting started in an occupation, acquiring legal rights for voting, sex, purchasing alcohol, driving licence, military service, and cohabitation.

◎ *Non-normative shifts* include parental divorce, family bereavement, illness (see below), natural disasters, war, incest, emigration, disruption of peer network, risk-taking behaviours, 'disadvantage' (because of gender, class, regional or ethnic discrimination), physical and/or mental handicap.

According to Kloep and Hendry (1999):

> Although all adolescents have to cope with the psychosocial challenges associated with their maturing body, new relationships with parents and peers, with school and the transitions toward employment, a growing number encounter additional problems like family disruption, economic deprivation or social or cultural changes ...

A normative shift may become non-normative, if, say, there are other circumstances that cause a normal developmental 'task' to become more difficult. An example would be the unusually early or late onset of puberty.

Anna told us that Josh is a bright boy and, although he has no idea what he wants to do, he's going into the sixth form and is expected to go to university. These would all be normative shifts for Josh. She also confided that she was a single mother, having been divorced a year ago: a non-normative shift for both her and Josh.

PUBERTY: THE SOCIAL AND PSYCHOLOGICAL MEANING OF BIOLOGICAL CHANGES

PUBERTY AND BODY IMAGE

Adjusting to puberty is one of the most important adjustments that adolescents have to make (Coleman and Hendry, 1990). Even as a purely biological phenomenon, puberty is far from being a simple, straightforward process. While all adolescents experience the same bodily changes (see Box 17.1 and Figure 17.1), the sequence of changes may vary within individuals (*intraindividual asynchronies*: Alsaker, 1996). For example, for some girls menstruation may occur very early on in puberty, while for others it may occur after most other changes (e.g. growth spurt, breast development) have taken place.

Major changes in puberty

Physiologically, puberty begins when the seminal vesicles and prostate gland enlarge in the male, and the ovaries enlarge in the female. Both males and females experience the

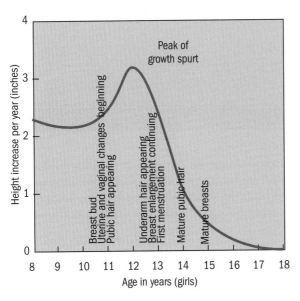
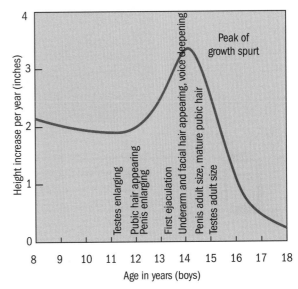

Figure 17.1 The development of secondary sex characteristics. The curved lines represent the average increase in height from 8 to 18 years of age. The characteristics shown may occur earlier or later in a person's development, but usually occur in the order shown (based on Tanner, 1978, and Tanner & Whitehouse, 1976). Reproduced with the permission of the copyright holders, Castlemead Publications.

adolescent growth spurt. Male *secondary sex characteristics* include growth of pubic and then chest and facial hair, and sperm production. In females, breast size increases, pubic hair grows and menstruation begins.

Anna said Josh had grown rapidly from 12 to 14; he is now 6'2" and physically mature. The need to physically adjust to his new body could explain Anna's comment that Josh is awkward, always breaking things.

Box 17.1 Adolescents' brains

- According to some neuroscientists, the brain undergoes some fundamental restructuring during adolescence, just as it does during the earliest years of childhood. While the *plasticity* of the infant's and young child's brain is widely accepted (see Gross, 2005), this has traditionally been seen as stopping at puberty.

- However, two MRI studies, one *longitudinal* (which followed up the same set of youngsters over several years: Giedd *et al*., 1999), the other *cross-sectional* (which compared a group of 14-year-olds with a group in their mid-twenties: Sowell *et al*., 1999), suggest otherwise.

- Areas of the cortex that deal with more basic functions, such as sensory and motor processing, do indeed stabilise in early childhood. But the parietal and frontal lobes, which are specialised for visuospatial and 'executive functions' (e.g. planning and self-control) respectively, show a *growth surge* between the ages of 10 and 12.

- This sudden 'bulking up' is then followed by an equally dramatic *reduction* in size, which continues right through the teenage years and into the early twenties. The grey-matter density decreases, indicating that the number of synaptic connections have become fewer (consistent with the theory that a mature brain involves the 'pruning' of connections in order to strengthen those that remain). It stops only when these areas have reached their adult proportions.

- This late shrinkage is taken to be a sign of maturation.

- According to Rapoport (in Connor, 2004), 'One could speculate that some of the more immature aspects of adolescent behaviour may be due to the lack of maturity of some parts of the frontal lobes of the brain.'

(Based on McCrone, 2000)

Anna said Josh had become 'a stranger' over the last year. Previously good-natured, he'd become defiant, and often didn't come home at night, saying he was sleeping at friends' houses. When he was at home, he was anti-social and uncooperative, and he had recently become subject to unpredictable mood swings. Anna's worried he's taking drugs.

According to Davies and Furnham (1986), the average adolescent isn't only sensitive to, but also critical of, his or her changing physical self. Because of gender and sexual development, young people are inevitably confronted, perhaps for the first time, by cultural standards of beauty in evaluating their own body images (via the media and the reactions of others). This may produce a *non-normative shift* in the form of dieting practices, leading to eating disorders (see Gross, 2005). Young people may be especially vulnerable to teasing and exclusion if they're perceived by their peers as over- or under-weight (Kloep and Hendry, 1999).

I'd noticed Josh had acne, and asked Anna when it had started. She said it had been gradual and she guessed over a year ago. She knew he was self-conscious about it and had bought him all the special skin preparations that were advertised. She'd tried to 'joke him out of it'.

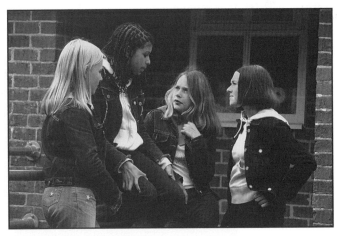

The need to not be different

ASK YOURSELF …
- Do you consider puberty to be a more difficult transition for boys or girls *in general*?

- Why?

GENDER DIFFERENCES

While puberty may be a normative, maturational shift, it may be a more difficult transition for girls than boys. This is because of the *subjective meaning* of bodily change (what it means for the individual), which mirrors the *socio-cultural significance* of puberty (its significance for society). According to the *cultural ideal hypothesis* (CIH) (Simmons and Blyth, 1987), puberty will bring boys *closer* to their physical ideal (an increase in muscle distribution and lung capacity produces greater stamina, strength and athletic capacities), while girls move *further away* from theirs.

For girls, who begin puberty on average two years ahead of boys, it's normal to experience an increase in body fat and rapid weight gain, thus making their bodies less like the western cultural ideal of the thin, sylph-like supermodel. In addition, they have to deal with menstruation, which is negatively associated with blood and physical discomfort (Crawford and Unger, 1995).

However, the onset of menstruation is regarded as a clear delineation of girls' sexual maturity, almost a rite of passage?

THE IMPORTANCE OF TIMING

If the CIH is valid, it follows that *early maturing boys* will be at an *advantage* relative to their 'on-time' and late-maturing peers (they'll be moving faster towards the male ideal). By the same token, *early maturing girls* will be at a *disadvantage* (they'll be moving faster away from the female ideal). As Bergevin *et al.* (2003) put it:

> … girls who enter puberty early relative to other girls are typically far ahead of virtually all boys. Likewise, boys who enter puberty late are far behind most boys and behind almost all girls. These two sets of adolescents, early-maturing girls and late-maturing boys, are those who are clearly most out of step with their peers …

Indeed, according to Alsaker (1996), '... pubertal timing is generally regarded as a more crucial aspect of pubertal development than pubertal maturation itself'. In other words, it's not the *fact* of puberty that matters as much as *when* it occurs, and it matters mainly in relation to body image and self-esteem.

According to his mother, Josh's puberty was early but not traumatic; for Josh it also brought with it clumsiness and acne, which wasn't good for his self-esteem.

> ### Box 17.2 The falling age of puberty onset
>
> - One in six girls reaches puberty by the age of eight, compared with 1 in 100 a generation ago. Also, 1 in 14 eight-year-old boys has pubic hair (an early indicator of puberty), compared with 1 in 150 of their fathers' generation.
>
> - Bristol University's Institute of Child Health tracked the development of 1150 children from birth. It's the first study of puberty in Britain since the 1960s (see Figure 17.1). Not only are children starting puberty earlier, but it's lasting longer. The reasons are unclear, but likely causes are higher oestrogen levels in mothers, diet, lifestyle and pollution. There could also be a genetic link, since the mothers of girls who begin puberty earlier also matured earlier.
>
> - Separate research has found that the average age of menarche has fallen below 13 in Britain for the first time. It's now 12 years 10 months, compared with 13 years 6 months in 1969.
>
> - These findings mean that children could be developing sexually before they have the emotional maturity to deal with the possible consequences.
>
> (Based on Peek, 2000)

ASK YOURSELF ...
- A common finding is that early-maturing girls and late-maturing boys suffer lower self-esteem. Why do you think this might be?

When they searched Josh's pockets for some identification, they found cigarettes, a lighter and a packet of condoms – so it looks as though Josh may already be sexually active.

◎ One popular explanation is the *deviancy hypothesis* (DH), according to which those who are 'off-time' in physical maturation are socially deviant compared with peers of the same age and gender (Wichstrom, 1998). Since girls begin puberty on average two years before boys, early-maturing girls are the first to enter this deviant position, followed by late-maturing boys.

◎ An alternative explanation is the *developmental readiness hypothesis* (DRH) (Simmons and Blyth, 1987). In the case of early or sudden puberty, too little time will have been spent on ego development during latency, with early-maturing girls once more being most affected. (This explanation is similar to Coleman's *focal theory* – see page 328.)

◎ As far as the CIH is concerned, the suggestion that the pubertal girl moves further away from the western stereotyped female ideal may *not* be true. *Both* boys and girls move closer to their ideals, provided they don't put on excessive weight (Wichstrom, 1998).

According to Wichstrom, the CIH is sensitive to changes in time and context. For example, in Norway there may be less emphasis on stereotypical male stature compared with the USA and UK. Perhaps also the embarrassment and negative affect experienced by American girls when starting their periods and becoming sexually responsive are less prevalent among Norwegian girls, due to relatively greater openness about adolescent sexuality (Wichstrom, 1998).

Anna said she had tried to talk to Josh about sex once or twice, but they were both embarrassed. He said they had sex education at school and 'knew all about it'. Sister explained there was a system for referral to the school nurse where Josh could have help if he wanted it.

ADOLESCENTS IN HOSPITAL

ASK YOURSELF ...
- What are some of the major problems that adolescent patients are likely to experience compared with children on the one hand, and adults on the other? (You may find it useful to look back at Piaget's theory (Chapter 15) and research into altered body image/ABI (Chapter 16).)

CRITICAL DISCUSSION 17.1 Adolescents in hospital: do they have special needs?

- Young people who need hospital care can find themselves admitted to either adult or children's wards. This is despite recommendations by the Platt Report (1959), the British Paediatric Association (1985) and the WHO (1986) to provide specialised wards designed to meet the needs of teenagers (Gillies, 1992).

- Hospitals concentrate on addressing young people's physical problems but tend to neglect their emotional needs. Also, there's no special training in caring for adolescents, so health professionals tend to be less aware of their needs and their rights as individuals. Part of the nurse's role is to help patients settle into the often unfamiliar and potentially threatening environment of a hospital ward; this is a particularly difficult role if little is known about the patient's needs, which the available facilities fail to meet (Gillies, 1992).

- Acute or chronic illness, hospitalisation and terminal admission all affect adolescent developmental issues (Kuykendall, 1989). In relation to body image, Kuykendall gives the example of a 14-year-old girl with spina bifida and hydrocephalus who'd had her shunt revised throughout her life without any complications. Everyone assumed that this very sophisticated patient would be able to handle the latest lengthening of the catheter perfectly well, because she'd had it done so many times before. But in hospital she became hysterical and at home she became reclusive.

- Adolescents are highly sensitive about their appearance, and any deformity or imperfection can cause feelings of shame and disgust (Tait *et al.*, 1982, in Burt, 1995). Adolescents with cancer may be particularly vulnerable to the effects of a disrupted body image. In addition, nurses may be reluctant to discuss sexual matters with the adolescent patient, and may contribute to adolescents with cancer being ignored as sexual beings (Burt, 1995; see also Chapter 16).

- Weller (1985, in Farrelly, 1994) identifies a number of special needs of adolescents in hospital.

- Adolescents' ability to think about situations they've not actually experienced can induce anxiety and depression (see Chapter 16). For example, they can imagine what might happen in their lives as a result of hospitalisation, such as in terms of their college and occupational prospects, and the possible long-term effects of giving up school. Denholm (1987, in Farrelly, 1994) reports that the anticipation of missing school, falling behind and then the need to make up the missed school work can produce significant anxiety. Muller *et al.* (1988, in Farrelly, 1994) confirm that it can be acutely distressing if hospitalisation disrupts exams.

- Similarly, adolescents understand that an amputation has implications for the future, often inducing depression. In contrast, a young child who has a leg amputated goes home and still talks about becoming a fireman when he grows up (Kuykendall, 1989).

- Adolescents have a relatively adult picture of life and death. Although they may find it difficult to discuss, adolescents who are seriously ill will be thinking about death (MacKenzie, 1988, in Farrelly, 1994). They may display a great deal of anger at the prospect of dying before achieving their ambitions, which may prove a barrier to communication (Brook, 1986, in Farrelly, 1994; see also Chapter 20).

- Lack of privacy as another problem for adolescents in hospital. Wards often provide little privacy, which, together with physical examinations, treatments and maintaining hygiene, can embarrass these young people, who are already acutely aware of their bodies.

At 16, Josh should be treated as an adult. Section 8 of the Family Law and Reform Act 1969 says that, at 16, minors can give valid consent to treatment – treatment covers all nursing care (Dimond, 2003). But the adult ward isn't a suitable place for Josh – he's in a bay with three elderly men; one is confused and incontinent. There are no distractions like games, TV or computers as there are on the children's ward; however, he would be equally out of place there. We need a ward for adolescents!

As Gillies (1992) points out, adolescence involves developing a sense of independence, by making decisions and having increased responsibility for their everyday lives (see below). But hospitalisation can threaten this role by 'infanticising' teenagers: they can revert from being increasingly independent at home to being dependent in hospital. Many in-patients have chronic conditions that may result in readmission. Some often take medicines at home or need special care, such as stoma care or regular physiotherapy. Having become used to performing self-care at home, including being responsible for their own medications, readmission to hospital restricts that independence – especially in relation to medication. Relaxing the regulations and guidelines could mean more continuity for those adolescents considered to be responsible (Gillies, 1992).

Josh's behaviour at home indicates he is trying to assert his independence; so, although his mother understandably wishes to take charge, we should defer to his wishes as far as possible.

THEORIES OF ADOLESCENCE

HALL'S THEORY: ADOLESCENCE AS STORM AND STRESS

This is probably the earliest formal theory of adolescence. Hall (1904) saw adolescence as a time of 'storm and stress' (or *Sturm und Drang*) and there is some evidence suggesting that emotional reactions are more *intense* and *volatile* during adolescence compared with other periods of life (see Gross, 2005). However, a more important indicator of storm and stress is mental disorder.

Studies of mental disorder

Several studies have found that *early-maturing girls* score higher on measures of depressive feelings and sadness (e.g. Alsaker, 1992; Stattin and Magnusson, 1990), although this was true only when the measures were taken before or simultaneously with changing schools (Petersen *et al.*, 1991). They've also been reported to have more psychosomatic (psychophysiological) symptoms (e.g. Stattin and Magnusson, 1990), to display greater concerns about eating (e.g. Brooks–Gunn *et al.*, 1989), and to score higher on measures of emotional disturbance (e.g. Brooks–Gunn and Warren, 1985).

As far as *early-maturing boys* are concerned, the evidence is much more mixed (Alsaker, 1996). While early maturation is usually found to be advantageous, it's also been found to be associated with more psychopathology (e.g. Petersen and Crockett, 1985), depressive tendencies and anxiety (e.g. Alsaker, 1992).

Based on their study of a large, representative sample of 14–15 year olds (more than 2000), Rutter *et al.* (1976) concluded that:

◎ there's a rather modest peak in psychiatric disorders in adolescence

◎ although severe clinical depression is rare, some degree of inner turmoil may characterise a sizeable minority of adolescents; while it's not a myth, neither should it be exaggerated

◎ a substantial proportion of those adolescents with psychiatric problems had had them since childhood. Also, when problems did first appear during adolescence, they were mainly associated with stressful situations (such as parents' marital discord) – 'adolescent turmoil is fact, not fiction, but its psychiatric importance has probably been overestimated in the past' (Rutter *et al.*, 1976).

In western societies, while some adolescents may display affective disturbances or disorders, it's a relatively small minority who'll show clinical depression or report 'inner turmoil' (Compas *et al.*, 1995). Instead, the majority worry about everyday issues, such as school and examination performance, finding work, family and social relationships, self-image, conflicts with authority, and the future generally (Gallagher *et al.*, 1992).

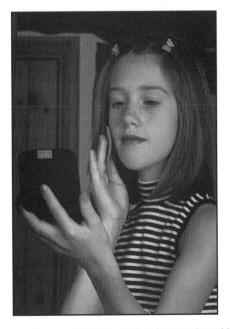

Pre-teens are growing up faster than ever before, and early-maturing girls are most at risk of mental disorder and delinquency

Anna's concerns about Josh support Gallagher et al.'s (1992) findings. She said Josh is 'the anxious type' – he worried a great deal about his recent GCSE exams. Since she and his father split up, Josh has become increasingly angry and resentful; she feels he blames her. He's concerned about his appearance and constantly challenges her authority.

ERIKSON'S THEORY: IDENTITY CRISIS

Erikson (1963) believed that it's human nature to pass through a genetically determined sequence of *psychosocial stages*, spanning the whole lifespan. Each stage involves a struggle between two conflicting personality outcomes, one of which is positive (or *adaptive*), while the other is negative (or *maladaptive*). Healthy development involves the adaptive outweighing the maladaptive.

The major challenge of adolescence is to establish a strong sense of *personal identity*. The dramatic onset of puberty – combined with more sophisticated intellectual abilities (see Chapter 16) – makes adolescents particularly concerned with finding their own personal place in adult society.

In western societies adolescence is a *moratorium*, an authorised delay of adulthood, which frees adolescents from most responsibilities and helps them make the difficult transition from childhood to adulthood. Although this is meant to make the transition easier, it can also have the opposite effect. Most of the societies studied by cultural anthropologists have important public ceremonies to mark the transition from childhood to adulthood. This is in stark contrast to western, industrialised nations, which leave children to their own devices in finding their identity. Without a clearly defined procedure to follow, this process can be difficult – both for adolescents and for their parents (see *Generation gap* below).

If Josh does go to university, his adolescence will be prolonged until he's nearly 22.

Does society create identity crisis?

As well as the perceived absence of 'rites of passage' in western society, a problem for both adolescents and their parents is the related lack of consensus as to where adolescence begins and ends, and precisely what adolescent rights, privileges and responsibilities are. For example, the question 'When do I become an adult?' elicits a different response from a teacher, doctor, parent, or police officer (Coleman, 1995).

The 'maturity gap' refers to the incongruity of achieving biological maturity at adolescence without simultaneously being awarded adult status (Curry, 1998). According to Hendry and Kloep (1999):

> ... young people, as they grow up, find themselves in the trap of having to respond more and more to society's demands in a 'responsible' adult way while being treated as immature and not capable of holding sound opinions on a wide range of social matters.

One possible escape route from this trap is *risk-taking behaviour* (see page 322). As well as having to deal with the question 'Who am I?', the adolescent must also ask 'Who will I be?' Erikson saw the creation of an adult personality as achieved mainly through choosing and developing a commitment to an occupation or role in life. The development of *ego identity* (a firm sense of who one is and what one stands for) is positive and can carry people through difficult times.

ASK YOURSELF ...
- Can you think of any inconsistencies or contradictions that adolescents face between different aspects of their development?

- How do they perceive their social status?

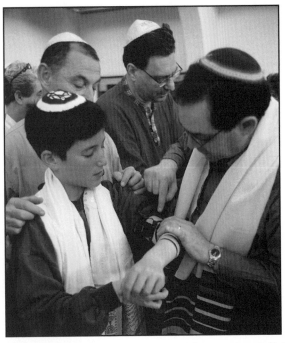

The Jewish bar mitzvah marks the 13-year-old boy's entry into manhood. But to the rest of society, he's still just a teenager

When working with psychiatrically disturbed soldiers in the Second World War, Erikson coined the term *identity crisis* to describe the loss of personal identity which the stress of combat seemed to have caused. Some years later, he extended the use of the term to include 'severely conflicted young people whose sense of confusion is due ... to a war within themselves'.

Evidently, Josh has no career plan or work 'identity' to aim for, so to stay at school for another two years may seem pointless.

Role confusion

Failure to integrate perceptions of the self into a coherent whole results in *role confusion*, which, according to Erikson, can affect several areas of life:

◎ *Intimacy*: a fear of commitment to, or involvement in, close relationships arises from a fear of losing one's identity. This may result in stereotyped and formalised relationships, or isolation.
◎ *Time perspective*: the adolescent is unable to plan for the future or retain any sense of time. This is associated with anxieties about change and becoming an adult.
◎ *Industry*: difficulty in channelling resources in a realistic way into work or study, both of which require commitment. As a defence, the adolescent may find it impossible to concentrate, or become frenetically engaged in a single activity to the exclusion of all others.
◎ *Negative identity*: engaging in abnormal or delinquent behaviour (such as drug-taking, or even suicide) as an attempt to resolve the identity crisis. This extreme position, which sets such adolescents apart from the crowd, is preferable to the loneliness and

isolation that come with failing to achieve a distinct and more functional role in life ('a negative identity is better than no identity').

Related to Erikson's claims about negative identity is *risk-taking behaviour*. Hendry (1999) asks if risk-taking is '… part of the psychological make-up of youth – a thrill-seeking stage in a developmental transition – a necessary rite of passage en route to the acquisition of adult skills and self-esteem …'.

Anna worries because Josh spends hours obsessively playing computer games, which may indicate he's lonely. He may have started drinking and smoking in order to find a group identity.

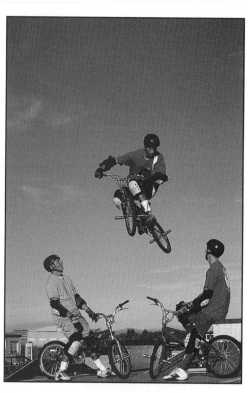

Thrill seeking: a rite of passage into adulthood?

Many teenagers seek out excitement, thrills and risks as earnestly as in childhood, perhaps to escape a drab existence, or to exert some control over their own lives and to achieve *something*. Two ways of achieving this are through drugs and sex. Traditionally, what parents of teenagers have most feared is that their children will engage in (particularly unprotected) sex and (especially hard) drugs (see Chapter 7 and Gross, 2005).

Anna is frantically worried about both of these, but at least Josh seemed to be aware of the need for protection in sex. His mood swings might indicate he has been experimenting with drugs, although none was found on him. Anna seemed relieved when Sister told her Josh would be referred to the School Nurse. I was curious to know more about that.

CRITICAL DISCUSSION 17.2 The biopsychosocial aspects of unwanted teenage pregnancy (based on Hughes, 2003)

- Adolescents are becoming sexually active at an increasingly younger age. According to the Family Planning Association, almost one in five young women say they have had sex before the age of 16 (Maner and Rees, 1998, in Hughes, 2003). Much of this activity is risky, contraceptive use is often erratic and may result in unwanted pregnancies.

- The UK has the highest teenage birth rate in western Europe, with Wales having a consistently higher rate than England. In 2000, the conception rate in Wales for under-18s was 47.3 per cent per 1000 females (actually lower than the 1998 peak).

- Abortion remains a common approach to dealing with unwanted pregnancies and is ideally performed in the first trimester.

- There are many biological, psychological and social reasons why women opt to terminate a pregnancy. For example, in some socio-cultural settings pre-marital sexual activity is taboo, using contraception is forbidden among unmarried youth, and abortion is viewed as the only solution to pre-marital pregnancy (WHO, 2002, in Hughes, 2003).

- Jolly (2002, in Hughes, 2003) argues that sexual health must depend on an understanding of why teenagers engage in unprotected sex, and stresses that social disadvantage and poverty are associated with increased risk-taking.

- Pre- and post-operative visiting by a perioperative nurse can provide emotional support to teenagers undergoing surgical termination, although nurses' attitudes and behaviours vary considerably. These teenagers are subject to many sources of stress, but evidence suggests that their psychological state improves post-operatively (Gilchrist, 1995, in Hughes, 2003). Although there may be feelings of regret, sadness and guilt, severe negative reactions are uncommon in the immediate and short-term aftermath of a first-trimester termination (Zolese and Blacker, 1992, in Hughes, 2003). (But see Chapter 20 for a discussion of longer-term grief reactions.)

- Adolescents undergoing surgical termination are often anxious and frightened, and for the majority it will be their first experience of an operating theatre. The role of the perioperative nurse is to reduce anxiety and provide biological and psychological care. Prolonged anxiety levels delay recovery and increase the risk of physiological complications (see Chapter 3).

From my diary (17): Year 2/School Nurse

When Josh (see my diary entry, above) was discharged from my ward following a head injury, he was referred to his School Nurse. As I'm interested in health education, I arranged to spend two days at his school. Nadine, the specialist nurse heading the health team, explained they have developed a comprehensive health education programme at primary and secondary level. They also run a drop-in centre for advice and counselling. Nadine explained that the provision of School Nurses depends on funding and the Health Trust's priorities. As unplanned pregnancy is a significant problem, her Health Trust had opted into a programme instigated by Exeter University called Added Power And Understanding in Sex Education (A PAUSE). This aims to improve sex and relationship education, and emphasises peer support. I was interested to discover Josh was involved in this.

Talking to Nadine about Josh, I discovered most of his friends had left school after GCSEs. In the sixth form, he has to fit into a relatively new group, so his involvement in A PAUSE may help.

For some, delinquency may be the solution to role confusion: it could actually be *adaptive* as a way of facilitating self-definition and expressing autonomy (Compas *et al.*, 1995).

According to Bergevin *et al.* (2003):

> ... One of the challenges of the self in adolescence is with identifying the ways that one is unique and how one is similar to others. Maintaining a sense of individuality while trying to fit into the group is an important task for adolescents. Emphasising differences can lead to loneliness and alienation, while emphasising similarities may impede the development of autonomy.

Such conflict seems to be largely absent in societies where the complete transition to adulthood is officially approved and celebrated at a specific age, often through a particular ceremony. These enable both the individual and society to adjust to change and enjoy a sense of continuity (Price and Crapo, 1999; see Gross, 2005).

ASK YOURSELF ...

- Do you agree with Price and Crapo's comments about female circumcision?

- Is our condemnation of such practices simply a reflection of western values, or are there universal principles and standards that apply regardless of who's being judged and who's doing the judging?

KEY STUDY 17.1 Initiation into adulthood in non-western cultures

- Brown (1963) described 'rites of passage' for girls in 43 societies from all major regions of the world. They most commonly occur where young girls continue to live and work in their mothers' home after marriage, but they also sometimes occur even when young women permanently leave home, and here they involve genital operations or extensive tattooing. These dramatically help the girl understand that she must make the transition from dependent child to a woman, who'll have to fend for herself in a male-dominated environment (Price and Crapo, 1999).

- In recent years, *infibulation* (the most extreme form of female circumcision) has become a global human rights issue. Its purpose is to preserve the virginity of young girls before marriage, and to tame the disturbing power of women. In many traditional Islamic countries, especially Sudan, Ethiopia and Somalia, millions of young girls continue to undergo painful and risky genital operations.

  Although the act of infibulation may, from a western perspective, deindividualise and depersonalise women:

  > ... it acts as a transition or a rite of passage to a greater female adult collective; one where women hold relatively few advantages in a male-dominated world. It may in fact be one of the few positive status markers for women in traditional Islamic societies ... (Price and Crapo, 1999)

Although we're not supposed to impose our own values on people from other cultures, I find this difficult to accept. Shouldn't everyone have the right to informed consent? According to Katherine Dempski (2001), the three elements that constitute informed consent are:

- the patient or client needs to have all the necessary information
- the consent needs to be given voluntarily, and
- the patient or client has to be competent (in Tschudin 2003 p. 173)

But Tschudin (2003, p. 176) also says, 'children under the age of 16 years are not able to give consent', so, in our own culture, legally it is parents who decide what is done to children. Except Nadine told me about The Frazer Guidelines (DfEE 2000) which state that 'competent' under 16's can decide for themselves about contraceptive treatment. It's very complicated . . . is the issue the consent – or the act itself?

According to Coleman and Roker (1998), an important trend in adolescence research is an increasing focus on identity development among ethnically diverse populations, such as young black women (e.g. Robinson, 1997) and mixed-race young people (Tizard and Phoenix, 1993). Coleman and Roker (1998) believe that notions of identity and identity formation are likely to become more central to the study of adolescence as this life stage becomes longer and more fragmented, and entry into adulthood becomes more problematic.

A number of students, especially Asian girls, self-harm. Nadine suggested 'culture clash' could be a cause of cutting and anorexia nervosa. Many of them start smoking in an effort to control their weight.

Studies of self-esteem

Tests of Erikson's theory have typically used measures of self-concept (especially *self-esteem*) as indicators of crisis. Girls' dissatisfaction with their appearance begins during puberty, along with a decline in self-esteem (Crawford and Unger, 1995). Comparisons between *early- and late-maturing girls* indicate that dissatisfaction with looks is associated with the rapid and normal weight gain that's part of growing up (Attie and Brooks-Gunn, 1989; Blyth *et al.*, 1981).

Early maturers have a less positive body image, despite the fact that they date more and earlier. Also, sexual activity is more problematic for adolescent girls (as it is for females in general): there are persisting double standards regarding sex (as reflected in the terms 'slag' and 'stud' for sexually active females and males respectively), together with differential responsibility for contraception and pregnancy (see above).

However, Offer *et al.* (1988) deny there's any increase in disturbance of the self-image during early adolescence. For Coleman and Hendry (1990), although such disturbance is more likely in early than late adolescence, only a very small proportion of the total adolescent population is likely to have a negative self-image or very low self-esteem.

By contrast, *early-maturing boys* feel more attractive (Tobin-Richards *et al.*, 1983) and tend to be more satisfied with their bodies, looks and muscle development (Blyth *et al.*, 1981; Simmons and Blyth, 1987). However, Alsaker (1996) refers to two studies, which have found a correlation between pubertal boys' dissatisfaction with their bodies and the development of pubic and body hair. She asks whether this reflects some contemporary images of men in advertisements, and a new trend for men to shave their bodies and be *less* hairy.

Most of these (and other similar) studies have been conducted in the USA, UK and other English-speaking countries. But a study of a very large, nationally representative Norwegian sample found that the global self-esteem of both late-maturing boys and girls suffered, while early and on-time maturers (of both sexes) enjoy equally high self-esteem (Wichstrom, 1998).

The fact that Josh has acne must detract from his positive self-image.

SOCIOLOGICAL APPROACHES: GENERATION GAP

Sociologists see *role change* as an integral aspect of adolescent development (Coleman, 1995). Changing school or college, leaving home and beginning a job all involve new

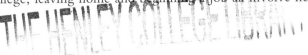

sets of relationships, producing different and often greater expectations. These expectations themselves demand a substantial reassessment of the self-concept and speed up the socialisation process. Some adolescents find this problematic because of the wide variety of competing socialising agencies (such as the family, mass media and peer group), which often present *conflicting* values and demands (see discussion above of the identity crisis).

Sociologists also see socialisation as being more dependent on the adolescent's *own generation* than on the family or other social institutions (*auto-socialisation*: Marsland, 1987). As Marsland says, 'The crucial meaning of youth is withdrawal from adult control and influence compared with childhood ...'

Young people withdraw into their peer groups, and this withdrawal is (within limits) accepted by adults. What Marsland is describing here is the *generation gap*.

Josh's withdrawal into his peer group wasn't acceptable to Anna; she said she disapproved of the fact that most of his friends were allowed far too much freedom for their age.

Parent–adolescent relationships

According to Hendry (1999), 'Adolescence as a transition from childhood to adulthood requires changes from child–parent relationships to young-adult–parent relationships ...'

Failure to negotiate new relationships with parents, or having highly critical or rejecting parents, is likely to make adolescents adopt a negative identity (Curry, 1998). Also, parents who rated their own adolescence as stormy and stressful reported more conflict in their relationships with adolescent children and were less satisfied with their family (Scheer and Unger, 1995). Parents of adolescents in general are often going through a time of transition themselves, reappraising their life goals, career and family ambitions, and assessing whether they've fulfilled their expectations as parents.

> **ASK YOURSELF ...**
> • While adolescents and their parents are, by definition, different generations, does this necessarily and inevitably mean that there's a generation gap – that is, that there will be conflict between them because they occupy 'different worlds'?

Anna understandably found it hard to cope with Josh's mood swings and open defiance. At the age of 38, she has lost the stability of what Erikson (1950) calls the intimacy and generativity stages, and is having to establish a new identity for herself as a single mother and returning to work. This is anticipating the 'midlife crisis' described by Levinson at the ages of 40–45.

However, for most adolescents relationships with parents become more equal and reciprocal, and parental authority comes to be seen as open to discussion and negotiation (e.g. Coleman and Hendry, 1990; Hendry *et al.*, 1993). The study by Hendry *et al.* (1993) also suggests that relationships with mothers and fathers don't necessarily change in the same ways and to the same extent (see Gross, 2005).

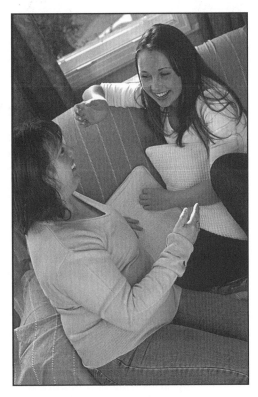

Generational harmony – not generation gap

Studies conducted in several countries have found that young people get along well with their parents (e.g. Hendry *et al.*, 1993; Kloep and Tarifa, 1993), adopt their views and values, and perceive family members as the most important 'significant others' in their lives (McGlone *et al.*, 1996). Furthermore, most adolescents who had conflicts with their parents already had poor relationships with them before puberty (Stattin and Klackenberg, 1992).

Disagreements between young people and their parents are similar everywhere in Europe. According to Jackson *et al.* (1996) disagreements can arise because:

◎ parents expect greater independence of action from their teenagers
◎ parents don't wish to grant as much autonomy as the adolescent demands (with young women having more conflict than young men over independence)
◎ parents and adolescents have different personal tastes and preferences.

Despite this potential for conflict, evidence suggests that competence as an independent adult can best be achieved within the context of a secure family environment, where exploration of alternative ideas, identities and behaviour is allowed and actively encouraged (Barber and Buehler, 1996). So, while detachment and separation from the family are necessary and desirable, young people don't have to reject their parents in order to become adults in their own right (Hill, 1993; Ryan and Lynch, 1989; see also Chapter 14).

While in hospital and upset, Josh turned to his mother for comfort, behaving for a short while like a younger child.

Peer relationships

Adolescent *friendship groups* (established around mutual interests) are normally embedded within the wider network of *peer groups* (which set 'norms', provide comparisons and pressures to conform to 'expected' behaviours). Friendship groups reaffirm self-image, and enable the young person to experience a new form of intimacy and learn social skills (such as discussing and solving conflicts, sharing and self-assertion). They also offer the opportunity to expand knowledge, develop a new identity, and experiment away from the watchful eyes of adults and family (Coleman and Hendry, 1990).

Generally, peers become more important as providers of advice, support, feedback and companionship, as models for behaviour and as sources of comparison with respect to personal qualities and skills. But while peer groups and friendship groups become important points of reference in social development and provide social contexts for shaping day-to-day values, they often *support* traditional parental attitudes and beliefs. Hence, peer and friendship groups can work in concert with, rather than in opposition to, adult goals and achievements (Hendry, 1999).

This is why A PAUSE has peer-led sessions in the programme in Year 9.

COLEMAN'S FOCAL THEORY: MANAGING ONE CHANGE AT A TIME

According to Coleman and Hendry (1990), the picture that emerges from the research as a whole is that while adolescence is a difficult time for some, for the majority it appears to be a period of relative stability. Coleman's (1980) *focal theory* is an attempt to explain how this is achieved.

The theory is based on a study of 800 6-, 11-, 13-, 15- and 17-year-old boys and girls. Attitudes towards self-image, being alone, heterosexual and parental relationships, friendships and large-group situations all changed as a function of age. More importantly, concerns about different issues reached a peak at different ages for both sexes.

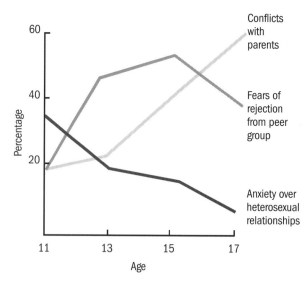

Figure 17.2 Peak ages of the expression of different themes. These data are for boys only (from Coleman & Hendry, 1990)

Particular sorts of relationship pattern come into *focus* (are most prominent) at different ages, although no pattern is specific to one age. The patterns overlap and there are wide individual differences.

Coleman believes that adolescents are able to cope with the potentially stressful changes as well as they do by dealing with one issue at a time. They spread the process of adaptation over a span of years, attempting to resolve one issue first before addressing the next. Because different problems and relationships come into focus and are dealt with at different points during the adolescent years, the stresses resulting from the need to adapt don't all have to be dealt with together.

According to Coleman and Hendry (1990), it's those adolescents who, for whatever reason, must deal with *more than one issue* (or normative shift) at a time who are most likely to experience difficulties. If normative shifts coincide with non-normative ones, the situation is even more problematic (Hendry and Kloep, 1999).

Josh had to cope with his new body, his acne, his voice breaking and his father leaving the family within a short time span. While focused on his GCSEs he seemed all right, but as soon as that goal was achieved he seemed to lose direction.

Coleman's original findings have been successfully replicated by Kroger (1985) with large North American and New Zealand samples. Others have successfully tested hypotheses derived from the theory. For example, Simmons and Blyth (1987) predicted that if change (such as puberty)

◎ occurred at too young an age (causing the individual to be developmentally 'off-time')
◎ was marked by sharp discontinuity (i.e. sudden change) or
◎ involved accumulation of significant and temporally close issues (important shifts occurred together)

then adjustment would be more difficult. Their results strongly supported their predictions.

CONCLUSIONS

Adolescence involves a number of important transitions from childhood to adulthood, including puberty. The potential for storm and stress in western societies is increased by the lack of clear definitions regarding when adulthood is reached. This makes the task of attaining an adult identity, as well as relationships with parents, more difficult compared with non-industrialised societies.

However, adolescence in western societies isn't as problem-ridden as the popular stereotype would have it. If any serious problems do arise, they're directly linked to *rapid social change* (Dasen, 1999), with the associated extension of adolescence and youth. Young people aren't given a productive role to play when entering adult society (Segall *et al.*, 1999).

While most of the major theories of adolescence paint a picture of adolescence as an *inherently* difficult developmental stage, the evidence suggests that this isn't necessarily so. Certain groups may be more vulnerable than others (such as early-maturing girls), but the majority seem to cope well. According to Coleman's theory, it *isn't* adolescence itself that's stressful but the timing and combination of the transitions faced by young people.

My experience with Josh in hospital showed me the need for extra sensitivity to the troubled emotions of teenagers at a time of crisis. To care for them properly we need to appreciate the complexity of their needs; theories of adolescence reveal the physical and social as well as the psychological elements affecting teenagers.

I'm pleased I followed up on Josh's discharge. My short placement at the school showed me how much adolescence (like other developmental stages) varies between individuals, families and cultures. It also reminded me that as health professionals, we have to be aware of the law regarding young people and to work within it. And the question of consent raised a difficult philosophical issue!

I was made very aware of how social, economic and public health policies, particularly investment in health promotion, can affect the provision of support that Josh and many other adolescents need. Although we do recognise their special status, it isn't always possible to provide ideal facilities for their care.

CHAPTER SUMMARY

◎ Adolescence involves **multiple transitions**. Compared with previous generations, it begins sooner and ends later. Various 'adulthood-postponing' changes have coincided with increased freedom at earlier ages.

◎ These transitions or **shifts** can be categorised as **normative maturational**, **normative society-dependent** and **non-normative**. Normative shifts can become non-normative, as when puberty begins unusually early or late.

◎ **Puberty** involves the **adolescent growth spurt** and the development of **secondary sex characteristics** (both sexes). While girls typically enter puberty two years before boys, there are important individual differences within each sex (such as **intraindividual asynchronies**).

◎ Adolescents evaluate their changing body images in terms of cultural standards of beauty, especially as these relate to weight. According to the **cultural ideal hypothesis** (CIH), girls move further away from their physical ideal and **early-maturing girls** will face a double disadvantage. **Early-maturing boys** will move fastest towards their physical ideal.

◎ Some of the particular problems faced by **adolescents in hospital** include **lack of privacy** and a renewed **dependence** on adults for the care and management of their illness.

◎ Hall's **recapitulation theory** saw adolescence as a time of **storm and stress**. While mood swings are more common during adolescence, rates of **mental disorder** are higher only in early-maturing girls and adolescents with problems prior to puberty. The evidence for **off-time** maturation in boys is more mixed.

◎ According to Erikson, adolescence involves a conflict between **ego identity** and **role confusion**. In western societies, adolescence is a **moratorium**, intended to help ease the transition to adulthood. However, the lack of clear definitions of adulthood may contribute to the adolescent **identity crisis**.

◎ Role confusion can take the form of **negative identity**, related to which is **risk-taking behaviour**. These problems are largely absent in societies which mark the transition to adulthood by **initiation ceremonies**.

◎ While **self-esteem** may decline in early adolescence, especially in girls, this affects only a very small proportion of all adolescents.

◎ **Sociological approaches** stress **role change**, the **conflicting** values and demands of different socialising agencies, and **auto-socialisation**, which produces the **generation gap**.

◎ Renegotiating relationships with parents is necessary, and while there are inevitable disagreements, adult status is probably best achieved within the context of a **secure family environment**.

◎ **Friendship groups** (as 'sub-groups' of the wider **peer group**) assume much greater significance during adolescence, such as helping to shape basic values. But these values are often **consistent** with parents' values, goals and achievements.

◎ According to Coleman's **focal theory**, most adolescents cope as well as they do by spreading the process of adaptation over several years. Having to deal with more than **one issue at a time** is stressful, especially if changes occur too early or suddenly.

ADULTHOOD 18

INTRODUCTION AND OVERVIEW

Assuming that we enjoy a normal lifespan, the longest phase of the life cycle will be spent in adulthood. Until recently, however, personality changes in adulthood attracted little psychological research interest. Indeed, as Levinson *et al.* (1978) have observed, adulthood is '… one of the best-kept secrets in our society and probably in human history generally'.

This chapter attempts to reveal some of these secrets by examining what theory and research have told us about personality change in adulthood, including the occurrence of crises and transitions.

Many theorists believe that adult concerns and involvements are patterned in such a way that we can speak about *stages* of adult development. However, evidence concerning the predictability of changes in adult life (or what Levinson, 1986, calls *psychobiosocial transitions*) is conflicting. Three kinds of influence can affect the way we develop in adulthood (Hetherington and Baltes, 1988):

1. *Normative age-graded influences* are biological (such as the menopause) and social changes (such as marriage and parenting) that normally occur at fairly predictable ages.
2. *Normative history-graded influences* are historical events that affect whole generations or *cohorts* at about the same time (examples include wars, recessions and epidemics).
3. *Non-normative influences* are idiosyncratic transitions, such as divorce, unemployment and illness.

Levinson's (1986) term *marker events* refers to age-graded and non-normative influences. Others prefer the term *critical life events* to describe such influences, although it's probably more accurate to describe them as *processes*. Some critical life events, such as divorce, unemployment and bereavement, can occur at any time during adulthood (bereavement is discussed in Chapter 20). Others occur late in adulthood, such as retirement (see Chapter 19). Yet others tend to happen early in adulthood, such as marriage (or partnering) and parenting.

From my diary (14): Second year/Medical Ward

Mr Briggs (Frank), a 49-year-old police officer, was transferred at short notice from the Coronary Care Unit (CCU) as they needed the bed on the ward. He had an acute myocardial infarction (AMI) two days ago, so went into a high-dependency bed. He was on oxygen, his pain being controlled by diamorphine. His wife, Denise, had been with him almost continuously and was very anxious about him. He was devastated by this illness; when his father died of a heart attack at 62, Frank gave up smoking, reduced

ASK YOURSELF …
- What do you understand by the term 'adulthood'?
- What does it mean to be an adult?

his weight and monitored his cholesterol levels, although he was still a fairly heavy social drinker. Sister asked that we should be sensitive to the patient's and the family's need for reassurance and explanation. This worried me, as I was aware I knew very little about caring for a patient with AMI. As I arrived to do his observations, his wife was trying to arrange his pillows more comfortably. Obviously, she hadn't succeeded because he said angrily he wished she'd leave him alone. Denise looked tearful and left the ward. Frank looked upset but said nothing. I didn't know whether to ignore it, stay with him or go after his wife.

ERIKSON'S THEORY: ACHIEVING INTIMACY AND GENERATIVITY

As we saw in Chapter 17, Erikson believes that human development occurs through a sequence of *psychosocial stages*. As far as early and middle adulthood are concerned, Erikson described two primary developmental crises (the sixth and seventh of his psychosocial stages – see Table 18.1, page 335).

The first involves the establishment of *intimacy*, which is a criterion of having attained the psychosocial state of adulthood. By intimacy, Erikson means the ability to form close, meaningful relationships with others without 'the fear of losing oneself in the process' (Elkind, 1970). Erikson believed that a prerequisite for intimacy was the attainment of *identity* (the reconciliation of all our various roles into one enduring and stable personality: see Chapter 17). Identity is necessary, because we cannot know what it means to love someone and seek to share our life with them until we know who we are and what we want to do with our lives. Thus, genuine intimacy requires us to give up some of our sense of separateness, and we must each have a firm identity to do this.

Intimacy needn't involve sexuality. Since intimacy refers to the essential ability to relate our deepest hopes and fears to another person, and in turn to accept another's need for intimacy, it describes the relationship between friends just as much as that between sexual partners (Dacey, 1982). By sharing ourselves with others, our personal identity becomes fully realised and consolidated. Erikson believed that if a sense of intimacy isn't established with friends or a partner, then *isolation* (a sense of being alone without anyone to share with or care for) would result. We normally achieve intimacy in young adulthood (our twenties and thirties), after which we enter middle age (our forties and fifties). This involves the attainment of *generativity*, the positive outcome of the second developmental crisis.

Jenkins and Rogers (1995, in Alexander et al., 2006) recommend a planned move from CCU, with staff taking time to discuss the patient's feelings of fear and vulnerability. Frank's transfer was unexpected and this may have added to his tension. Denise's anxiety may have been expressed behaviourally by 'fussing' and Frank's by anger.

According to Thompson and Webster, 'Spending time with relatives, both when they are visiting and when they are alone, may allow worries and fears to be expressed' (in Alexander et al., 2006:27). I was pleased that after I'd finished doing Frank's observations I reassured him and went to find Denise. Between her concerns, she told me Frank is a 'workaholic'; they'd been married for 25 years and have 2 children: Tom is 23 and also a policeman and Bridget is 19 and at university. So their parents appear to have successfully completed the stages of intimacy and generativity.

Table 18.1 Comparison between Erikson's and Freud's stages of development (based on Erikson, 1950; Thomas, 1985)

No. of stage	Name of stage (psychosocial crisis)	Psychosocial modalities (dominant modes of being and acting)	Radius of significant relationships	Human virtues (qualities of strength)	Freud's psychosexual stages	Approx. ages
1	Basic trust vs basic mistrust	To get. To give in return	Mother or mother figure	Hope	Oral	0–1
2	Autonomy vs shame and doubt	To hold on. To let go	Parents	Willpower	Anal	1–3
3	Initiative vs guilt	To make (going after). To 'make like' (playing)	Basic family	Purpose	Phallic	3–6
4	Industry vs inferiority	To make things (completing). To make things together	Neighbourhood and school	Competence	Latency	6–12
5	Identity vs role confusion	To be oneself (or not to be). To share being oneself	Peer groups and outgroups. Models of leadership	Fidelity	Genital	12–18
6	Intimacy vs isolation	To lose and find oneself in another	Partners in friendship, sex, competition, cooperation	Love		20s
7	Generativity vs stagnation	To make be. To take care of	Divided labour and shared household	Care		Late 20s–50s
8	Ego integrity vs despair	To be, through having been. To face not being	'Humankind', 'my kind'	Wisdom		50s and beyond

335

Both Frank's children visited during the day and showed loving concern for their father, indicating a mutual caring relationship. Denise is a teacher, so both parents have socially responsible jobs.

EVALUATION OF ERIKSON'S THEORY

◎ The sequence from identity to intimacy may not accurately reflect present-day realities. In recent years, the trend has been for adults to live together before marrying, so they tend to marry later in life than people did in the past (see below). Many people struggle with identity issues (such as career choice) at the same time as dealing with intimacy issues.

◎ Additionally, some evidence suggests that females achieve intimacy *before* 'occupational identity'. The typical life course of women involves passing directly into a stage of intimacy without having achieved personal identity. Sangiuliano (1978) argues that most women submerge their identities into those of their partners, and only in mid-life do they emerge from this and search for separate identities and full independence. There's also a possible interaction between gender and *social class*. For example, working-class men see early marriage as a 'good' life pattern: early adulthood is a time for 'settling down', having a family and maintaining a steady job. By contrast, middle-class men and women see early adulthood as a time for exploration, in which different occupations are tried. Marriage tends to occur after this, and 'settling down' doesn't usually take place before 30 (Neugarten, 1975).

◎ Another example of how Erikson's stages may not apply to everyone is the case of 'baby fathers', the name given to young black men who have children with a number of women and wear this as a 'badge of honour' (Alibhai-Brown, 2000).

◎ Erikson's psychosocial stages were meant to be *universal*, applying to both genders in all cultures. However, he acknowledged that the sequence of stages is different for a woman, who suspends her identity as she prepares to attract the man who will marry her. Men achieve identity before achieving intimacy with sexual partners, whereas, for women, Erikson's developmental crises appear to be fused. As Gilligan (1982) has observed, 'The female comes to know herself as she is known, through relationships with others.'

◎ All the above evidence suggests that it's almost certainly impossible to describe universal stages for adults. Moreover, there's evidence of a growing prolongation of adolescence (see Chapter 17 and Gross, 2005).

Denise said she'd happily given up work (her words, not mine!) when she married Frank – he was ambitious, his job involved shift work and they wanted to start a family. In contrast, her son Tom and his girlfriend are living together, both working full-time, and have no intention of getting married or having a family yet. However, the developmental task of achieving intimacy is the same.

LEVINSON *ET AL.*'S 'SEASONS OF A MAN'S LIFE'

Perhaps the most systematic study of personality and life changes in adulthood began in 1969, when Levinson *et al.* (1978) interviewed 40 men aged 35 to 45. Transcripts were made of the five to ten tape-recorded interviews that each participant gave over several months. Levinson *et al.* looked at how adulthood is actually *experienced*.

In *The Seasons of a Man's Life*, Levinson *et al.* (1978) advanced a *life-structure theory*, defining life structure as the underlying pattern or design of a person's life at any given time. Life structure allows us to 'see how the self is in the world and how the world is in the self', and evolves through a series of *phases* or *periods* which give overall shape to the course of adult development. Adult development comprises a sequence of *eras* which overlap in the form of *cross-era transitions*. These last about five years, ending the outgoing era and initiating the incoming one. The four eras are pre-adulthood (age 0–22), early adulthood (17–45), middle adulthood (40–65) and late adulthood (60 onwards).

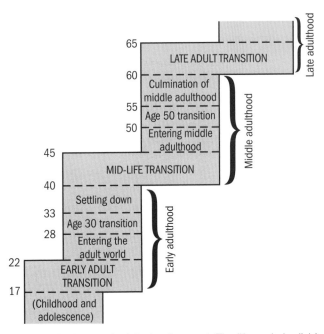

Figure 18.1 Levinson *et al.*'s theory of adult development. The life cycle is divided into four major eras that overlap in the form of cross-era transitions (from Levinson *et al.*, 1978, *The Seasons of a Man's Life*. New York: A.A. Knopf, a division of Random House, Inc. Reprinted by permission of SLL/Sterling Lord Literistic, Inc. © 1975 by Daniel J. Levinson)

The phases or periods alternate between those that are stable (or *structure-building*) and those that are transitional (or *structure-changing*). Although each phase involves biological, psychological and social adjustments, family and work roles are seen as central to the life structure at any time, and individual development is interwoven with changes in these roles.

According to Levinson et al.'s (1978) theory, Frank spent his early adulthood stage 'structure building' his career, marriage and family. Now he's experiencing mid-life transition into middle adulthood.

THE ERA OF EARLY ADULTHOOD

Early adult transition (17–22) is a developmental 'bridge' between adolescence and adulthood. Two key themes of the early adult transition are *separation* and the formation of *attachments* to the adult world.

◎ *External separation* involves moving out of the family home, increasing financial independence, and entering more independent and responsible roles and living arrangements.

◎ *Internal separation* involves greater psychological distance from the family, less emotional dependence on the parents, and greater differentiation between the self and family. Although we separate from our parents, Levinson *et al.* argue that we never complete the process, which continues throughout life.

◎ *Attachment* involves exploring the world's possibilities, imagining ourselves as part of it, and identifying and establishing changes for living in the world before we become 'full members' of it.

Frank's daughter, Bridget, is in Levinson et al.'s early adult transition stage; she is living in digs and independent – except financially, Denise says!

Between the ages of 22 and 28, we *enter the adult world*. This is the first *structure-building* (rather than *structure-changing*) phase and hence is referred to as the *entry life structure for early adulthood*. In it, we try to fashion '… a provisional structure that provides a workable link between the valued self and adult society'.

In the *novice phase*, we try to define ourselves as adults and live with the initial choices we make concerning jobs, relationships, lifestyles and values. However, we need to create a balance between 'keeping our options open' (which allows us to explore possibilities without being committed to a given course) and 'putting down roots' (or creating stable life structures).

Our decisions are made in the context of our *dreams*: the 'vague sense' we have of ourselves in the adult world and what we want to do with our lives. We must overcome disappointments and setbacks, and learn to accept and profit from successes, so that the dream's 'thread' doesn't get lost in the course of 'moving up the ladder' and revising the life structure. To help us in our efforts at self-definition, we look to *mentors*, older and more experienced others, for guidance and direction. Mentors can take a formal role in guiding, teaching and helping novices to define their dreams. Alternatively, a mentor's role may be informal, providing an advisory and emotionally supportive function (as a parent does).

ASK YOURSELF …
- What qualities would your ideal mentor possess?
- What qualities do you think s/he would like to find in a mentee?

According to Levinson <u>et. al.</u>, Frank's son Tom is in the novice phase of early adulthood. He'd decided at school he wanted to be a policeman, like his father. Frank was no doubt an informal mentor to Tom at this stage; however, formal mentoring is finding its place in the police service as well as in teaching and nursing (Morton-Cooper and Palmer, 2003, in Downie and Basford, 2003). These authors suggest that the many characteristics of an effective mentor can be drawn together under a framework of three important personal attributes: competence, demonstrating personal confidence and a commitment to the development of others. Adam is an excellent mentor; he's highly skilled, decisive and is always teaching, challenging and encouraging me.

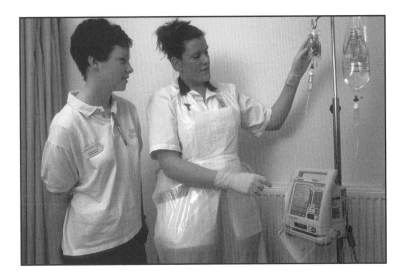

The age-30 transition (28–33) provides an opportunity to work on the flaws and limitations of the first life structure, and to create the basis for a more satisfactory structure that will complete the era of young adulthood. Most of Levinson *et al.*'s participants experienced *age-30 crises* which involved stress, self-doubt, feelings that life was losing its 'provisional quality' and becoming more serious, and time pressure. Thus, the participants saw this as being the time for change, if change was needed. However, for a minority the age-30 transition was crisis-free.

Box 18.2 Settling down

- The *settling down* (or *culminating life structure for early adulthood*: 33–40) *phase* represents consolidation of the second life structure. This involves a shift away from tentative choices regarding family and career towards a strong sense of commitment to a personal, familial and occupational future.

- Paths for success in work and husband and father roles are mapped out and, instead of just beginning to find out what's important and what our opinions are, we see ourselves as responsible adults.

- The settling down phase comprises two sub-stages: *early settling down* (33–36) and *becoming one's own man* (BOOM) (36–40). In the latter, men strive to advance and succeed in building better lives, improve and use their skills, be creative, and in general contribute to society.

- A man wants recognition and affirmation from society, but he also wants to be self-sufficient and free of social pressure and control. Although a 'boy–man' conflict may be produced, this can represent a step forward. This sub-stage may also see him assume a mentor role for someone younger (see above).

Adam is in this 'BOOM' phase, which may explain his commitment and enthusiasm for his mentoring role.

THE ERA OF MIDDLE ADULTHOOD

ASK YOURSELF ...
- What do you think is meant by the 'mid-life crisis'?

- Do you think it's a real phenomenon?

The *mid-life transition* (40–45) involves terminating one life structure, initiating another, and continuing the process of *individuation* started during the BOOM sub-stage. This is a time of soul-searching, questioning, and assessing the real meaning of the life structure's achievement. It's sometimes referred to as the *mid-life crisis*, although Levinson *et al.* didn't actually use this term. For some people, the change is gradual and fairly painless. But for others, it's full of uncertainties.

The crisis stems from unconscious tensions between attachment and separation, the resurfacing of the need to be creative (which is often repressed in order to achieve a career), and retrospective comparisons between dreams and life's reality.

Most participants in Levinson *et al.*'s study hadn't reached age 45. Following interviews two years after the main study was concluded, some were chosen for more extensive study. But the evidence for the remaining phases is much less detailed than for the earlier ones.

In *entering middle adulthood* (or *early life structure for middle adulthood*: 45–50), we've resolved (more or less satisfactorily) whether what we've committed ourselves to really is worthwhile. It's again necessary to make choices regarding a new life structure. Sometimes, these choices are defined by *marker events* such as divorce, illness, occupational change, or the death of a loved one. However, the choices may also be influenced by less obvious but significant changes, such as shifts in the enthusiasm for work or in the quality of marriage. As before, the resulting life structure varies in how satisfying it is and how connected it is to the self. It may not be intrinsically happy and fulfilling. The restructuring consists of many steps, and there may be setbacks in which options have to be abandoned ('back to the drawing board').

Denise said Frank missed the children when they left home (a normative shift) and had 'thrown himself into work'; he was hoping for promotion to chief inspector. His illness – what Levinson calls a 'marker event' – could severely disrupt his plans.

Is there a 'mid-life crisis'?

Just as the 'identity crisis' is part of the popular stereotype of adolescence (see Chapter 17), Levinson *et al.* have helped to make the 'mid-life crisis' part of the common-sense understanding of adult development. Like Erikson, Levinson *et al.* see crisis as *inevitable*. As they note, 'It is not possible to get through middle adulthood without having at least a moderate crisis in either the mid-life transition or the age-50 transition.' They also see crisis as *necessary*. If we don't engage in soul searching, we'll '… pay the price in a later developmental crisis or in a progressive withering of the self and a life structure minimally connected to the self'.

The view that crisis is both inevitable and necessary (or *normative*, to use Erikson's term) is controversial. People of all ages suffer occasional depression, self-doubt, sexual uncertainty and concerns about the future. Indeed, there appears to be an increasingly wide age range and a growing number of people who decide to make radical changes in their lifestyle, both earlier and later than predicted by Levinson *et al.*'s theory.

According to Tredre (1996), the concept of a mid-life crisis is too narrow. We need to think in terms of early-, mid- and late-life crises: people of all age groups and walks of life are 'feeling the itch'. One response to this is *downshifting*, which refers to voluntarily opting out of a pressurised career (and often an exceptionally well-paid job) in the pursuit of a more fulfilling way of life.

This may be an option for Frank. But from what Denise said he would find it very hard to let go of the authority and status of the work he enjoys, for less stressful employment. Denise's mid-life transition stage coincided with her children's growing independence, so she decided to train as a teacher. She finds it rewarding but also stressful.

Box 18.3 Identity crisis and the life cycle

- Marcia (1998) also believes that the concept of a mid-life crisis is misleading and too narrow. He argues that 'adolescing' (making decisions about one's identity) occurs *throughout* the lifespan, whenever we review or reorganise our lives. At the very least, we might expect identity crises to accompany (in Erikson's terms) intimacy–isolation, generativity–stagnation and integrity–despair (see Chapter 19).

- Just as puberty and other changes in early adolescence disrupt the partial identities of childhood, so the demands of intimacy require a reformulation of the initial identity achieved at late adolescence. Similarly, the generative, care-giving requirements of middle age differ from those of being with an intimate partner. The virtues of fidelity, love and care (see Table 18.1), which derive from positive resolution of young and middle adulthood, don't emerge without a struggle. According to Marcia (1998), 'Periods of adolescing are normal, expectable components of life cycle growth.'

- However, while crises aren't limited to specific times in our lives, those associated with middle (and old) age are especially difficult.

For further discussion of the mid-life crisis, including the question of whether there's a male menopause, see Gross (2005).

The seasons of a woman's life

Levinson *et al.*'s research was carried out on an all-male sample. In *The Seasons of a Woman's Life* (1997), Levinson and Levinson presented their findings for 45 women (aged 35 to 45), comprising 15 homemakers (full-time housewives/mothers), 15 business women and 15 academics. The broad pattern of developmental periods based on the original male sample was confirmed. But men and women have been shown to differ in terms of their *dreams*.

> **Box 18.4 Women's dreams and 'gender-splitting'**
>
> • Levinson (1986) argues that a *'gender-splitting'* phenomenon occurs in adult development. Men have fairly unified visions of their futures, which tend to be focused on their careers. But women have 'dreams' which are more likely to be split between a career and marriage.
>
> • This was certainly true of academics and business women, although the former were less ambitious and more likely to forego a career, whereas the latter wanted to maintain their careers but at a reduced level. Only the homemakers had unified dreams (to be full-time wives and mothers, as their own mothers had been).
>
> • The family plays a 'supportive' role for men. Women's dreams were constructed around their relationships with their husbands and families, which subordinated their personal needs. So, part of *her* dream is *his* success. For Durkin (1995), this difference in women's and men's priorities may put women at greater risk '... of disappointment and developmental tension as their investment in others' goals conflicts with their personal needs'.
>
> • Women who give marriage and motherhood top priority in their twenties tend to develop more individualistic goals for their thirties. However, those who are career-oriented early on in adulthood tend to focus on marriage and family concerns later.
>
> • Generally, the transitory instability of the early thirties lasts longer for women than for men, and 'settling down' is much less clear-cut. Trying to integrate career and marriage/family responsibilities is very difficult for most women, who experience greater conflicts than their husbands are likely to.

Both Denise and I put our careers second to caring for children. Denise's change of role, when her children left home, was normative; mine, at 28, was triggered by divorce and non-normative. Or did my age-30 transition trigger the divorce?

Gender-splitting is relevant to discussion of marriage/partnering and parenthood (see below).

THE VALIDITY OF STAGE THEORIES OF ADULT DEVELOPMENT

ASK YOURSELF ...
• Do you think it's appropriate to describe adulthood in terms of distinct stages?

◎ Erikson's and Levinson *et al.*'s theories of adult development emphasise a 'ladder-like' progression through an inevitable and universal series of stages/phases. But this view of adult development as 'stage-like' has been criticised on the grounds that it underestimates the degree of *individual variability* (Rutter and Rutter, 1992). Many members of the mainstream working-class population don't grow or change in systematic ways. Instead, they show many rapid fluctuations, depending on things like relationships, work demands and other life stresses that are taking place (Craig, 1992).

◎ Stage theories also imply a *discontinuity* of development. But many psychologists believe there's also considerable *continuity* of personality during adult life.

From what I've seen, and what Denise has told me, I think Frank is ambitious, tetchy and driven. This describes what is known as a 'Type A behaviour pattern personality'; such people appear to respond more to stress than other 'types' (Fletcher, 1995; see Chapter 5).

◎ Current views of adult development stress the transitions and milestones that mark adult life, rather than a rigid developmental sequence (Baltes, 1983; Schlossberg, 1984). This is commonly referred to as the *life-events approach*. Yet, despite the growing unpredictability of changes in adult life, most people still unconsciously evaluate their transitions according to a *social clock*, which determines whether they're 'on time' with respect to particular life events – such as getting married (see Schlossberg *et al.*, 1978). If they're 'off time', either early or late, they're *age-deviant*. Like other types of deviancy, this can result in social penalties, such as amusement, pity or rejection.

◎ While all cultures have social clocks that define the 'right' time to marry, begin work, have children, and so on, these clocks vary greatly *between* cultures (Wade and Tavris, 1999). Because of the sheer diversity of experiences in an adult's life, Craig (1992) doesn't believe it's possible to describe major 'milestones' that will apply to nearly everyone.

Both Denise and I are 'age-deviant' regarding our careers. But in our culture this particular social clock (Wade and Tavris, 1999) is changing; there are so many mature students in nursing now I don't feel deviant!

CRITICAL DISCUSSION 18.1 What is an adult? Re-setting the social clock

- Just as social clocks are 'set' at different times in different cultures for different life changes, in western societies the clock becomes 're-set' over time.

- For example, 40–50 years ago, a stable job and income could be achieved (by men) by age 21, so this was seen as the time to 'settle down'. If a woman wasn't married by the time she was 25, she was 'on the shelf', and if still single by 29, she was an 'old maid'.

- Common beliefs about the appropriate age for child-bearing put pressure on women to become mothers by their early twenties, and pregnancy after 26 was seen as 'late' (Apter, 2001). These patterns are drastically different now.

- As both cause and effect of these changes, our whole understanding of what it means to be adult is changing. In *The Myth of Maturity* (2001), Apter argues that it's taking young people far longer to achieve adult status than it used to. She refers to 18–24-year-olds as 'thresholders', because they're only *on the brink* of achieving self-sufficiency and autonomy (commonly cited adult qualities). They're like 'apprentices to adulthood'.

- A total of 58 per cent of 22–24-year-olds and 30 per cent of 24–30-year-olds (still) live with their parents. Leaving home isn't a single event, but a prolonged *process*: 40 per cent of female, and 50 per cent of male, thresholders who leave home will subsequently return.

- There are a thousand different routes from adolescence to adulthood, each involving uncertainty and risk (Apter, 2001).

ASK YOURSELF …
- Would you describe yourself as a thresholder?

- Are many of your peers thresholders?

ASK YOURSELF …
- Identify some arguments for and against marriage, as compared with 'living together' (cohabitation).

MARRIAGE

Since over 90 per cent of adults in western countries marry at least once, marriage is an example of a *normative age-graded influence* (see Introduction and Overview). Marriage is an important transition for young adults, because it involves a lasting personal commitment to another person (and so is a means of achieving Erikson's *intimacy*), financial responsibilities and, perhaps, family responsibilities.

But social norms are changing; marriage usually follows living together (see above) as Tom and his partner do, and often follows having children.

THE BENEFITS OF MARRIAGE

It's long been recognised that mortality is affected by marital status. Married people tend to live longer than unmarried people, are happier, healthier and have lower rates of various mental disorders than the single, widowed or divorced. The greater mortality of the unmarried relative to the married has generally been increasing over the past two to three decades, and it seems that divorced (and widowed) people in their twenties and thirties have particularly high risks of dying compared with other people of the same age (Cramer, 1995).

> ### CRITICAL DISCUSSION 18.2 Do men get more from marriage than women?
>
> - Bee (1994) argues that the greatest beneficiaries of marriage are men, partly because they're less likely than women to have close confidants outside marriage, and partly because wives provide more emotional warmth and support for husbands than husbands do for wives.
>
> - Marriage is less obviously psychologically protective for women, not because a confiding and harmonious relationship is any less important for them (indeed, if anything it's more important), but because:
>
>   (a) many marriages don't provide such relationships, and
>
>   (b) other consequences of marriage differ between the sexes.
>
>   (The 'advantage' of marriage for men is reflected in the higher rates of men's re-marriage following divorce: see text below.)
>
> - Although our attitudes towards education and women's careers have changed, Rutter and Rutter (1992), echoing Levinson's concept of 'gender-splitting' (see Box 18.4), have proposed that:
>
>   > The potential benefits of a harmonious relationship may, for a woman, be counterbalanced by the stresses involved in giving up a job or in being handicapped in a career progression or promotion through having to combine a career and parenthood.
>
>   This is discussed further on pages 347–348.

For a discussion of the effects of divorce, see Gross, 2005.

I'm not happy that the incidence of coronary heart disease in women is increasing. A study by Hayes et al. (1980, in Ogden, 2004) showed that having a higher number of children increased the risk of CHD in working women, but not in non-working women.

ASK YOURSELF ...

- Why – or how – might marriage produce these beneficial effects? Look back at your answers to the previous 'Ask Yourself ...' box. Did any of the arguments for marriage include its psychological/emotional benefits?

- Are there any reasons for believing that either men or women derive greater benefits?

PARENTHOOD

For most people, parenthood and child-rearing represent key transitions. According to Bee (1994), 90 per cent of adults will become parents, mostly in their twenties and thirties. But parenthood varies in meaning and impact more than any other life transition. It may occur at any time from adolescence to middle age, and for some men may even occur in late adulthood! Parenthood may also be planned or unplanned, wanted or unwanted, and there are many motives for having children.

Traditionally, parenthood is the domain of the married couple. However, it may involve a single woman, a homosexual couple (see page 348), a cohabiting couple or couples who adopt or foster children. In recent decades there's been a marked rise in the number of teenage pregnancies (see Critical Discussion 17.2), and even more recently, the phenomenon of 'minimal parenting' (as in donor insemination – see Chapter 14).

Equally, though, the increasing importance of careers for women has also led to more and more couples postponing starting a family, so that the woman can become better established in her career (see Box 18.4). For example, women's average age at the birth of their first child was almost 30 in 2003 – compared with 23 in the 1960s (Groskop, 2004). Consequently, there's a new class of middle-aged parents with young children (Turnbull, 1995).

PREGNANCY AND CHILDBIRTH

Pregnancy, childbirth and parenthood require massive physiological and psychological adjustments on the part of the woman. Even under normal circumstances, the transition to motherhood may be problematical, especially if the woman's prior expectations don't meet with reality (Hillan, 1991).

CRITICAL DISCUSSION 18.3 What do women know about childbirth? (based on Churchill, 1995)

- The report *Changing Childbirth* (1993, in Churchill, 1995) provided the blueprint for a change in midwifery and obstetric practice to a more woman-centred approach, potentially helping to resolve the conflict between lay and professional views and experience of childbirth.

- The main recommendations of the report were that women should be provided with adequate information to enable decision-making regarding care, and that continuity of care (provided primarily by midwives) is essential for communication between health care professionals and patients.

- The notion of consent to medical intervention becomes a nonsense if women aren't adequately informed. For example, women may be manipulated by the professional's concentration on delivery as a potential disaster, feel forced into the hospital's 'surgical agenda', or feel pressurised into conforming to the expectations of the patient role in what could be, after all, an emergency situation. These are ethical as much as practical issues.

- It is the responsibility of health care professionals to provide women and their partners with information that's both accurate and accessible, enabling them to participate in the decision-making process and to feel that they have taken a meaningful role in the birth of their child.

- Churchill cites evidence from both the UK and the USA, which shows that many women are dissatisfied with the amount of information they receive during childbirth and that this affects their perceptions and sense of participation in the birth process.
- *Changing Childbirth* places midwives at the centre of the information-providing process. Vocal midwives have for many years been advocating a more dominant and less subservient role for women in the delivery process. They can facilitate communication between women and their doctors, and ensure that women's needs aren't ignored or suppressed.

This is emphasising the advocacy role of nurses. Advocacy is about 'influencing those who have power on behalf of those who do not' (Teasdale, 1998: 1).

Oakley (1980, in Hillan, 1991) found that the most normal of births can involve elements of loss for the mother: of self-confidence, body image (see Chapter 16) and previous employment. Many women worry that their baby may be abnormal, and about how well they'll cope with motherhood.

In addition to these 'normal' stressors, the woman who has had a Caesarean section (CS) has to cope with the physical and psychological impact of anaesthesia and major surgery, which may have occurred on top of a long and exhausting labour (Hillan, 1991). The very use of 'section' distinguishes a Caesarean from other types of abdominal surgery (Oakley, 1983, in Hillan, 1991). For example, a common consequence of major surgery is depression, yet the same assumption isn't made about a CS. At the same time, the woman who's undergone a Caesarean delivery is often expected to cope with the demands of her new baby, and this may involve activities that are normally forbidden to patients who've had abdominal surgery.

Hillan cites several studies that show a range of negative responses to delivery by CS, including:

◎ a sense of failure at not being able to deliver the baby normally
◎ a sense of guilt at putting the baby in danger and depriving her partner of the shared experience of birth, and
◎ a sense of anger and disappointment at having been deprived of a normal birth.

She also cites studies which suggest that three factors in particular may moderate some of these negative responses. These are:

1. preparation for the CS – women who experience an emergency CS have less positive perceptions of the delivery method than those delivered either vaginally or by elective CS

2. the type of anaesthesia used: women who have an epidural and so remain conscious throughout feel more in control of the situation and benefit from early contact with the baby. A general anaesthetic may produce a gap in the woman's recollections and she may find it difficult to identify the baby as her own

3. the presence of the father in the operating theatre – when partners are present, women express greater satisfaction with the delivery experience. Many hospitals in the UK and the USA allow fathers to be present in the operating theatre for delivery (see Chapter 14).

Nicky, a young single mother I met on my community placement (see diary entry page 255) who was failing to bond with her second baby, had all these negative experiences: a Caesarean section under general anaesthetic, her baby was in intensive care for 24 hours and the father was absent.

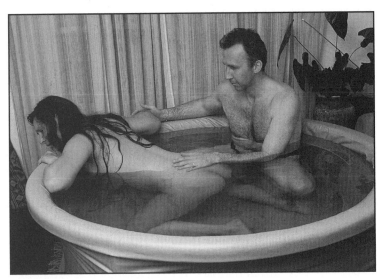

Being at the birth of his child can help counteract a father's feelings of being excluded during the pregnancy – and afterwards. It can also help him to form an emotional bond with the baby

WOMANHOOD AND MOTHERHOOD

According to Kremer (1998), in the postindustrial/postmodern world of the twenty-first century we're still influenced by beliefs and attitudes regarding work and the sexes (or 'gendered employment profiles') inherited from an earlier time. For example, the *motherhood mystique/mandate* refers to the belief that women are born and reared to be, first and foremost, mothers: while the 'fatherhood mandate' is hardly, if ever, mentioned (see Chapter 14). Another example is the stereotype of men as inherently more committed to work than women, whose attitudes towards it are less positive than men's.

The motherhood mandate has at least three important implications:

1. Motherhood is 'natural'. Berryman (in Lacey, 1998) maintains that motherhood is still seen as synonymous with womanhood:

> Parenthood is seen as a central, key role in women's lives in a way that it isn't for men. Women who don't become mothers are seen as psychologically inadequate – wanting in some way. But there is plenty of evidence that motherhood doesn't come naturally to all women; it is a skill that many women have to learn.

For example, Berryman maintains that, because smaller families and fewer siblings are now the norm, many women today have little experience of children when they start their own families – and the reality can come as a shock. This belief that mothering comes 'naturally' is so deep-rooted that women who don't bond immediately with their babies feel inadequate or guilty, or perhaps both. However, there are indications that attitudes towards having children are changing. There will be 107,000 fewer children in the UK in 2020 than in 2006, and in 2005 22 per cent of women aged 35 hadn't yet had children. Seven million people live alone in the UK, twice as many as in 1973 (Hinsliff and Martin, 2006).

2. Most people would probably consider it to be 'unnatural' (or 'wicked') for a mother to leave her children, even if they're left in the care of their father, who she believes will

look after them better than she could herself. However, the number of absent mothers targeted by the (now defunct) Child Support Agency (CSA) trebled between 1995 and 1998, with over 37,000 being approached to pay child maintenance. One in 20 absent parents is a woman (Lacey, 1998). Either there are a lot more 'unnatural' or 'wicked' women out there than was previously thought, or the motherhood mandate needs serious revision.

3. It's 'unnatural' or simply 'wrong' for a mother of young children to go out to work. Related to this is the stereotype concerning women's attitudes towards paid employment. Is there any foundation for this stereotype (see Gross, 2005)?

Nicky needed help to develop mothering skills; I learned mine from my extended family. The third point is the source of many of my, and my colleagues', guilt. But are we 'unnatural' or simply victims of a traditional perspective in a changing world?

LESBIAN AND GAY PARENTING

In the context of advocating that psychologists should study homosexual relationships in their own terms (and not by comparison with heterosexual ones), Kitzinger and Coyle (1995) suggest that we might want to ask how the children of lesbian/gay couples understand and talk about their parents' relationships, and how they can develop positive views about homosexuality in a heterosexual culture. Homosexual couples have always been involved in parenting through partners' previous heterosexual relationships. The recent increase in fostering/adoption of children by gay men, and the ongoing 'lesbian baby boom', mean that many more homosexual couples are parents than used to be the case.

According to Kitzinger *et al.* (1998), research into lesbian/gay parenting was initially concerned with whether or how far the children of lesbians and (to a lesser extent) gay men could be distinguished psychologically from those of heterosexuals. On balance, this research suggested that these children were no more 'at risk' than children raised in heterosexual families.

For example, Taylor (1993) found no evidence that children reared in gay/lesbian families were more disturbed or had greater gender identity confusion than those reared in heterosexual families. Barrett and Robinson (1994) reviewed the impact of gay fathering on children. They stress the need to take into account that these children are likely to have experienced parental divorce and to show the psychological distress that often accompanies it. Although these children may be isolated, angry and in need of help sorting out their feelings about homosexuality in general, they're in little danger of being sexually abused, and adjust well to their family situations. While the relationships with their fathers may be stormy at first, they also have the potential for considerable honesty and openness.

Increasingly, psychologists are researching areas directly rooted in the concerns of lesbian/gay parents themselves, including coming out to one's children, and managing different co-parenting arrangements (such as a lesbian mother with her female lover, her ex-husband, a gay male sperm donor, or a gay male co-parent; Kitzinger *et al.*, 1998).

CONCLUSIONS

Although some of the most influential and popular explanations of personality change in early and middle adulthood have adopted *stage approaches*, critics argue that adult development doesn't occur in predictable and ordered ways. An alternative, yet *complementary*, approach is to assess the impact of *critical life events*. These include two major *normative age-graded* influences, marriage/partnering and parenthood.

In the case of parenthood, the changing roles of men and women have been shown to be crucial, especially women's participation in the labour market. This means that to appreciate the impact of various life events, they must be examined in the broader context of social norms, which, at least in western countries, are constantly shifting. The chapter has also illustrated the *mutual influence* of different life events involving family and relationships.

Levinson's theory of development has made me aware how a critical life event such as illness can be life changing for many people other than the patient. For Frank, the future he anticipated is, at best, less predictable and may be threatened. His leadership role, at work and in the family, has suddenly changed to a highly dependent one. He may need to become less ambitious – or even decide to take early retirement from his high-stress occupation. The change to his career plans may depress him at a time when his wife is establishing hers.

Reflecting on the individual life experiences of Frank's family shows that what is considered 'normal' at each stage can change over a generation. Frank's wife devoted her early adulthood to caring for the family, an example of Levinson's (1986) 'gender-splitting' phenomenon; she now has her own satisfying career. Frank's illness may lead to conflict between her own goals and her investment in her husband's needs (Durkin, 1995).

While concern for Frank's condition must take immediate priority, in the overall caring situation we must consider him in the context of the unique psychosocial factors that make up his lived experience.

CHAPTER SUMMARY

◎ In Erikson's **psychosocial theory**, the task of **young adulthood** is to achieve **intimacy** and to avoid **isolation**. The central task of **middle adulthood** is the attainment of generativity and avoidance of **stagnation**.

◎ Many people struggle with issues of identity and intimacy **at the same time**, and women tend to achieve intimacy **before** 'occupational identity', submerging their identity into those of their partners.

◎ Levinson *et al.* were concerned with how adulthood is actually **experienced**. Their **life-structure theory** identifies **phases/periods** that are either stable (**structure-building**) or transitional (**structure-changing**). A sequence of eras overlaps in the form of **cross-era transitions**.

◎ **Early adult transition** is a developmental bridge between adolescence and adulthood, and **entry life structure for early adulthood** is the first structure-building phase.

◎ Levinson *et al.* see **crisis** as both inevitable and necessary (**normative**). But people of all ages suffer crises (**'adolescing'**), and a growing number of people are deciding to make radical changes in their lifestyles (**downshifting**), both earlier and later than 'mid-life'.

◎ While men have fairly unified, career-focused visions of the future, women's **dreams** are split between career and marriage/family responsibilities (**gender-splitting**).

- The **age-30 transition** generally lasts longer for women than for men, and **'settling down'** is much less clear-cut. Trying to integrate career and marriage and family responsibilities is very difficult for most women.
- The view that adult development is **'stage-like'** has been criticised on the grounds that it underestimates **individual variability**. Stage theories also imply a **discontinuity** of development.
- **Marriage** and **parenting** are **normative, age-graded influences**. These are also called **marker events** or **critical life events**.
- **Married people** tend to live longer, and are happier, healthier and have lower rates of mental disorder than unmarried people. Men benefit most from marriage, and the potential benefits of marriage for women may be counterbalanced by gender-splitting.
- **Parenthood** has greater variability in meaning and impact than any other life transition.
- It's vital that women receive sufficient information about **childbirth** so that they are able to participate fully in the process. This applies especially in the case of birth by **Caesarean section (CS)**.
- The **motherhood mystique/mandate** can make women who don't bond immediately with their babies feel inadequate. But women are increasingly postponing having children, or deciding not to have children at all.
- The motherhood mandate also implies that it's unnatural for mothers to leave their children, and that it's wrong for a mother of young children to go out to work.
- Many more **lesbian/gay couples** are parents than used to be the case. Early research examined whether the children of such parents were more 'at risk' than those raised in heterosexual families, but more recently the emphasis has shifted to issues such as co-parenting arrangements.

LATE ADULTHOOD

19

While 'growing up' is normally seen as desirable, 'growing old' has far more negative connotations. This negative view is based on the *decrement model*, which sees ageing as a process of decay or decline in physical and mental health, intellectual abilities and social relationships.

An alternative to the decrement model is the *personal growth model*, which stresses the potential advantages of late adulthood (or 'old age'), such as increased leisure time, reduced responsibilities, and the ability to concentrate only on matters of high priority (Kalish, 1982). This much more positive view is how ageing has been studied within the *lifespan approach*.

In this chapter we consider some of the theories and research concerned with *adjustment to late adulthood*. It begins by looking at what's meant by the term 'old', which turns out to be more complex than it might seem. *Stereotyped beliefs* about what elderly people are like are an inherent part of prejudiced attitudes towards them. Research into some of the cognitive and social changes that occur in late adulthood bring these stereotypes and prejudice into sharp focus. *Retirement* (a *normative, age-graded influence*) is often taken to mark the 'official' start of old age (see Gross, 2005).

From my diary (15): Year 2/Teaching Block

Today I attended the Arthritis Club to see Alfred Green, the subject of my case study of an elderly person showing client-led assessment of needs. I met Alfred (he asked me to use his first name) during my first year community placement; he was caring for his wife who'd had a stroke two years previously and has since died. He's suffering from osteoarthritis of his left hip which has worsened recently. I noticed he hobbled painfully to the tea table, where Joan, the regular Health Care Assistant (HCA), was putting out cups of tea.

As Alfred sat down, Joan took his stick and put it in the corner (out of his reach). She pushed the plate of biscuits towards him, which Alfred refused, indicating his waistline. Joan then patted him on the head and told him he was a 'very good boy' as though he were a child. She moved on – oblivious to his reaction.

Alfred looked very angry and pushed back his chair to get up. I quickly fetched his stick and tried to help him but he shook my hand away and struggled to his feet. I suggested we go to a quiet corner for our chat. When he was settled I offered to get us some tea (and remembered to ask how he liked it)!

ASK YOURSELF ...
- How old is old?

- Is 'old' simply a matter of chronological age? (Not the same question.)

THE MEANING OF 'OLD'

People today are living longer and retaining their health better than any previous generation (Baltes and Baltes, 1993). The proportion of older people in the British population has increased dramatically in recent years. In 1961, 2 per cent of the population (one million people) were aged 80 or over. By 1991, this figure had risen to 4 per cent (two million people). The number of centenarians in the UK has risen from 271 (in 1951), to 1185 (1971), to 4400 (1991). In 1997, the number stood at 8000 with projections of 12,000 (2001) and 30,000 (2030) (McCrystal, 1997). Figures for the USA show that the number of centenarians doubled between 1990 and 2000, and may increase more than eleven-fold by 2050 (Brown, 2000).

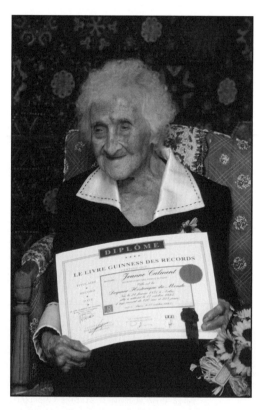

The oldest person who ever lived: Jeanne Calment died in 1997 at the age of 122

Because of this *demographic imperative* (Swensen, 1983), developmental psychologists have become increasingly interested in our later years. But what do we mean by 'old'? Kastenbaum's (1979) *'The ages of me'* questionnaire assesses how people see themselves at the present moment in relation to their ages (see Box 19.1).

Box 19.1 Kastenbaum's 'The ages of me' questionnaire

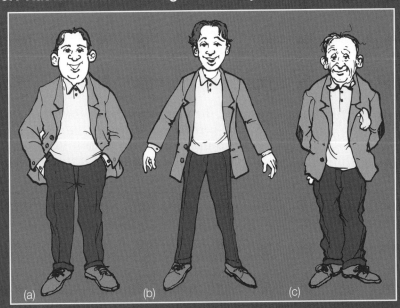

Figure 19.1 While (c) might depict someone's chronological age, (a) might correspond to his biological age and (b) might represent his subjective age

- My **chronological age** is my actual or official age, dated from my time of birth. My chronological age is …

- My **biological age** refers to the state of my face and body. In other people's eyes, I look as though I am about … years of age. In my own eyes, I look like someone of about … years of age.

- My **subjective age** is indicated by how I feel. Deep down inside, I really feel like a person of about … years of age.

- My **functional age**, which is closely related to my **social age**, refers to the kind of life I lead, what I am able to do, the status I believe I have, whether I work, have dependent children and live in my own home. My thoughts and interests are like those of a person of about … years of age, and my position in society is like that of a person of about … years of age.

(Adapted from Kastenbaum, 1979)

Alfred is 71 and looks younger; he's very trim, with an energetic manner and is usually affable. But his osteoarthritic hip is indicative of bodily ageing (i.e. his biological age). This limits his activity, which affects his functional, and no doubt his social, age. His condition is painful, which may affect his subjective age. When I asked him how he was, he said he was fine except when he was treated like a six-year-old! So although the age perceptions seem interrelated, Alfred's negative feelings seemed to stem more from his functional age and the attitude of others.

ASK YOURSELF ...

• How old are you according to Kastenbaum's questionnaire?

• Which measure of age is most significant in defining current health care policy?

Few people, irrespective of their chronological ages, describe themselves *consistently* (that is, they tend to give *different* responses to the different questionnaire items). For example, people over 20 (including those in their 70s and 80s) usually describe themselves as feeling younger than their chronological ages. We also generally consider ourselves to be *too* old.

AGEISM

It seems, then, that knowing a person's chronological age tells us little about the sort of life that person leads or what s/he is like. However, one of the dangerous aspects of ageism is that chronological age is assumed to be an accurate indicator of all the other ages. According to Comfort (1977), ageism is:

> ... the notion that people cease to be people, cease to be the same people or become people of a distinct and inferior kind by virtue of having lived a specified number of years ... Like racism, which it resembles, it is based on fear.

Similarly, Bromley (1977) argues that most people react adversely to the elderly because they seem to deviate from our concept of 'normal' human beings. As part of the 'welfarist approach' to understanding the problems of an ageing society (Fennell *et al.*, 1988), 'they' (i.e. elderly people) are designated as different, occupying another world from 'us' – a process that for all perceived minorities tends to be dehumanising and sets lower or different standards of social value or individual worth (Manthorpe, 1994).

Using collective terms, whatever they are, for older patients suggests stereotyping, and that ageism is entrenched in our way of thinking.

THE EFFECTS OF STEREOTYPING

Box 19.2 Can stereotypes make you ill?

- In April 2000, the charity Age Concern highlighted the plight of Jill Baker, a cancer patient in her 60s. She was shocked to discover that, despite still being in a generally good state of health, a junior doctor she'd never met had put 'not for resuscitation' on her records.

- According to Ebrahim (in Payne, 2000), 'Medical students still rejoice in their stereotypes of "geriatric crumbly" and "GOMER" (get out of my emergency room) patients.'

- Ebrahim cites US evidence showing that 'do not resuscitate' orders are commonly used for people with HIV, blacks, alcohol misusers, and non-English speakers, suggesting that doctors have stereotypes of who isn't worth saving.

- In the UK, 1 in 20 people aged over 65 had been refused treatment by the NHS, with 1 in 10 over-50s believing they were treated differently (i.e. worse) because of their age (based on an Age Concern survey).

Having read all this I'm uncomfortably aware of how easy it is to make stereotypical assumptions about patients.

Adler (2000) cites American research by Levy and her colleagues showing that stereotypes can affect how the elderly think about themselves in ways that can be detrimental to their mental and physical health. In one study, elderly participants spent a few minutes concentrating on a computer-based reaction-time test. Age-related words were subliminally presented on the screen (too quickly to be consciously registered) and were either negative (e.g. 'senile, 'forgetful', diseased'), or positive (e.g. 'wise', 'astute', 'accomplished').

The participants were subsequently asked if they'd request an expensive but potentially life-saving medical treatment, without which they'd die within a month. Most of those who'd 'seen' the positive words (evoking a positive stereotype) chose the life-saving treatment, but most of those who were exposed to negative words declined.

In another study, participants were challenged with a series of maths problems following ten minutes' exposure to positive or negative words. The latter showed signs of stress – heart rate, blood pressure and skin conductance all increased, and stayed high for over 30 minutes. In contrast, those exposed to positive words sailed through the challenge stress free.

Since many studies have linked chronic stress to disease (see Chapter 5), Levy suspects that repeated triggering of negative stereotypes over a period of several years may be making elderly people ill (Adler, 2000).

Joan's remarks obviously affected Alfred negatively; he was very upset – I could almost see his BP rising!

Stereotypes of older people – 'the elderly' – are more deeply entrenched than (mis)conceptions of gender differences. It's therefore not surprising that people are overwhelmingly unenthusiastic about becoming 'old' (Stuart-Hamilton, 1997). According to Jones (1993), everyone over retirement age is seen as forming a strange homogeneous mass, with limited abilities, few needs and few rights:

> What other section of the population that spans more than 30 years in biological time is grouped together in such an illogical manner? ... As a consequence, older people suffer a great deal ... As for experience and wisdom, these qualities are no longer valued in this fast-moving high-technology world. They are devalued by the community, as well as by their owners. (Jones, 1993)

Basing his treatment on Alfred's chronological age makes no more sense than assuming all young people are equally fit. He was a talented tennis player when young and worked as manager of a large sports shop. He was extremely well informed about his condition – he'd researched it on the Internet. He watched his weight, followed a recommended 'arthritis' diet and did his limited exercises daily, although he finds weight-bearing ones painful now. 'I've resorted to playing computer games and Sudoku instead,' he said, sounding apologetic.

BODILY CHANGES AND ADVANCED OLD AGE

According to Coleman and O'Hanlon (2004), the lack of research interest in advanced old age (AOA) has produced an imbalance in theories of ageing. A major focus of recent developmental accounts has been on the concept of 'successful ageing' (Rowe and Kahn, 1998). But one effect of this has been to stigmatise further the *very* old. If successful ageing includes the avoidance of disease and disability, preservation of

355

cognitive abilities and an active life, then sooner or later many people will fail the test. As Tobin (1999) puts it, 'What comes after successful ageing?' One of the major lifespan theorists, Erikson, towards the end of his long life, questioned whether there might be a stage beyond *ego integrity* (versus *despair* – see page 366).

Strawbridge *et al.* (1998, in Coleman and O'Hanlon, 2004) have proposed that 'frailty' (a functional loss in at least two of: physical and nutritional status; cognitive functioning; sensory functioning) is much more useful than 'disability' in relation to late life. They found that only 20 per cent in the 65–74 age group were frail, compared with 32 per cent of 75–84-year-olds and 49 per cent of the over-85s. This is consistent with the clinical observation that half of the 'very old' (i.e. 85 and over) need practical help. So, 85 seems to be a convenient age to define late life (AOA) at the present time in most western societies. It's also worth noting that this age group are 'survivors': they represent just 25 per cent of their original birth cohort (while those over 95 represent a mere 3 per cent) (Smith and Baltes, 1997).

A Finnish interview study by Heikkinnen (2000, in Coleman and O'Hanlon, 2004) found that, by 85, most participants felt they'd crossed a line into old age:

> Deteriorating health, deteriorating sense perception (particularly eyesight and hearing), frailty, pain, impaired memory, mobility problems and loss of human relations (particularly the loss of spouse through death), were the vulnerability factors that … formed the boundary conditions for experienced ageing. (Heikkinnen, 2000, in Coleman and O'Hanlon, 2004)

By 85, life had to be structured more and more around physical needs. 'Bodiliness' had become a critical concern.

Frail is the last word I'd use to describe Alfred. He doesn't consider himself a problem – he has a problem, that's all. He's on the waiting list for a hip replacement; when it's dealt with I'm sure he'll be back to 'successfully ageing'.

ASK YOURSELF ...
• Do nurses have a role to play in the lives of those who are 'successfully ageing'?

RESEARCH QUESTION
• Why can't we generalise from cross-sectional studies?

COGNITIVE CHANGES IN LATE ADULTHOOD

Until recently, and consistent with the *decrement model* (see Introduction and Overview), it was commonly believed that intellectual capacity peaked in the late teens or early twenties, levelled off, and then began to decline fairly steadily during middle age and more rapidly in old age.

The evidence on which this claim was based came from *cross-sectional studies* (studying different age groups at the same time).

However, we cannot draw firm conclusions from such studies, because the age groups compared represent different generations with different experiences (the *cohort effect*). Unless we know how 60-year-olds, say, performed when they were 40 and 20, it's impossible to say whether or not intelligence declines with age.

An alternative methodology is the *longitudinal study*, in which the same people are tested and retested at various times during their lives. Several such studies have produced data contradicting the results of cross-sectional studies, indicating that at least some people retain their intellect well into middle age and beyond (Holahan and Sears, 1995). However, the evidence suggests that there are some age-related changes in different kinds of intelligence and aspects of memory.

Alfred seems as alert as he ever was, but how can I tell? This highlights the difficulty in establishing 'baseline' measures for psychological as well as physiological observations.

CHANGES IN INTELLIGENCE

Although psychologists have always disagreed about the definition of intelligence, there's general acceptance that it's *multi-dimensional* (composed of several different abilities). An important – and very relevant – distinction is that between crystallised and fluid intelligence.

◎ *Crystallised intelligence* results from accumulated knowledge, including a knowledge of how to reason, language skills and an understanding of technology. This type of intelligence is linked to education, experience and cultural background, and is measured by tests of general information.

◎ *Fluid intelligence* is the ability to solve novel and unusual problems (those not experienced before). It allows us to perceive and draw inferences about relationships among patterns of stimuli and to conceptualise abstract information, which aids problem-solving. Fluid intelligence is measured by tests using novel and unusual problems not based on specific knowledge or particular previous learning.

Crystallised intelligence *increases* with age, and people tend to continue improving their performance until near the end of their lives (Horn, 1982). Using the *cross-longitudinal method* (in which *different* age groups are *retested* over a long period of time), Schaie and Hertzog (1983) reported that fluid intelligence *declines* for all age groups over time, peaking between 20 and 30.

Explaining changes in intelligence

Intelligence (IQ) tests are typically heavily loaded with *fluid* intelligence questions at the expense of crystallised, and they are also usually *timed*. This implies that tests of general intelligence are biased against older people (see below). But tests of crystallised intelligence are, arguably, biased *in favour* of older people (there's usually *no* time limit). However, removing the time limit from tests of fluid intelligence doesn't remove the age difference – but it does reduce it. So, the preservation of crystallised intelligence in later life is, in part, illusory (Stuart-Hamilton, 2000).

Physiological changes (such as cardiovascular and metabolic dysfunction) can have serious effects on physiological processes in the brain; in turn, these can lower intellectual performance. For example, *response times* (RTs) are a good indicator of how efficiently the nervous system operates. Not only do we get slower as we get older, but this slowing is strongly correlated with IQ test scores: the slower the RTs, the lower the test score (the *general slowing hypothesis* – Stuart-Hamilton, 2003).

The prime cause of the decline in intelligence in elderly people is a slowing of nervous system processes (Stuart-Hamilton, 2003). Some argue that an even better indication of change is the state of the *sensory systems* (as measured by vision and hearing). A composite index composed of measures of sensory efficiency correlates impressively with IQ test scores (Baltes and Lindenberger, 1997, in Stuart-Hamilton, 2003). Alternative measures of intellectual activity (such as problem-solving or memory: see below) are highly correlated with IQ (Rabbitt, 1993).

ASK YOURSELF ...
- Does slower necessarily mean less intelligent?
- Why should Alfred be encouraged to pursue his latest hobbies?

The demands of retirement are not usually the same as those of a work environment, so if Alfred takes a bit longer to solve his puzzles or complete his games, does it matter? What does matter to him is his ability to function independently.

CHANGES IN MEMORY

Some aspects of memory appear to decline with age, possibly because we become less effective at processing information (which may underlie cognitive changes in general – Stuart-Hamilton, 1994). On *recall* tests, older adults generally perform more poorly than younger adults. But the reverse is sometimes true, as shown by the performance of older contestants on the TV quiz show *Mastermind*. On *recognition* tests, the differences between younger and older people are less apparent, and may even disappear. As far as everyday memory is concerned, the evidence indicates that elderly people do have trouble recalling events from their youth and early lives (Miller and Morris, 1993).

Alfred complained that his short-term memory has deteriorated, which I expected. But I thought older people enjoyed talking about their past lives because they had little to look forward to. Was that another stereotypical assumption?

Dementia

Significant memory deficits are one feature of dementia (mental frailty). Fortunately, severe dementia affects only a minority of elderly people, in contrast with physical frailty (see above). Sometimes, they coincide, as in late-onset Parkinson's disease (Coleman and O'Hanlon, 2004). The onset of physical disability, suddenly (as in a stroke) or more generally (as with osteoarthritis), represents one form of pathway into late life. Dementia represents a very different pathway:

> ... The many disabling consequences arising from mental frailty make dementia the major health problem of later life in modern western society. It is the most age-related of all the disabling conditions affecting older people ... (Coleman and O'Hanlon, 2004)

The rate of dementia changes with age in a strikingly consistent way. The average rate is 5.6 per cent at age 75–79, 10.5 per cent at 80–84, and 39 per cent at 90–95 (Black *et al.*, 1990, in Coleman and O'Hanlon, 2004). However, other studies have found rates varying from 40–70 per cent for the 90–95 age group (Hofman *et al.*, 1991, in Coleman and O'Hanlon). It's unclear whether the rate continues to increase in centenarians. But with so many more people surviving into their nineties, overall prevalence is increasing. According to Coleman and O'Hanlon,

> Dementia has now become the major reason for receiving institutional care, and a challenge to the physically frail who need to be cared for in the same environment.

There are many types of dementia, including those induced by brain injuries, tumours, toxic states and infections, but the most common form is *Alzheimer's disease* (AD). AD accounts for about half of all cases of dementia, but only 5–15 per cent of over-65s and 20–40 per cent of over-80s are affected (Voss, 2002). Even very late in life cortical neurons seem capable of responding to enriched conditions by forming new functional connections with other neurons. This is supported by the finding that those who keep mentally active are those who maintain their cognitive abilities (Rogers *et al.*, 1990).

AD is one of the most debilitating and dreaded of the common diseases of ageing. It's estimated that, by 2010, over one million people in the UK will be affected. It used to be described more generally as 'senile dementia', but is now referred to as 'senile dementia of the Alzheimer's type'. People at the height of their intellectual powers can be struck down with it. Patients experience a frightening loss of sense of their own identity and access to their store of personal memories. Their brains shrink, and the neurons themselves change appearance – they develop 'tangles and plaques' (Rose, 2003).

According to Rogers et al. (1990) it's excellent that Alfred is playing computer games – he's doing a sort of cognitive keep fit! On the other hand, as Rose (2003) points out, it doesn't prevent intellectuals like Iris Murdoch being 'struck down' by Alzheimer's.

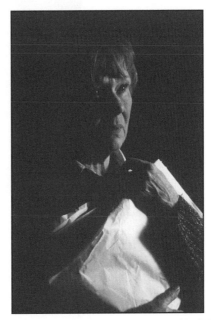

Judi Dench as Iris Murdoch, the gifted novelist and academic, in *Iris* (2001). She died from Alzheimer's disease

Is Alzheimer's a disease process or part of normal ageing?

Some researchers claim that Alzheimer's disease is an *accelerated form* of normal changes in the ageing brain, so that we'd all get the disease if we lived long enough. The opposing view is that cognitive decline isn't an inevitable part of ageing, but rather it reflects a *disease process* that is more likely to affect us as we get older (Smith, 1998).

Work by the Oxford Project to Investigate Memory and Ageing (OPTIMA) has used X-ray computerised tomography (CT) to examine the *medial temporal lobe*. While this tiny area comprises only 2 per cent of the volume of the whole cerebral cortex, it includes the *hippocampus*, a structure known to be crucial for memory. Also, the neurons of the medial temporal lobe connect with almost all other parts of the cortex, so any damage to this part of the brain is likely to have consequences for the functioning of the rest of the cortex.

X-ray CT images show that the medial temporal lobe is markedly smaller in people with dementia who eventually die of Alzheimer's disease than in age-matched controls without cognitive deficit. Repeated CT scans over periods of several years have found that shrinkage is slow in control participants (about 1–1.5 per cent per year), compared with an alarming rate of some 15 per cent per year in Alzheimer's patients (Smith, 1998).

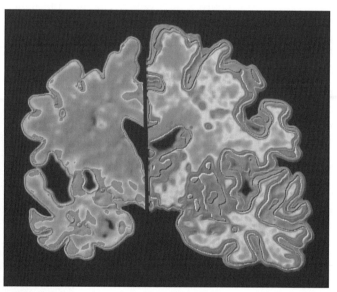

A CT scan of the brain of an Alzheimer's patient (left) and of a normal person (right)

These, and other supportive data, led the OPTIMA researchers to conclude that Alzheimer's disease is distinct from normal ageing, and that it cannot be simply an acceleration of normal ageing. Although cognitive decline does appear to increase with age for the population as a whole, if we rigorously exclude those with pathological changes (such as early Alzheimer's), then a majority may not show any significant decline. According to Smith (1998), 'We must abandon the fatalistic view that mental decline is an inevitable accompaniment of ageing.' Consistent with this conclusion is the belief that negative cultural stereotypes of ageing actually cause memory decline in the elderly (see Gross, 2005).

So, unless he is unlucky enough to suffer from Alzheimer's disease, Alfred's computer puzzles are a very positive way to maintain his cognitive functioning.

SOCIAL CHANGES IN LATE ADULTHOOD

SOCIAL DISENGAGEMENT THEORY (SDT)

According to Manthorpe (1994), Cumming and Henry's (1961) *social disengagement theory* (SDT) represented the first major attempt to produce a theory about individuals' relationships with society. Based on a five-year study of 275 50–90-year-olds in Kansas City, USA, Cumming and Henry claimed that, 'Many of the relationships between a person and other members of society are severed and those remaining are altered in quality.'

This social disengagement involves the *mutual withdrawal* of society from the individual (through compulsory retirement, children growing up and leaving home, the death of a spouse, and so on) and of the individual from society (Cumming, 1975). As people grow older, they become more solitary, retreat into the inner world of their memories, become emotionally quiescent, and engage in pensive self-reflection.

Cumming sees disengagement as having three components:

1. *shrinkage of life space* refers to the tendency to interact with fewer other people as we grow older, and to occupy fewer roles
2. *increased individuality* means that in the roles that remain, older people are much less governed by strict rules and expectations
3. *acceptance* (even embrace) *of these changes*, so that withdrawal is a voluntary, natural and inevitable process, and represents the most appropriate and successful way of growing old.

As far as society is concerned, the individual's withdrawal is part of an inevitable move towards death – the ultimate disengagement (Manthorpe, 1994). By replacing older individuals with younger people, society renews itself and the elderly are free to die (Bromley, 1988).

Manthorpe's (1994) view of old age predominantly as a progression towards death is a pessimistic one. Disengagement may be welcome for some, but surely that depends on whether it is a voluntary process or not. As his wife's carer Alfred couldn't socialise as much, but it didn't mean he wanted to withdraw from society. And to assume he's 'emotionally quiescent' seems to deny his feelings about the loss of his wife.

An evaluation of social disengagement theory

◎ Bee (1994) sees the first two components as difficult to dispute. However, the third is more controversial because of its view of disengagement as a natural, voluntary and inevitable process, rather than an imposed one.

◎ Bromley (1988) argues that such a view of ageing has detrimental *practical* consequences for the elderly, such as encouraging a policy of segregation, even indifference, and the very destructive belief that old age has no value. For Bromley, an even more serious criticism concerns whether everyone actually does disengage.

ASK YOURSELF ...
- What are the implications of SDT for the current emphasis on caring for elderly people in the community?

> ### KEY STUDY 19.1 Do all older people disengage? (Havighurst *et al.*, 1968)
>
> - Havighurst *et al.* followed up about half the sample originally studied by Cumming and Henry (1961).

- Although increasing age was accompanied by increasing disengagement, at least some remained active and engaged, and they tended to be the happiest. The fact that those who disengage the least are the happiest, have the highest morale and live the longest, contradicts SDT's view that withdrawal from mainstream society is a natural and inherent part of the ageing process (Bee, 1994).

- While some people may choose to lead socially isolated lives and find contentment in them, such disengagement doesn't appear to be necessary for overall mental health in old age.

- Havighurst *et al.* also identified several different *personality types*. These included:

  (a) *reorganisers*, who were involved in a wide range of activities and reorganised their lives to compensate for lost activities, and

  (b) the *disengaged*, who voluntarily moved away from role commitments.

- Consistent with SDT, the latter reported low levels of activity but high 'life satisfaction'. However, the disposition to disengage is a *personality dimension* as well as a characteristic of ageing (Bromley, 1988).

- SDT focuses on *quantitative* changes, such as the reduced number of relationships and roles in old age. But for Carstensen (1996), it's the *qualitative* changes that are crucial:

  > Although age is associated with many losses, including loss of power, social partners, physical health, cognitive efficiency, and, eventually, life itself – and although this list of losses encompasses the very things that younger people typically equate with happiness – research suggests that older people are at least as satisfied with their lives as their younger counterparts.

Havighurst et. al. and Bromley's (1968) comments are convincing. I'd say Alfred is a reorganiser; he didn't voluntarily 'disengage', it was forced on him by circumstances. Eysenck's 'introvert' personality type (see Chapter 6) might well be happier alone; Alfred has an outgoing personality and is already involved in organising funds for the Stroke Association.

The importance of friendships

Although many of these losses are beyond the older person's control (Rosnow, 1985), such as retirement (see below), *friendships* are voluntary, non-institutionalised and relatively enduring relationships which offer comfort and stability. Informal support from friends (and other primary relationships) also reduces dependency on social security agencies, the helping professions and other formal organisations (Duck, 1991; Rainey, 1998). It's the choice element that differentiates friendships from other types of relationships (Baltes and Baltes, 1986), providing older people with control over at least one life domain (Rainey, 1998).

Maintaining close relationships with others is often a significant factor in determining whether older people feel a sense of belonging to the social system. This may become more important with age, because society withdraws from older adults both *behaviourally* (compulsory retirement) and *attitudinally* (attributing diminishing powers, abilities and qualities to elderly people). Both relatives and friends are crucial for determining how life is experienced by older people. Overall, individual adaptation to old age on all levels has been shown to be highly dependent on personal tolerance of stress and life events, and on the availability of informal social support networks (Duck, 1991). These findings regarding the role of friendships and other relationships are consistent with *socio-emotional selectivity theory* (see below).

When I asked Alfred if he enjoyed the weekly meetings at the Arthritis Club he laughed and said, 'Not a lot, but it gets me out, and helps pass the time.' He has little physical contact with his family, so he may well be lonely, which would explain why he goes to the club every week.

ACTIVITY (OR RE-ENGAGEMENT) THEORY (AT)

The major alternative to SDT is *activity* (or *re-engagement*) *theory* (AT) (Havighurst, 1964; Maddox, 1964). Except for inevitable biological and health changes, older people are essentially the same as middle-aged people, with the same psychological and social needs. Decreased social interaction in old age is the result of the withdrawal of an inherently ageist society from the ageing person, and happens against the wishes of most elderly people. The withdrawal *isn't* mutual.

Optimal ageing involves staying active and managing to resist the 'shrinkage' of the social world. This can be achieved by maintaining the activities of middle age for as long as possible, and then finding substitutes for work or retirement (such as leisure or hobbies) and for spouses and friends upon their death (such as grandchildren). It's important for older adults to maintain their role counts, to ensure they always have several different roles to play.

Alfred's roles changed dramatically in retirement. He lost his work role of manager, but became secretary of the bowling club. He gave that up to become a carer; he told me that learning to be a housekeeper and nurse had been hard. Now he's also lost the role of husband and carer. However, he's become active in fundraising for the Stroke Association – he doesn't seem to want to 'disengage'.

An evaluation of activity theory

RESEARCH QUESTION

- Can you think of any objections to activity theory?
- Is it realistic?
- Does it repeat any of the mistakes of SDT?

◉ According to Bond *et al.* (1993), AT can be criticised for being

> … unrealistic because the economic, political and social structure of society prevents the older worker from maintaining a major activity of middle age, namely, 'productive' employment.

The implication seems to be that there really is no substitute for paid employment (at least for men – see below). According to Dex and Phillipson (1986), society appears to measure people's worth by their ability to undertake paid labour, and the more autonomous people are in their working practices, the more respect they seem to deserve. When someone retires, they not only lose their autonomy and right to work for money, but they also lose their *identity*: they cease to be a participant in society and their status is reduced to 'pensioner/senior citizen' or simply 'old person'.

◎ As noted in Key Study 19.1, some elderly people seem satisfied with disengagement, suggesting that AT alone cannot explain successful ageing.

◎ Just as disengagement may be involuntary (as in the case of poor health), so we may face involuntarily high levels of activity (as in looking after grandchildren). Both disengagement and activity may, therefore, be equally maladaptive. SDT might actually *under*estimate, and AT *over*estimate, the degree of control people have over the 'reconstruction' of their lives.

◎ Additionally, both theories see ageing as essentially the same for everyone. But each refers to a legitimate process through which people may come to terms with the many changes that accompany ageing; in other words, they represent *options* (Hayslip and Panek, 1989) and people will select the styles of ageing best suited to their personalities and past experiences or lifestyles. There's no single 'best way' to age (Neugarten and Neugarten, 1987). For Turner and Helms (1989), personality is the key factor, and neither theory can adequately explain successful ageing.

As a manager Alfred must be used to being in control, but at present his athritis prevents him from selecting a way of ageing that seems to fit his personality.

SOCIAL EXCHANGE THEORY (SET)

According to Dyson (1980), both SDT and AT fail to take sufficient account of the physical, social and economic factors which might limit people's choices about how they age. Age robs people of the capacity to engage in the reciprocal give-and-take that is the hallmark of social relationships, and thus weakens their attachment to others. In addition, Dowd (1975) argues that,

> Unlike the aged in traditional societies, older people in industrialised societies have precious few power resources to exchange in daily social interaction.

This inequality of power results in dependence on others and compliance with others' wishes. But for both Dyson and Dowd, there's a more positive aspect to this loss of power. Adjusting to old age in general, and retirement in particular, involves a sort of *contract* between the individual and society. The elderly give up their roles as economically active members of society, but in *exchange* they receive increased leisure time, take on fewer responsibilities, and so on. Although the contract is largely unwritten and not enforceable, most people will probably conform to the expectations about being old which are built into social institutions and stereotypes (see above).

Alfred told me he'd spent a great deal of money on paying for help, holidays and extra treats for his wife. He is no longer as financially secure and this may also limit his social activities.

SOCIO-EMOTIONAL SELECTIVITY THEORY (SST)

According to *socio-emotional selectivity theory* (SST) (Carstensen, 1991, 1992, 1993, 1996; Carstensen *et al.*, 1999), social contact is motivated by various goals, including basic survival, information-seeking, development of self-concept and the regulation of emotion. While these all operate throughout life, the importance of specific goals varies, depending on one's place in the life cycle. For example, when *emotional regulation* is the major goal, people are highly selective in their choice of social partners, preferring familiar others. This selectivity is at its peak in infancy (see Chapter 14) and old age: elderly people turn increasingly to friends and adult children for emotional support (see above).

Even independent Alfred needs emotional support. If he was getting this from his family and friends, would he bother to come to the Arthritis Club?

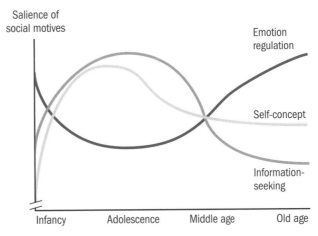

Figure 19.2 Idealised illustration of the lifespan trajectory (from Carstensen, Socioemotional selectivity: A life-span developmental account of social behaviour. In M.R. Merrens & G.C. Brannigan (eds) *The Developmental Psychologists: Research Adventures across the Life-Span*. Copyright 1996, reproduced with permission of the McGraw-Hill Companies.)

◎ According to SST, a major factor contributing to these changes in social motives is *construal of the future*, which is indicated by chronological age. When the future is perceived as largely open-ended, long-term goals assume great significance. But when the future is perceived as limited, attention shifts to the *present*. Immediate needs, such as emotional states, become more salient. So, contrary to SDT (which sees reduced social contact as being caused by emotional states becoming diluted and dampened down), SST predicts that emotional concerns will become *more* important in old age. Reduced social activity in old age is deliberately and actively chosen, because it benefits the elderly person (and so can be considered 'successful').

◎ Health is the other major factor that accounts for these changes. In many cases, healthy older people *don't* show these patterns of social activity (Carstensen, 1991).

Alfred's lack of social activity doesn't appear to be voluntary; it's been imposed on him by life events, his absent family and his own disability.

An evaluation of SST

If SST is correct, it would follow that when younger people hold expectations about the future that are similar to those of elderly people, they should make the same kinds of social choices as those typically made by the latter.

KEY STUDY 19.2 How a limited future can influence current concerns (Carstensen, 1996)

- Carstensen describes a study involving a group of healthy gay men, a group of HIV-positive, asymptomatic gay men, and a group of HIV-positive, symptomatic gay men. A group of young, middle-aged and old men representing the general population served as a control group.

- The social preferences of the healthy gay men were similar to those of the young men from the control group. Those of the asymptomatic group mimicked those of the middle-aged controls, while those of the symptomatic group were strikingly similar to those of the oldest control participants. In other words:

  > The closer the men were to the end of their lives, the greater weight they placed on affective qualities of prospective social partners ... changes in social preferences appear to be altered in much the same way when futures are limited by age as when futures are limited by disease ... (Carstensen, 1996)

- According to Carstensen (1996), the findings relevant to SST taken together paint quite an optimistic picture. Age-related reduction in social contact appears to be highly selective (rather than reflecting a reduced capacity), such that interaction is limited to those people who are most familiar and can provide the greatest emotional security and comfort. This is an excellent strategy when time and social energy need to be invested wisely.

Alfred has lost his most significant affective relationship and his arthritic hip prevents him from compensating for that. I suspect when he's recovered from his operation he'll take up bowling again.

PSYCHOSOCIAL THEORY

Another alternative to SDT and AT is Erikson's *psychosocial theory* (see Chapters 17 and 18). A more valid and useful way of looking at what all elderly people have in common might be to examine the importance of old age as a stage of development, albeit the last (which is where its importance lies).

Erikson's theory suggests that in old age, there's a conflict between *ego-integrity* (the positive force) and *despair* (the negative force). As with the other psychosocial stages, we cannot avoid the conflict altogether, which occurs as a result of biological, psychological and social forces. The task is to end this stage, and hence life, with greater ego-integrity than despair, and this requires us to take stock of our life, reflect on it and assess how worthwhile and fulfilling it has been.

The characteristics of ego-integrity

◎ We believe that life does have a purpose and makes sense.
◎ We accept that, within the context of our lives as a whole, what happened was somehow inevitable and could only have happened when and how it did.
◎ We believe that all life's experiences offer something of value and that we can learn from everything that happens to us. Looking back, we can see how we have grown psychologically as a result of life's ups and downs, triumphs and failures, calms and crises.

◎ We see our parents in a new light and understand them better, because we've lived through our own adulthood and have probably raised children of our own.

◎ We realise that we share with all other human beings, past, present and future, the inevitable cycle of birth and death. Whatever the historical, cultural and other differences, we all have this much in common. In the light of this, death 'loses its sting'.

Fear of death is the most conspicuous symptom of despair. In despair, we express the belief that it's too late to undo the past and turn the clock back in order to right wrongs or do what hasn't been done. Life isn't a 'rehearsal'; this is the only chance we get.

That's what Alfred said when he took his wife on her last holiday – that he didn't want there to be anything to regret.

Reminiscence and the life review

According to Coleman and O'Hanlon (2004), *reminiscence* is the process of recalling past events and experiences. It illustrates the practical relevance of developmental theory, especially Erikson's concept of ego integrity. Encouraging older people to reminisce is now seen as a natural activity and very much part of care work (which wasn't so 30 years ago). But it owes an even greater debt to Butler's (1963) *life review* (LR), which refers to a more focused consideration of one's past life as a whole.

Butler, a practising psychotherapist, proposed that LR is a normative process that all people undergo as they realise their lives are coming to an end. But, while this may be beneficial, a failure to resolve troublesome memories may produce feelings of despair. Also, Coleman and O'Hanlon cite research which suggests that well-being in later life isn't dependent on reminiscence, and that LR requires high levels of inner skills that most older people may not possess. Reminiscence in adulthood seems to be more often used to reassert previous patterns of self-understanding (such as in response to threat or challenge) than to create the new understanding arising from LR.

Butler's LR reflects the Judaeo-Christian concern with repentance and release from guilt, but it also implies the search for meaning through reflection on one's life experience. A longitudinal study begun in the late 1920s showed that although LR wasn't associated with self-ratings of life satisfaction in those in their late sixties to mid-seventies, it was positively related to ratings of creativity, spirituality and generativity (Wink, 1999, in Coleman and O'Hanlon, 2004). Coleman and O'Hanlon consider these to be much more socially relevant than subjective well-being.

Wink and Schiff (2002, in Coleman and O'Hanlon, 2004) believe that LR is an adaptive response to ageing in those who've encountered marked difficulties in their lives; for the majority, it's *not* a necessary adaptation. Indeed, Butler originally described LR as a means to achieving self-change, but this is a difficult and anxiety-provoking task, especially for those (the majority) who are reasonably satisfied with their lives and aren't seeking self-growth.

While none of these theories seems just right, they all contribute to understanding the complexities of caring for an older person. Reading this has made me very wary of making assumptions about what an older person thinks and wants; there's no single 'best way' to age (Neugarten and Neugarten, 1987).

Alfred, with very little external support, has managed his recent years very successfully, adapting to changed circumstances and learning new roles. He gave up a great deal, without resentment, to care for his wife, respecting her dignity and independence. It seems right that he should be able to expect the same for himself.

Hayslip and Panek (1989) state that people will select styles of ageing best suited to their personalities and past experiences or lifestyles, and Alfred is a good example of this; he is the only one who knows what he needs from us. Turner and Helms (1989) suggest that personality is the key factor in how people age, but surely Alfred's beliefs, life events, financial situation and, perhaps most of all, his health status are relevant. The matter of his operation seems very important now.

CONCLUSIONS

According to Voss (2002):

> 'Older people may not feel old; they may not feel any different than they did during their younger years. They simply face life from an angle that bears the shadow of death more acutely than before. This provides them with an insight unavailable to others and the wisdom not yet achieved by those trying to help them. Acknowledging this is an invaluable part of promoting the respect that older people deserve as fellow human beings … we should … help older adults to welcome integrity and wisdom, in whatever form, at the conclusion of their winter years.

CHAPTER SUMMARY

◎ While 'growing up' has positive connotations, 'growing old' has negative ones, reflecting the **decrement model**. An alternative, more positive view is the **personal growth model**.

◎ One feature of **ageism** is the assumption that **chronological age** is an accurate indicator of **biological**, **subjective**, **functional** and **social age**. **Stereotypes** of the elderly are deeply rooted in rapidly changing western societies, where their experience and wisdom are no longer valued.

◎ The claim that intelligence declines fairly rapidly in old age is based on **cross-sectional studies**, which suffer from the problem of the **cohort effect**. **Longitudinal studies** indicate that while **crystallised intelligence** increases with age, **fluid intelligence** declines for all age groups over time.

◎ Some aspects of **memory** decline with age, perhaps due to less effective **information-processing**. Older adults generally perform more poorly than younger adults on **recall** tests, but the differences are much smaller when **recognition** tests are used.

◎ Evidence from the **OPTIMA project** suggests that **dementia** (such as **Alzheimer's disease**) isn't an accelerated form of normal ageing. Rather, it appears to reflect a **disease process** which is more likely to affect us as we get older.

◎ **Negative cultural stereotypes** of ageing actually cause memory decline in the elderly and may become **self-fulfilling prophecies**.

◎ The most controversial claim made by **social disengagement theory** (SDT) is that the elderly accept and even welcome disengagement, and that this is a natural and inevitable process.

◎ SDT emphasises the **quantitative** changes to the exclusion of the **qualitative** changes, which may become more important with age. The latter include **friendships**, which are under the older person's control and provide essential informal support.

◎ **Activity or re-engagement theory** (AT) claims that older people are psychologically and socially essentially the same as middle-aged people. The withdrawal of society and the individual isn't mutual, and optimal ageing involves maintaining the activities of middle age for as long as possible.

◎ According to **social exchange theory** (SET), older people in industrialised societies have few power resources to exchange in everyday social interaction, making them dependent on others. But the elderly relinquish their roles as economically active members of society in exchange for increased leisure time and fewer responsibilities.

◎ **Socio-emotional selectivity theory** (SST) maintains that for the elderly, **emotional regulation** assumes major importance, making them highly selective as regards social partners. This change in social motives is largely determined by **construal of the future**.

◎ According to Erikson's **psychosocial theory**, old age involves a conflict between **ego-integrity** and **despair**. The task of ageing is to assess and evaluate life's value and meaning. Despair is characterised by a fear of death.

◎ The process of **reminiscing** has been influenced both by Erikson's concept of ego-integrity and Butler's **life review**.

DEATH AND DYING

20

INTRODUCTION AND OVERVIEW

The loss, through death, of loved ones (*bereavement*) can occur at any stage of the life cycle (a *non-normative influence*). However, it becomes more likely as we get older. Some losses are more 'non-normative' than others, such as the loss of a child. This can occur at any stage from conception through to childhood and adolescence, and beyond. Miscarriage, stillbirth and neonatal death are all forms of bereavement, as are terminations.

The psychological and bodily reactions that occur in people who suffer bereavement (whatever form it takes) are called *grief*. The 'observable expression of grief' (Parkes and Weiss, 1983) is called *mourning*, although this term is often used to refer to the social conventions surrounding death (such as funerals and wearing black clothes).

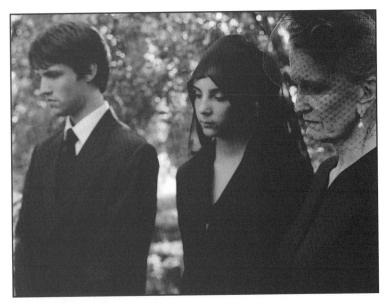

Mourners at a western funeral

But grief can 'begin' before the actual death, and those who are dying can also grieve for their own death. Nurses have a crucial role to play in helping patients with a terminal illness to accept their condition. They're in the privileged position of being able to listen to patients talking about their hopes and fears, and their experience, knowledge and skills may enable patients to explore their feelings and come to terms with their condition (Dean, 2002). The patients may be children, adolescents (see Chapter 17) or adults (including elderly adults – see Chapter 19).

From my diary (6): Year 1/Community Placement (District Nurse)

Today Sally (my mentor) and I visited Gail, a 35-year-old woman in the later stages of terminal illness. Her mother, Lydia, who is a retired nurse, is caring for her. Gail, who was propped up against her pillows making a feeble attempt to brush her hair, didn't answer our greeting. Sally picked up Gail's case notes and unobtrusively indicated to me the increased pain prescription. Lydia said that Gail was bathed and ready to get up when her syringe driver was changed. Gail muttered that she wasn't going to get up. Lydia said positively that of course she must, it wouldn't be good for her to stay in bed all day. Gail surprised me then by flinging her hairbrush on the floor and shouting angrily at her mother that there was no point and why didn't everyone leave her alone.

I felt uncomfortable and didn't know how to respond; I picked up the brush and gave it to Lydia, who smiled apologetically and began collecting the laundry. In spite of her apparent control, she looked distraught.

Sally sat on the bed and asked Gail calmly if she'd had a bad night. Gail fell back against the pillows and closed her eyes, saying every night was a bad night. Just then Gail's father (Ron) put his head round the door saying he'd made a cup of tea. I offered to fetch it; I was glad to escape from the room. In the kitchen, I asked him how he was coping and he said he was OK – it was Gail's mum who was bearing the brunt of it. He said jokingly that he was 'just the tea maker', but as he turned away I saw him blinking back tears. I took my mug off the tray and said I'd like to have my tea in the kitchen with him, if he didn't mind.

APPROACHES TO THE UNDERSTANDING OF GRIEF

According to Archer (1999), grief has been variously depicted as:

(a) a natural human reaction
(b) a psychiatric disorder, and
(c) a disease process.

All three approaches contain an element of truth. As far as (a) is concerned, grief is a *universal* feature of human existence, found in all cultures. But its form and the intensity of its expression vary considerably (see pages 384–386). As far as (b) is concerned, although grief itself has never been classified as a mental disorder, 'The psychiatric framework emphasises the human suffering grief involves, and therefore provides a useful balance to viewing it simply as a natural reaction' (Archer, 1999).

Regarding (c), although there may be increased rates of morbidity (health deterioration) or mortality (death) among bereaved people, these aren't necessarily directly caused by the grief process. For example, the effects of change in lifestyle (such as altered nutrition or drug intake), or increased attention to physical illness, which predated the bereavement, might be mistaken for the effects of grief itself. However, there's substantial evidence that bereaved spouses are more at risk of dying themselves compared with matched non-bereaved controls. This is true mainly for widowers (Stroebe and Stroebe, 1993), and especially for younger widowers experiencing an unexpected bereavement (Smith and Zick, 1996).

The fact that grief contributes to physical illness supports the biopsychosocial model of health. Gail was divorced five years ago and has no children; her parents will be the most affected by her death, so will the increased risk of illness apply to them?

STAGE OR PHASE ACCOUNTS OF GRIEF

According to Archer (1999), a widely held assumption is that grief proceeds through an orderly series of stages or phases, with distinct features. While different accounts vary in the details of particular stages, the two most commonly cited are those of Bowlby (1980) and Kübler-Ross (1969).

Box 20.1 Bowlby's phase theory of grief

According to Bowlby (1980), adult grief is an extension of a general distress response to separation commonly observed in young children (see Chapter 14). Adult grief is a form of *separation anxiety* in response to the disruption of an attachment bond.

- **Phase of numbing:** Numbness and disbelief, which can last from a few hours up to a week, may be punctuated by outbursts of extremely intense distress and/or anger.
- **Yearning and searching:** These are accompanied by anxiety and intermittent periods of anger, and can last for months or even years.
- **Disorganisation and despair:** Feelings of depression and apathy occur when old patterns have been discarded.
- **Reorganisation:** There's a greater/lesser degree of recovery from bereavement and acceptance of what has occurred.

Thinking about grief as the breaking of the attachment bond is enlightening. As Gail has become more dependent, she has returned increasingly to the more childlike, dependent behaviour characteristic of early attachment. When Gail dies, this could make Lydia's loss even more acute.

Kübler-Ross's stage theory: anticipatory grief

Kübler-Ross's (1969) stage account was based on her pioneering work with over 200 terminally ill patients. She was interested in how they prepared for their imminent deaths (*anticipatory grief*), and so her stages describe the *process of dying*. But she was inspired by an earlier version of Bowlby's theory (Parkes, 1995) and her stages were later applied (by other researchers) to *grief for others*. Her theory remains very influential in nursing and counselling, with both dying patients and the bereaved (Archer, 1999).

Box 20.2 Kübler-Ross's stages of dying

- **Denial ('No, not me'):** This prevents the patient from being overwhelmed by the initial shock. It may take the form of seeking a second opinion, or holding contradictory beliefs. Denial (or, at least, partial denial) is used by most patients not only at this early stage of their

---

illness, but also later on. It's as if they can contemplate the possibility of their own death for a defined time period, but then have to turn away from such thoughts so that they can carry on with life. Denial acts as a buffer system, allowing the patient time to develop other coping mechanisms. It can also bring isolation. The patient may fear rejection and abandonment in suffering and feel that nobody understands what the suffering is like. Avoidance by staff, for whatever reasons, can exacerbate this feeling of isolation in terminal illness (Parkinson, 1992).

- **Anger ('It's not fair – why me?'):** This may be directed at doctors, nurses, relatives, other healthy people who'll go on living, or God. This can be the most difficult stage for family and staff to deal with. They may react personally to the patient's anger and respond with anger of their own; this only increases the patient's hostile behaviour (Parkinson, 1992).

- **Bargaining ('Please God let me ...'):** This is an attempt to postpone death by 'doing a deal' with God (or fate, or the hospital), much as a child might bargain with its parents in order to get its own way. So, it has to include a prize for 'good behaviour' and sets a self-imposed 'deadline' such as a son or daughter's wedding; the patient promises not to ask for more time if this postponement is granted.

- **Depression ('How can I leave all this behind?'):** This is likely to arise when the patient realises that no bargain can be struck and that death is inevitable. S/he grieves for all the losses that death represents. This is *preparatory depression*, a form of preparatory grief that helps the patient to prepare him/herself for the final separation from the world. *Reactive depression* involves expressions of fear and anxiety and a sense of great loss – of body image (disfigurement – see Chapter 16), job, financial security, or ability to continue caring for children.

- **Acceptance ('Leave me be, I am ready to die'):** Almost devoid of feelings, the patient seems to have given up the struggle for life, sleeps more and withdraws from other people, as if preparing for 'the long journey'.

Kübler-Ross helps to explain the family's behaviour this morning. Gail's reaction seemed a mixture of anger and depression; I assume she had gone past the 'bargaining' phase. She wanted to be left alone, but it didn't seem like acceptance; she appeared troubled. Lydia may have been using denial as a coping mechanism and Ron was definitely sadly accepting. He confessed he felt inadequate to help either of them.

Almost all the patients she interviewed initially denied they had life-threatening illnesses, although only three remained in a constant state of denial (the rest drifted in and out). Denial was more common when someone had been given the diagnosis in an abrupt or insensitive way, or if they were surrounded by family and/or staff who were also in denial. Searching for a second opinion was a very common initial reaction, representing a desperate attempt to change the unpredictable world they'd just been catapulted into, back into the world they knew and understood (March and Doherty, 1999).

Depression is a common reaction in the dying. For example, Hinton (1975) reported that 18 per cent of those who committed suicide suffered from serious physical illnesses, with 4 per cent having illnesses that probably would have killed them within six months.

Elderly people who've lived full lives have relatively little to grieve for – they've gained much and lost few opportunities. But people who perceive lives full of mistakes and missed opportunities may, paradoxically, have *more* to grieve for as they begin to realise that these opportunities are now lost for ever. This resembles Erikson's despair (see page 367), as does *resignation*, which Kübler-Ross distinguished from acceptance.

The detachment and stillness of those who've achieved acceptance comes from calmness, while in those who've become resigned it comes from despair. The latter cannot accept death, nor can they deny its existence any longer (March and Doherty, 1999). Kübler-Ross found that there are a few patients who fight to the end, struggle and keep hoping, which makes it almost impossible for them to achieve true acceptance.

Hope (for a cure, a new drug or a miracle) is the constant thread running through all these stages and is necessary to maintain the patient's morale through the illness. Hope is rationalisation of suffering for some and a means of much-needed denial for others. Kübler-Ross found that if a patient stopped expressing hope, it was usually a sign of imminent death (Parkinson, 1992).

Lydia's concentration on practical matters might indicate her denial. As a nurse she must know Gail hasn't long to live; as a mother she may not be able to face Gail suggesting there is no hope left. Gail herself may be regretting her broken marriage and lack of children.

An important consideration within the process of dying is *awareness* of death. According to Glaser and Strauss (1968, in Parkinson, 1992), awareness is what each interacting person knows of the patient's defined status, combined with the patient's recognition of others' awareness of his/her defined status. They identify four awareness contexts:

1. *closed awareness* – the patient doesn't recognise s/he is dying, although everyone around does
2. *suspected awareness* – the patient suspects s/he may be dying and attempts to find out what the prognosis is
3. *mutual pretence awareness* – everyone knows the patient is dying but they all pretend they don't
4. *open awareness* – the patient, relatives and staff all admit that death is inevitable, and speak and act accordingly.

It's within these awareness contexts that interactions between patients, relatives and staff take place and can affect the management of the dying patient. Kübler-Ross favours the open awareness context, arguing that the question isn't 'Do I tell my patient?' but 'How do I share this knowledge with my patient?'. She suggests that whether the patient is told explicitly or not about the terminal illness, s/he will come to this awareness independently. If the news can be transmitted in an empathetic and hopeful manner before this stage is reached, the patient will have time to work through the different reactions, which will enable him/her to cope with this new situation and develop confidence in carers. It's also within open awareness that she has identified the stages described in Box 20.2. Patients can only ask 'Why me?' if they know their diagnosis/prognosis. In reality, the question is a statement of their deepest *spiritual pain* – 'I am hurting terribly' (Morrison, 1992; see Chapter 3).

Sally had told me Gail is aware there is no hope of recovery, as are her parents. Until now, there seems to have been 'mutual pretence awareness'. Was Gail's anger this morning perhaps the first step towards the open awareness stage?

AN EVALUATION OF STAGE THEORIES OF GRIEF

◎ Generally, stage models haven't been well supported by subsequent research. Both Bowlby's and Kübler-Ross's accounts were proposed before any prolonged, detailed follow-up studies of bereaved people had been undertaken (Archer, 1999).

◎ According to March and Doherty (1999), they represent generalisations from the experience of some individuals, and lack the flexibility necessary to describe the range of individual reactions. Grief *isn't* a simple, universal process we all go through (Stroebe *et al.*, 1993).

◎ Some researchers prefer to talk about the *components of grief*. Ramsay and de Groot (1977), for example, have identified nine such components, some of which occur early and others late in the grieving process.

Box 20.3 Ramsay and de Groot's nine components of grief

1. **Shock:** This is usually the first response, most often described as a feeling of 'numbness', which can also include pain, calm, apathy, depersonalisation and 'de-realisation'. It's as if the feelings are so strong that they're 'turned off'. This can last from a few seconds to several weeks.

2. **Disorganisation:** This can be the inability to do the simplest thing or, alternatively, organising the entire funeral and then collapsing.

3. **Denial:** Behaving as if the deceased were still alive is a defence against feeling too much pain. It's usually an early feature of grief, but one that can recur at any time. A common form of denial is searching behaviour (e.g. waiting for the deceased to come home, or having hallucinations of them).

4. **Depression:** This emerges as the denial breaks down but can occur, usually less frequently and intensely, at any point during the grieving process. It can consist of either 'desolate pining' (a yearning and longing, an emptiness interspersed with waves of intense psychic pain) or 'despair' (feelings of helplessness, the blackness of the realisation of powerlessness to bring back the dead).

5. **Guilt:** This can be both real and imagined, for actual neglect of the deceased when they were alive, or for angry thoughts and feelings.

6. **Anxiety:** This can involve fear of losing control of one's feelings, of going mad, or more general apprehension about the future (changed roles, increased responsibilities, financial worries, and so on).

7. **Aggression:** This can take the form of irritability towards family and friends, outbursts of anger towards God or fate, doctors and nurses, the clergy or even the person who's died.

8. **Resolution:** This is an emerging acceptance of the death, a 'taking leave of the dead and acceptance that life must go on'.

9. **Reintegration:** This involves putting acceptance into practice by reorganising one's life in which the deceased has no place. However, pining and despair may reappear on anniversaries, birthdays, and so on.

Ramsay and de Groot's (1977) is a more elaborate and flexible account of grief, which helps me to better understand Gail's parents' feelings, but Kübler-Ross's concept of 'anticipatory grief' is better for helping me understand Gail's feelings.

◎ However, many stage theorists have explicitly *denied* that the stages are meant to apply equally and rigidly to everyone. For example, Bowlby (1980) himself said that, 'These phases are not clear-cut, and any one individual may oscillate for a time back

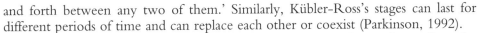
and forth between any two of them.' Similarly, Kübler-Ross's stages can last for different periods of time and can replace each other or coexist (Parkinson, 1992).

◎ Yet stages provide us with a framework or guidelines for understanding the experiences of bereaved and dying individuals, while at the same recognising that there's a huge variability in the ways individuals react. Stages don't prescribe where an individual 'ought' to be in the grieving process (March and Doherty, 1999).

Gail appeared to be alternating between different stages of anger and depression, which Bowlby (1980) said might happen.

NURSES, DEATH AND DYING

According to March (1995), 'Most nurses are confronted with the reality of death with a regularity that lay people would find shocking …'

Dying is a major crisis, which can be painfully distressing, unfamiliar and frightening (Baker, 1976, in Parkinson, 1992). In order to help patients and their families through this process, nurses need to develop awareness of their own attitudes and ability to face terminal illness and death, and their particular prejudices and convictions (Parkinson, 1992).

I experienced grief when my grandmother died, but she was old so it was a 'normative' loss. Gail is young; for her parents it will be a 'non-normative' loss. As this was my first experience of caring for a terminally ill patient, I felt helpless and inadequate; I didn't know what to say and, yes, I was distressed by Gail's anger.

TALKING TO DYING PATIENTS

Research suggests that a proportion of patients don't wish to talk about the terminal nature of their condition (Hunt and Meerabeau, 1993, in Dean, 2002). They may cope by avoiding having to focus on their prognosis (Rifkin, 2001, in Dean, 2002), or seeking escape in light-hearted conversation. In spite of these findings, authors have urged nurses, as a kind of blanket rule of good communication, to discuss with patients their feelings about their prognosis.

Dean proposes that nurses develop communication skills that not only allow them to talk sensitively about death and dying with patients but also give them the capacity to assess whether or not this is what the patient wants. Similarly, Parkinson (1992) maintains that providing opportunities to talk with patients so that they can express their fears, anger or depression should comprise a major focus of the nurse's work.

Webster (1981, in Dean) observed nurses communicating with dying patients in four English hospitals. They often displayed 'blocking' behaviour, avoiding intimate conversations by changing the subject, ignoring cues, making jokes or tailoring their responses to the least distressing aspect of the issues raised. Such light-hearted interactions allowed the nurses to sidestep potentially difficult conversations, keeping them on emotional 'safe ground'. Wilkinson (1991, in Dean) observed similar behaviour in 54 cancer nurses. Their blocking behaviours predominated over facilitative behaviours. For example, the psychosexual impact that gynaecological, bladder or bowel malignancy may have had on patients' lives was never discussed during the observed interactions. This was confirmed by Costello (2000, in Dean; see also Chapter 16).

I realise now that during our previous visit I'd 'sheltered' behind our conversation focusing on 'treatment' – pain control, etc. This time I had to face the real problem.

According to Hare and Pratt (1989, in March, 1995), until recently a death on the ward was a violent reminder of the failings of nursing/medicine. But major developments, such as growth of the hospice movement, suggest that the emphasis is changing from curing to caring. March maintains that 'Nursing appears to be redefining itself to include the wholehearted care of dying and bereaved people …'

Western culture generally has been moving since the 1960s towards open communication about death and dying, with paternalistic notions that patients would be too upset to discuss death slowly changing (Field and Copp, 1999, in Dean, 2002).

Hospice care is moving into general nursing; our local hospital has just appointed a palliative care consultant and a team of specialist nurses.

Communicating with dying children

Box 20.4 Children's understanding of death

- Evidence suggests that children develop a concept of death from an early age, and by the age of eight or nine this will be complete (Chesterfield, 1992).

- In Piaget's sensorimotor stage (birth to two – see Chapter 15), 'out of sight' is seen as the equivalent of death. Early games of peek-a-boo are often considered the first stage of learning about death (the word 'peek-a-boo' stems from the old English word meaning 'alive and dead'; Chesterfield, 1992).

- The egocentrism of the preoperational child (aged two to seven) means that s/he doesn't understand the finality of death, often seeing it as a kind of sleep. The toddler will attribute inanimate objects in general with life and will (animism). They often feel guilty because they believe that death is related to something they have wished for or done. They may show great interest in the practical aspects of death, such as what the dead person will eat. The clearest and most feared implication for younger children is separation from their attachment figures (see Chapter 14) and the belief that dead people/animals cannot move (Judd, 1993).

- During the concrete operational stage (ages seven to eleven), children recognise death as an immediate possibility that may happen to themselves as a consequence of 'badness'. Personification of death and a fear of the dark are common, and the ability to articulate feelings develops.

- In the formal operational stage (age 11–15), the adolescent may have an adult's cognitive abilities, but it's unlikely that s/he will have acquired the life skills or experience to cope with death as an adult would. The young person may regress at times of stress to egocentrism, magical thought, rages and dependency (see Chapter 17).

- According to Bowlby (1980), adults in western societies hold beliefs about life and death that are ambiguous and inconsistent, so it's no wonder that children's beliefs also vary widely. Anthony (1971) also maintains that children are influenced by beliefs about death that are generally accepted by their culture, especially adults' own animistic beliefs.

- According to Rochlin (1959, 1967, in Judd, 1993), children clearly know at a very early age about death as the extinction of all life. But they then use a range of defence mechanisms to avoid the full implications of this awareness (see Chapter 6). Children's use of denial omnipotence, magical thinking and actual independence all influence the extent of their fear

> or acceptance. This is all set against the very influential background of adults' oscillation between acceptance and denial:
>
> > … Adults' protective concern for children over issues around death clearly reflects their own fears and use of denial, in a society where the taboo may be lifting in a widespread social and intellectual sense, but not necessarily in a personal or private sense. (Judd, 1989, in Judd, 1993)

Knowing about Piaget's cognitive developmental stages and my week on the children's ward (see my diary entry on page 281) helps me understand this. For the young child, separation is as disturbing as death; no wonder they become so distressed. Taylor et al.'s (1999) advice (also in Chapter 15) to start from what the child knows, believes and understands seems the best idea.

ASK YOURSELF …
• Do you think children should be told that they are terminally ill?

• Should it be the parents' decision whether or not medical staff are honest with the child?

Children with a life-threatening illness sense that it's serious and that they might die or are dying, even if they're not explicitly told (Judd, 1993). Their anxiety levels are markedly higher than those of chronically ill children, even if undergoing the same number and duration of treatments (Spinetta *et al.*, 1973, in Judd, 1993). This anxiety and sense of isolation persists when the child isn't in hospital and even during periods of remission in children with leukaemia (Spinetta, 1975, in Judd, 1993).

The hospitalised dying child's awareness of death is more sharply focused when another child dies on the ward. If the child has the same illness, the link between that event and the dying child's imminent death is made more immediate. Judd (1993) believes that there's a more open and honest attitude on children's wards in most hospitals, where death and dying are often discussed openly in response to parents' questions and sometimes with the children, depending on the ethos of the unit.

Effective communication with dying children will be influenced by nurses' values, attitudes and beliefs, which in turn are influenced by past experience and religious, cultural and societal beliefs (Chesterfield, 1992). Chesterfield cites studies showing that doctors and nurses become skilled at withdrawal and distancing techniques; these strategies may help protect the practitioner from distress but inhibit effective communication with the dying child. The family may not want the child's impending death discussed openly, shielding the child from distress or because of their own fears (Lansdown and Benjamin, 1985; Lombardo and Lombardo, 1986, in Chesterfield). This mutual pretence – Kübler-Ross's mutual pretence awareness (see above) – can prove functional in maintaining hope and the roles of individual family members (Bluebond-Langner, 1978, in Chesterfield).

Nursing terminally ill children must be even more difficult than dealing with adult death. We're taught that our practice should be based on what research shows to be best practice applied to individual need, in this case the child would be the patient, but we would still have to take into account parents' values, cultural background and beliefs.

Clearly, the dying child needs an age- and developmentally appropriate opportunity to share its fears and concerns. This doesn't mean imposing a discussion, but involves attempting to be open to the child's willingness (or otherwise) to talk (Judd, 1993). If the child seems to be 'somewhere else' emotionally – but not depressed – this may be a very understandable way of achieving separation from the world around them. This should be tolerated and respected, rather than pressurising the child to be jolly or 'hang on' for the sake of others. As Judd points out, this choosing to withdraw may be the one area of control the child has left.

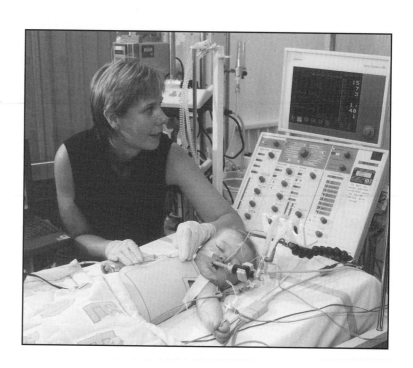

DIFFERENT KINDS OF BEREAVEMENT

The stage accounts of grief discussed above (Bowlby, 1980; Kübler-Ross, 1969) are both 'attachment models' (March, 1995). According to Parkes (1986), Bowlby's account applies to both dying and bereaved people:

> Most people who are dying have people around them who are mourning their death. The feelings and behaviour of dying and bereaved people are a function of the relationship between them and should not therefore be considered in isolation from each other. Indeed, one of the guiding principles of the new hospice movement is 'the unit of care is the family'.

Similarly, Kübler-Ross's account of the dying process can be applied to those who suffer the loss of a loved one. For people who have warning of an impending death, the process of grieving may be shorter and less complicated – they've grieved in advance (*anticipatory bereavement/grief*). But while this may be helpful for the long-term adjustment of the bereaved, it may cause problems for the dying patient:

> As loved ones come to accept the inevitability of death, they may begin to withdraw from the patient and begin to consider life after the patient's death. This ... may leave the dying patient feeling rejected and isolated ... (March, 1995)

But the reverse can also happen: the patient may begin to accept his/her own death and withdraw from loved ones, who remain overwhelmed by grief. The patient's withdrawal may only increase their grief (March, 1995).

According to Bowlby (1980):

> The loss of a loved person is one of the most intensely painful experiences any human being can suffer, and not only is it painful to experience, but also painful to witness, if only because we are impotent to help.

Similarly, Parkes (1972) states that:

> Pain is inevitable in such a case and cannot be avoided. It stems from the awareness of both parties that neither can give the other what he wants. The helper cannot bring back the person who's dead, and the bereaved person cannot gratify the helper by seeming helped.

The nurse's pain, like that of the relatives, may be more difficult to handle when there's been little or no time to prepare for the patient's death.

It is six months since Gail's ovarian cancer was diagnosed as terminal, so her parents have had time to adjust to her impending death. Driving back from Gail's, Sally asked me what had changed since our last visit. I said I thought Gail seemed angry and wanted to be left alone, and Lydia was keeping busy to avoid facing the fact Gail was dying. She agreed and said Gail's refusing to get up could mean she has stopped colluding with her mother's denial.

Death in A&E departments

The news of death can provoke an alarm reaction: the world suddenly becomes a threatening, unpredictable place. Anything that makes the loss unreal (such as a sudden, unexpected death and/or one that occurs in unusual or violent circumstances) is likely to make it more difficult to accept, which can produce a more prolonged and complicated grief reaction (Parkes and Weiss, 1983). Nurses in A&E are likely to have to deal with a higher proportion of such deaths than those working in other areas. Indeed, one-third of all deaths in hospital occur within the first few hours of a patient's arrival (Ewins and Bryant, 1992).

According to Smith (1997), although the hospice and palliative care movements have done much to prepare nurses as well as patients for death and for the terminal phase of conditions such as cancer and AIDS, many nurses in acute care still feel unprepared and unsupported. We live in a society where cardiovascular disease and accidents are major causes of mortality, and these deaths tend to occur in hospital with little or no warning for staff, let alone relatives or friends.

Wright (1996, in Smith, 1997) has looked at the issue of nurses coping with sudden death in A&E (and ICU, coronary care and paediatric ICU) in the USA. He concluded that the best mental health outcomes for relatives and staff depended on the foundations laid at the time of the patient's arrival in A&E. He now runs CRI-TEC (crisis training, education and counselling), a support service in the UK for those affected by sudden death. It provides courses for health professionals, the police and the fire brigade.

Staff caring for the newly bereaved should be able to provide support early on and help build a foundation for the relatives' recovery process (Cooke *et al.*, 1992, in Ewins and Bryant, 1992). But nursing and medical staff often feel inadequately prepared to meet relatives' needs. In A&E the situation is complicated by the fact that staff and relatives meet at a time of crisis, the meeting is usually brief, unexpected and may not have any follow-up. In contrast, a ward environment often allows time for a relationship and rapport to develop. The ethos of A&E is to save life, so when the patient dies this often leads to feelings of failure. But the input of highly trained and motivated nursing and medical staff, who understand the importance of bereavement care, can help relatives' psychological recovery (Ewins and Bryant, 1992).

I'm grateful my first experience of a patient dying is in such a calm and supportive situation. When it happens suddenly, I'll be better equipped to deal with it. But I imagine unexpected death would mean dealing more with the early shock, disorganisation and denial stages; I need to learn what to anticipate and how to respond in such a situation.

Death of a child

According to Raphael (1984):

> The loss of a child will always be painful, for it is in some way a loss of part of the self … In any society, the death of a young child seems to represent some failure of family or society and some loss of hope.

Inevitably, the parents will feel cheated of the child's life and future. Often the death is sudden and unexpected (from accident, injury or medical emergency). Much less often it's caused by progressive, debilitating or malignant conditions, which do allow anticipatory grief to take place. But whatever their nature, all childhood deaths are abhorrent and so are especially stressful.

Parents' relationship with their child begins long before birth. For each parent there's the fantasy child s/he will have, which builds on the pre-conception images of what a baby – this baby – will be. Of course, many pregnancies are unplanned or unwanted (initially or even throughout), which makes the relationship with the unborn baby highly ambivalent (Raphael, 1984). But, in all cases, the loss of a baby will need to be grieved for, at whatever stage of pregnancy this might occur.

Miscarriage (spontaneous abortion)

According to Raphael (1984), the level of the mother's grief will be affected by whether or not the baby was wanted. This can be true even with an early miscarriage (i.e. before the baby is viable). But after the baby's movements have been felt, it's more likely to be seen as the loss of a 'person'. The loss isn't 'nothing' or 'just a scrape' or 'not a life', but the beginning of a baby. The use of technical terms to describe the baby – products of conception, conceptus, embryo, foetus – might be perceived as an attempt to deny the existence of a baby the woman already loved, and thus to deny the reality of the grief she experiences for that baby (Buggins, 1995).

The sadness of the loss is often compounded by fear and panic, as in any emergency situation. There's rarely time to deal with these emotions, and many women report feelings of total helplessness (Sherr, 1989). Even if the mother doesn't have a very clear concept of her lost baby, as with other losses it can never be replaced (by another pregnancy). As Sherr says, 'Aspirations and dreams may still be met by a subsequent baby, but this is very different from adjusting to the loss of this particular baby …'

Termination (therapeutic or induced abortion)

To a woman and her family losing a much wanted baby, the term 'abortion' (even if qualified by 'spontaneous') can be deeply offensive (Buggins, 1995). In other words, 'abortion' is usually taken to denote 'termination'.

The Abortion Act 1967 defined therapeutic termination as one undertaken before the gestational age of 28 weeks. But advances in technology have greatly improved the chances of survival for premature babies, and a reduction to 24 weeks was approved by Parliament in 1990. The Abortion Act made it possible for a woman to have an abortion legally, provided two doctors independently agreed that the termination was necessary to prevent:

- the likelihood of the woman's death
- permanent illness (physical or psychological)
- damage to a woman's existing children
- abnormality in the baby.

The Act stopped far short of endorsing the idea that a woman has an absolute right to control her body. Practically, the law relies on individual doctors exercising discretion as to who qualifies for an abortion (Timpson, 1996, in Hughes, 2003).

Despite its legality, abortion is still a very 'live' moral issue. But the debate has also involved empirical concerns about the links between unwanted pregnancy, abortion and long-term mental health. Specifically, several authors have proposed that abortion may have adverse mental health effects owing to guilt, unresolved loss and lowered self-esteem (Fergusson *et al.*, 2006).

Fergusson *et al.* believe that, overall, the evidence is quite weak (i.e. inconclusive). They also note a number of confounding factors involved in many studies (factors that are associated with abortion and that could account for the mental health effects), such as the woman's circumstances at the time of pregnancy (including her age), whether or not the pregnancy was planned, and the stability of the relationship with her partner. In their study of young women aged 15–25 in New Zealand, they controlled for several pre-pregnancy factors (including social background, childhood and family history, mental health and personality).

The results suggest that those who had abortions were at a moderately increased risk of both concurrent and subsequent mental health problems compared with those who hadn't been pregnant or who'd been pregnant but hadn't had an abortion. These problems included depression, anxiety, suicidal behaviours and substance use disorders.

According to Raphael (1984) the pattern of grief is similar to that for miscarriage, but suppression or inhibition of grief is much more likely.

We don't know why Gail had no children; it's possible she's had miscarriages, or perhaps an abortion. If so, exploring her feelings about this might help her.

Stillbirth

According to Sherr (1989), a stillbirth occurs when a baby born after 27 weeks fails to breathe. Knowledge of the fact that there's no live baby at the end of the labour can magnify the experience of pain (see Chapter 3). The increased use of drugs may reflect the feeling that the labour is futile, but it's unclear whether parents want greater intervention or staff simply tend to take greater control and perceive the birth as a medical event in order to protect them from the reality. According to Sherr:

> Parents cannot 'wipe out' this baby – and may gain strength from the ritual of hello and farewell which will be the only interaction they will have with this child ... this is still their baby, even if it has died.

The baby shouldn't be whisked away or shielded from the parents, even if there's physical abnormality. Sherr believes it's much worse for parents to fear an imaginary baby than to view the real one: they seem to see the baby as beautiful no matter what.

If the stillbirth wasn't expected, the situation will be more traumatic for everyone, including the staff (Sherr, 1989). But if there's a congenital abnormality or intrauterine event that makes it obvious that the baby wasn't viable or that it's already died, there may be an opportunity for some anticipatory grieving (Raphael, 1984).

Neonatal death

This refers to babies in special care baby units (SCBUs) and neonatal intensive care units (NICUs), where the threat of death may hang over the parents, as well as babies who are full term and/or born healthy but then become ill later.

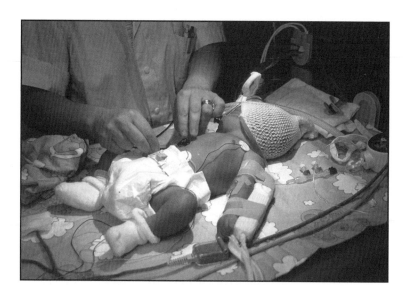

In the former, parents may have experienced some anticipatory grieving, but they grieve both for the expected healthy baby that they never had and the sick baby that they will soon have no more. Many babies will have spent their lives on SCBUs, and so will never have truly 'belonged' to their parents (Sherr, 1989). As Sherr observes, 'The environment of SCBU is in itself difficult. This … is a strange environment of incubators, ventilators, uniforms, tubes and high background noise.'

Many of the characteristics of grief following neonatal death are similar to those for stillbirth, except that in the former the parents have had some opportunity, however limited, to know and bond with their real child. The two have often been studied together as 'perinatal' death (Raphael, 1984).

Raphael describes adoption (the relinquishing of one's baby) and the birth of a baby with some abnormality or disability as losses that, like death, must be grieved for. She also discusses parents' grief for their children at ages from early childhood, through adolescence, up to adulthood.

So these feelings would all apply to Gail's parents too? It makes sense that, the longer the relationship with the child, the greater the sense of loss.

CULTURAL INFLUENCES ON REACTIONS TO BEREAVEMENT

Because of the huge individual variability, trying to distinguish 'normal' from 'abnormal' grief seems quite arbitrary (Schuchter and Zisook, 1993). According to Middleton *et al.* (1993), the validity of the concept of *pathological grief* must be considered in terms of *cultural norms*. Although grief is a universal response to major loss, its meaning, duration and how it's expressed are all culturally prescribed.

Inter- and intra-cultural differences

Cultures differ in how they define death and appropriate expressions of grief. According to Rosenblatt (1993),

> culture is such a crucial part of the context of bereavement that it is often impossible to separate an individual's grief from culturally required mourning.

For example, in cultures that believe 'do not grieve because grief will cause the ghost of the deceased to take you away' or 'do not grieve because the deceased has gone to a better life', it's difficult to assess accurately what appears to be muted or restrained grief. Similarly, when the 'rules' say 'cry' and people cry, how do we know the grief is genuine, deeply felt and likely to occur in the absence of the cultural demands for crying?

The Jewish rites of mourning are believed to be of therapeutic benefit, enabling the expression, rather than the repression, of grief. For the first few days following a burial, mourners are expected to be distressed and their despair is recognised and supported by relatives and friends who come to pay their respects.

By contrast, the Hindu, Sikh, Muslim and Buddhist religions all discourage too much weeping (Firth, 1993). The Hindus believe that weeping makes a river, which the soul of the deceased has to cross, and Sikhs believe the deceased has gone to God. However, the expression of grief is less inhibited in villages on the Indian sub-continent compared with Sikhs and Hindus living in Britain. Similarly, wailing is still very common among Muslims in Muslim countries (Firth, 1993).

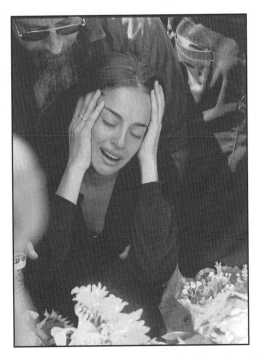

The degree to which weeping is acceptable or encouraged at funerals varies between religious and cultural groups

Compared with western women, Japanese women accept their husbands' death with composure and resignation. They believe strongly in an afterlife and that their ancestors are always with them. Their beliefs mitigate feelings of complete loss and, to this extent, they have less to grieve about. The long-lasting grief and depression observed among the bereaved in the UK is partly a result of the lack of rituals and beliefs, as well as the lack of an externally based end to the grieving process (March and Doherty, 1999).

According to Firth (1993), all the major religions of the world teach that there's some sort of continuity or survival after death. They also comfort and reassure the bereaved by helping to make sense of death and personal loss, providing shape and meaning to the grieving process. Mourning lasts for a clearly defined period in different cultures, providing 'milestones'. These allow the bereaved a gradual time to let go of the deceased and adjust to the psychological and social changes in their lives.

As well as differences between cultures, there are important differences *within* culturally diverse countries, such as the USA and the UK. For example, WASP (white Anglo-Saxon Protestant) Americans tend to 'psychologise' their emotional pain (e.g. depression), while people in many ethnic minority groups tend to 'somatise' theirs (e.g. bodily symptoms: Kleinman and Kleinman, 1985).

Discussing the visit, Sally said we have to deal with things as they arise – and, as always, according to each individual's need. She said we must put Gail first, but must also respond to the family's needs; from now on, they'll all need more emotional support. She'd offered Gail the service of a Macmillan nurse, whom she was also going to consult about managing Gail's increased pain. She also asked if Gail would like to see a priest.

Then she told me I'd done well to notice Gail's father was upset and I'd handled it well, which pleased me as it means I'm becoming more observant of emotional need. I wish I'd read all this before going this morning – but I feel that, by remembering the importance of listening, I did help a bit anyway.

CHAPTER SUMMARY

◎ **Bereavement** is a **non-normative influence**, but it becomes more likely as we get older.
◎ **Grief** has been portrayed as a **natural, universal human reaction** to bereavement, a **psychiatric disorder** and a **disease process**.
◎ The two most commonly cited **stage theories** of grief are those of Bowlby and Kübler-Ross. While both can be applied to the dying and the bereaved, Kübler-Ross's theory is an explicit account of **anticipatory grief** and describes the **process of dying**.
◎ Kübler-Ross distinguishes **acceptance** from **resignation**; the latter is similar to Erikson's concept of **despair**. **Hope** is a theme running through all the stages.
◎ Kübler-Ross favours the **open awareness context**, in which the patient, relatives and staff all admit that death is inevitable, and interact accordingly.
◎ Stage theories have been criticised on the grounds that grief isn't a simple, universal process which is the same for everyone. However, stages provide a **framework** for understanding bereaved people's experiences, which display a **huge variability**.
◎ Also, many stage theorists have explicitly denied that the stages are meant to apply equally and rigidly to everyone.
◎ Nurses' ability to help dying patients deal with their feelings will be influenced by

awareness of their own attitudes towards death and dying. They sometimes sidestep potentially difficult conversations, keeping interactions emotionally 'safe'.

◎ These withdrawal and distancing techniques are also used by staff dealing with **dying children**. But children with a life-threatening illness usually sense that they might be dying and they need an age- and developmentally appropriate opportunity to share their fears.

◎ Nurses in **A&E** are likely to have to deal with a higher proportion of sudden/unexpected deaths, which may occur in unusual or violent circumstances. Many nurses in acute care feel unprepared and unsupported.

◎ The **death of a child** can take the form of **miscarriage (spontaneous abortion)**, **termination (therapeutic/induced abortion)**, **stillbirth** or **neonatal death** (babies in **SCBUs/NICUs**). Each is a bereavement that needs to be grieved for, but termination is more likely to cause mental health problems in the mother.

◎ Although grief is a universal response to major loss, its meaning, duration and expression are all **culturally prescribed**. Cultures differ in how they define death, and it's often impossible to separate an individual's grief from culturally required mourning.

◎ All the world's major religions teach that there's some kind of **afterlife**. They also comfort the bereaved by helping to make sense of death and by providing 'milestones' that allow a gradual time to adjust to life without the deceased.

REFERENCES

Abrams, D., Wetherell, M., Cochrane, S., Hogg, M.A. and Turner, J.C. (1990) Knowing what to think by knowing who you are: self-categorisation and the nature of norm formation. *British Journal of Social Psychology, 29,* 97–119.

Adler, A. (1927) *The Practice and Theory of Individual Psychology.* New York: Harcourt Brace Jovanovich.

Adler, R. (2000) Pigeonholed. *New Scientist, 167*(2258), 389–391.

Adorno, T.W., Frenkel-Brunswick, E., Levinson, J.D. and Sanford, R.N. (1950) *The Authoritarian Personality.* New York: Harper & Row.

Ahmed, K. (2004) Official: £20bn cost of Britain's binge drinking. *Observer,* 14 March, 3.

Ahuja, A. (2000) Drugs blow your mind. *The Times,* 15 June, 5.

Ainsworth, M.D.S., Bell, S.M.V. and Stayton, D.J. (1971) Individual differences in Strange Situation behaviour of one-year-olds. In H.R. Schaffer (ed.) *The Origins of Human Social Relations.* New York: Academic Press.

Ainsworth, M.D.S., Blehar, M.C., Waters, E. and Wall, S. (1978) *Patters of Attachment: A Psychological Study of the Strange Situation.* Hillsdale, NJ: Lawrence Erlbaum Associates Inc.

Ajzen, I. (1988) *Attitudes, Personality and Behaviour.* Milton Keynes: Open University Press.

Ajzen, I. (1991) The theory of planned behaviour. *Organisational Behaviour & Human Decision Processes, 50,* 179–211.

Ajzen, I. and Fishbein, M. (1970) The prediction of behaviour from attitudinal and normative beliefs. *Journal of Personality & Social Psychology, 6,* 466–487.

Ajzen, I. and Fishbein, M. (1977) Attitude–behaviour relations: a theoretical analysis and review of empirical research. *Psychological Bulletin, 24,* 888–918.

Alexander, M.F., Fawcett, J.N. and Runciman, P.J. (eds) (2006) *Nursing Practice Hospital and Home* (3rd edn). London: Churchill Livingstone.

Alibhai-Brown, Y. (2000) We are black men. That means we make babies. *Guardian,* 13 April, 8.

Allen, V. and Levine, J.M. (1968) Social support, dissent and conformity. *Sociometry, 31,* 138–149.

Allen, V. and Levine, J.M. (1971) Social support and conformity: the role of independent assessment of reality. *Journal of Experimental Social Psychology, 7,* 48–58.

Allport, G.W. (1935) Attitudes. In C.M. Murchison (ed.) *Handbook of Social Psychology.* Worchester, MA: Clark University Press.

Allport, G.W. (1947) *The Use of Personal Documents in Psychological Science.* London: Holt, Rinehart & Winston.

Allport, G.W. (1954) *The Nature of Prejudice.* Reading, MA: Addison-Wesley.

Allport, G.W. (1955) *Theories of Perception and the Concept of Structure.* New York: Wiley.

Allport, G.W. (1968) The historical background of modern psychology. In G. Lindzey and E. Aronson (eds) *Handbook of Social Psychology,* Vol. 1 (2nd edn). Reading, MS: Addison-Wesley.

Alsaker, F.D. (1992) Pubertal timing, overweight, and psychological adjustment. *Journal of Early Adolescence, 12,* 396–419.

Alsaker, F.D. (1996) The impact of puberty. *Journal of Child Psychology & Psychiatry, 37*(3), 249–258.

Altman, A.I. and Taylor, D.A. (1973) *Social Penetration: The Development of Interpersonal Relationships.* New York: Holt, Rinehart & Winston.

American Psychiatric Association (2000) *Diagnostic and Statistical Manual of Mental Disorders* (4th edn, revised). Washington: American Psychiatric Association.

Amir, Y. (1969) Contact hypothesis in ethnic relations. *Psychological Bulletin, 71,* 319–342.

Amir, Y. (1994) The contact hypothesis in intergroup relations. In W.J. Lonner and R.S. Malpass (eds) *Psychology and Culture.* Boston: Allyn & Bacon.

Antaki, C. (1984) Core concepts in attribution theory. In J. Nicholson and H. Beloff (eds) *Psychology Survey, No. 5.* Leicester: British Psychological Society.

Anthony, S. (1971) *The Discovery of Death in Childhood and After.* Harmondsworth: Penguin.

Apter, T. (2001) *The Myth of Maturity.* New York: Norton.

Archer, J. (1999) *The Nature of Grief: The Evolution and Psychology of Reactions to Loss.* London: Routledge.

Arendt, H. (1965) *Eichmann in Jerusalem: A Report on the Banality of Evil.* New York: Viking.

Argyle, M., Alkema, F. and Gilmour, R. (1972) The communication of friendly and hostile attitudes by verbal and non-verbal signals. *European Journal of Social Psychology, 1,* 385–402.

Aronson, E. (1980) *The Social Animal* (3rd edn). San Francisco: WH Freeman.

Aronson, E. (1988) *The Social Animal* (5th edn). New York: Freeman.

Aronson, E. (1992) *The Social Animal* (6th edn). New York: Freeman.

Aronson, E. (2000) The jigsaw strategy: reducing prejudice in the classroom. *Psychology Review, 7*(2), 2–5.

Aronson, E. and Carlsmith, J.M. (1963) Effect of the severity of threat on the devaluation of forbidden behaviour. *Journal of Abnormal & Social Psychology, 6,* 584–588.

Aronson, E. and Mills, J. (1959) The effect of severity of initiation on liking for a group. *Journal of Abnormal & Social Psychology, 6,* 584–588.

Aronson, E., Bridgeman, D.L. and Geffner, R.F. (1978) The effects of a cooperative classroom structure on student behaviour and attitudes. In D. Bar-Tal and L. Saxe (eds) *Social Psychology of Education*. New York: Wiley.

Asch, S.E. (1946) Forming impressions of personality. *Journal of Abnormal and Social Psychology*, 41, 258–290.

Asch, S.E. (1951) Effect on group pressure upon the modification and distortion of judgements. In H. Guetzkow (ed.) *Groups, Leadership and Men*. Pittsburgh, PA: Carnegie Press.

Asch, S.E. (1952) *Social Psychology*. Englewood Cliffs, NJ: Prentice Hall.

Asch, S.E. (1955) Opinions and social pressure. *Scientific American*, 193, 31–35.

Aschoff, J. (1979) Circadian rhythms: general features and endocrinological aspects. In D.T. Krieger (ed.) *Endocrine Rhythms*. New York: Raven Press.

Atkinson, R.L., Atkinson, R.C., Smith, E.E. and Bem, D.J. (1990) *Introduction to Psychology* (10th edn). New York: Harcourt Brace Jovanovich.

Attie, I. and Brooks-Gunn, J. (1989) Development of eating problems in adolescent girls: a longitudinal study. *Developmental Psychology*, 25, 70–79.

Baker, A. (2000) 'Even as I bought it I knew it wouldn't work'. In A. Baker (ed.) *Serious Shopping: Essays in Psychotherapy and Consumerism*. London: Free Association Books.

Baltes, M.M. and Baltes, P.B. (1986) *The Psychology of Control and Ageing*. Hillsdale, NJ: Erlbaum.

Baltes, P.B. (1983) Life-span developmental psychology: observations on history and theory revisited. In R.M. Lerner (ed.) *Developmental Psychology: Historical and Philosophical Perspectives*. Hillsdale, NJ: Erlbaum.

Baltes, P.B. and Baltes, M.M. (1993) *Successful Ageing: Perspectives from the Behavioural Sciences*. Cambridge: Cambridge University Press.

Bandura, A. (1971) *Social Learning Theory*. Englewood Cliffs, NJ: Prentice Hall.

Bandura, A. (1977) Self-efficacy: toward a unifying theory of behaviour change. *Psychological Review*, 84, 191–215.

Bandura, A. (1986) *Social Foundations of Thought and Action*. Englewood Cliffs, NJ: Prentice Hall.

Banks, C. (1991) Alleviating anticipatory vomiting. *Nursing Times*, 87(16), 42–43.

Barber, B.K. and Buehler, C. (1996) Family cohesion and enmeshment: different constructs, different effects. *Journal of Marriage & the Family*, 58(2), 433–515.

Baron, R.A. and Byrne, D. (1991) *Social Psychology* (6th edn). Boston: Allyn & Bacon.

Barrett, R. and Robinson, B. (1994) Gay dads. In A.E. Gottfried and A.W. Gottfried (eds) *Redefining Families*. New York: Plenum Press.

Barron, A. (1990) The right to personal space. *Nursing Times*, 86(27), 28–32.

Bartlett, D. (1998) *Stress: Perspectives and Processes*. Buckingham: Open University Press.

Bassett, C. (2002) Nurses' and students' perceptions of care: a phenomenological study. *Nursing Times*, 94(34), 32–34.

Baumeister, R.F. (1982) A self-presentational view of social phenomena. *Psychological Bulletin*, 91, 3–26.

Baumeister, R.F. (1998) The self. In D.T. Gilbert, S.T. Fiske and G. Lindzey (eds) *Handbook of Social Psychology* (4th edn). New York: McGraw-Hill.

Baumeister, R.F., Smart, L. and Boden, J.M. (1996) Relation of threatened egotism to violence and aggression: the dark side of high self-esteem. *Psychological Review*, 103, 5–33.

Becker, M.H. (ed.) (1974) The health belief model and personal health behaviour. *Health Education Monographs*, 2, 324–508.

Becker, M.H. and Rosenstock, I.M. (1984) Compliance and medical advice. In A. Steptoe and A. Mathews (eds) *Health Care and Human Behaviour*. London: Academic Press.

Becker, M.H. and Rosenstock, I.M. (1987) Comparing social learning theory and the health belief model. In W.B. Ward (ed.) *Advances in Health Education and Promotion*. Greenwich, CT: JAI Press.

Becker, M.H., Maiman, L.A., Kirscht, J.P., Haefner, D.P. and Drachman, R.H. (1977) The health belief model and prediction of dietary compliance: a field experiment. *Journal of Health & Social Behaviour*, 18, 348–366.

Bee, H. (1994) *Lifespan Development*. New York: HarperCollins.

Bee, H. (2000) The Developing Child (9th edition). Boston: Allyn & Bacon.

Beecher, H.K. (1956) Relationship of significance of wound to the pain experienced. *Journal of the American Medical Association*, 161, 1609–1613.

Bell, S.M. and Ainsworth, M.D.S. (1972) Infant crying and maternal responsiveness. *Child Development*, 43, 1171–1190.

Bem, D.J. (1965) An experimental analysis of self-persuasion. *Journal of Experimental & Social Psychology*, 1, 199–218.

Bem, D.J. (1967) Self-perception: an alternative interpretation of cognitive dissonance phenomena. *Psychological Review*, 74, 183–200.

Bem, D.J. (1972) Self-perception theory. In L. Berkowitz (ed.) *Advances in Experimental Social Psychology*, Vol. 6. New York: Academic Press.

Bergevin, T., Bukowski, W.M. and Miners, R. (2003) Social development. In A. Slater and G. Bremner (eds) *An Introduction to Developmental Psychology*. Oxford: Blackwell Publishing.

Berry, J.W. (1994) *Cross-Cultural Health Psychology*. Keynote address presented to the International Conference of Applied Psychology. Madrid (July).

Berry, J.W. (1998) Acculturation and health: theory and research. In S.S. Kazarian and D.R. Evans (eds) *Cultural Clinical Psychology: Theory, Research and Practice*. New York: Oxford University Press.

Billig, M. (1976) *Social Psychology and Intergroup Relations*. London: Academic Press.

Blackman, D.E. (1980) Images of man in contemporary behaviourism. In A.J. Chapman and D.M. Jones (eds) *Models of Man*. Leicester: British Psychological Society.

Blackmore, C. (1989) Altered images. *Nursing Times*, 85(12), 36–39.

Blyth, D.A., Simmons, R.G., Bulcroft, R., Felt, D., Vancleave, E.F. and Bush, D.M. (1981) The effects of physical development on self-image and satisfaction with body-image for early adolescent males. *Research in Community & Mental Health*, 2, 43–73.

Boden, M. (1980) Artificial intelligence and intellectual imperialism. In A.J. Chapman and D.M. Jones (eds) *Models of Man*. Leicester: British Psychological Society.

Bond, J., Coleman, P. and Peace, S. (eds) (1993) *Ageing in Society: An Introduction to Social Gerontology*. London: Sage.

Bond, R.A. and Smith, P.B. (1996) Culture and conformity: a meta-analysis of studies using Asch's (1952b, 1956) line judgement task. *Psychological Bulletin*, 119, 111–137.

Borke, H. (1975) Piaget's mountains revisited: changes in the egocentric landscape. *Developmental Psychology*, 11, 240–243.

Bowlby, J. (1951) *Maternal Care and Mental Health*. Geneva: World Health Organization.

Bowlby, J. (1969) *Attachment and Loss. Vol. 1: Attachment*. Harmondsworth: Penguin.

Bowlby, J. (1973) *Attachment and Loss. Vol. 2: Separation*. Harmondsworth: Penguin.

Bowlby, J. (1980) *Attachment and Loss, Vol. 3: Loss, Sadness and Depression*. London: Hogarth Press.

Bowlby, J., Ainsworth, M., Boston, M. and Rosenbluth, D. (1956) The effects of mother–child separation: a follow-up study. *British Journal of Medical Psychology*, 24(3/4), 211–247.

BPS (British Psychological Society) (2004) *So You Want to be a Psychologist?* Leicester: British Psychological Society.

Bradley, L.A. (1995) Chronic benign pain. In D. Wedding (ed.) *Behaviour and Medicine* (2nd edn). St Louis, MO: Mosby-Year Book.

Bredin, M. (1999) Mastectomy, body image and therapeutic massage: a qualitative study of women's experience. *Journal of Advanced Nursing*, 29(5), 1113–1120.

Brehm, J.W. (1956) Post-decision changes in the desirability of alternatives. *Journal of Abnormal & Social Psychology*, 52, 384–389.

Brewer, M.B. (1999) The psychology of prejudice: ingroup love or outgroup hate? *Journal of Social Issues*, 55, 429–444.

Brewer, M.B. and Brown, R.J. (1998) Intergroup relations. In D.T. Gilbert, S.T. Fiske and G. Lindzey (eds) *Handbook of Social Psychology* (4th edn, Vol. 2). New York: McGraw-Hill.

Brislin, R. (1981) *Cross-Cultural Encounters: Face-to-Face Interaction*. Elmsford, NY: Pergamon.

Brislin, R. (1993) *Understanding Culture's Influence on Behaviour*. Orlando, FL: Harcourt Brace Jovanovich.

British National Formulary (2005) London: British Medical Association & The Royal Pharmaceutical Society of Great Britain.

Bromley, D.B. (1977) Speculations in social and environmental gerontology. *Nursing Times (Occasional Papers)*, 21 April, 53–56.

Bromley, D.B. (1988) *Human Ageing: An Introduction to Gerontology* (3rd edn). Harmondsworth: Penguin.

Bronfenbrenner, U. (1960) Freudian theories of identification and their derivatives. *Child Development*, 31, 15–40.

Brooking, J. (1991) Doctors and nurses: a personal view. *Nursing Standard*, 6(12), 24–28.

Brooks-Gunn, J. and Warren, M.P. (1985) The effects of delayed menarche in different contexts. Dance and non-dance students. *Journal of Youth & Adolescence*, 14, 285–300.

Brown, H. (1985) *People, Groups and Society*. Milton Keynes: Open University Press.

Brown, H. (1996) Themes in experimental research on groups from the 1930s to the 1990s. In M. Wetherell (ed.) *Identities, Groups and Social Issues*. London: Sage, in association with the Open University.

Brown, J.K. (1963) A cross-cultural study of female initiation rites. *American Anthropologist*, 65, 837–853.

Brown, K. (2000) How long have you got? *Scientific American Presents: The Quest to Beat Ageing*, 11(2), 8–15.

Brown, P. (1988) Punching the body clock. *Nursing Times*, 84(44), 26–28.

Brown, R. (1965) *Social Psychology*. New York: Free Press.

Brown, R. (1986) *Social Psychology* (2nd edn). New York: Free Press.

Brown, R.J. (1988) Intergroup relations. In M. Haewstone, W. Stroebe, J.P. Codol and G.M. Stephenson (eds) *Introduction to Social Psychology*. Oxford: Blackwell.

Brown, R., Marsas, P., Masser, B., Vivian, J. and Hewstone, M. (2001) Life on the ocean wave: testing some intergroup hypotheses in a naturalistic setting. *Group Processes & Intergroup Relations*, 4, 81–98.

Brubaker, C. and Wickersham, D. (1990) Encouraging the practice of testicular self-examination: a field application of the theory of reasoned action. *Health Psychology*, 9, 154–163.

Bruner, J.S. (1966) *Towards a Theory of Instruction*. Cambridge, MA: Harvard University Press.

Bruner, J.S. (1990) *Acts of Meaning*. Cambridge, MA: Harvard University Press.

Buggins, E. (1995) Mind your language. *Nursing Standard*, 10(1), 21–22.

BullyOnLine, www.bullyonline.com

Burke, J. and Asthana, A. (2004) So getting stoned is no longer a big deal – or is it? *Observer*, 18 January, 9–10.

Burnard, P. (1987) Meaningful dialogue. *Nursing Times*, 83(20), 43–45.

Burnard, P., Edwards, D., Fothergill, A., Hannigan, B. and Coyle, D. (2000) When the pressure's too much. *Nursing Times*, 96(19), 28–30.

Burns, R.B. (1980) *Essential Psychology*. Lancaster: MTP Press.

Burr, V. (2003) *Social Constructionism* (2nd edn). Hove, East Sussex: Routledge.

Burt, K. (1995) The effect of cancer on body image and sexuality. *Nursing Times*, 91(7), 36–37.

Bushman, B. (1984) Perceived symbols of authority and their influence on compliance. *Journal of Applied Social Psychology*, 14, 501–508.

Buss, A.H. (1992) Personality: primate heritage and human distinctiveness. In R.A. Zucker, A.I. Rabin, J. Aronoff and S.J. Frank (eds) *Personality Structure in the Life Course: Essays on Personality in the Murray Tradition*. New York: Springer.

Butler, R.N. (1963) The life review: an interpretation of reminiscence in the aged. *Psychiatry*, 26, 65–76.

Calne, S. (1994) Dehumanisation in intensive care. *Nursing Times*, 27(90), 31–33.

Carlson, N.R. and Buskist, W. (1997) *Psychology: The Science of Behaviour* (5th edn). Needham Heights, MA: Allyn & Bacon.

Carson, J., Fagin, L., Brown, D., Leary, J. and Bartlett, H. (1997) Self-esteem and stress in mental health nurses. *Nursing Times*, 93(44), 55–58

Carstensen, L.L. (1991) Selectivity theory: social activity in life-span context. *Annual Review of Gerontology & Geriatrics*, 11, 195–217.

Carstensen, L.L (1992) Social and emotional patterns in adulthood: support for socioemotional selectivity theory. *Psychology & Ageing*, 7, 331–338.

Carstensen, L.L. (1996) Socioemotional selectivity: a life span developmental account of social behaviour. In M.R. Merrens and G.C. Brannigan (eds) *The Developmental Psychologists: Research Adventures Across the Life Span*. New York: McGraw-Hill.

Carstensen, L.L., Isaacowitz, D.M. and Charles, S.T. (1999) Taking time seriously: a theory of socioemotional selectivity. *American Psychologist*, 54, 165–181.

Cattell, R.B. (1965) *The Scientific Analysis of Personality*. Harmondsworth: Penguin.

Chaiken, S. (1987) The heuristic model of persuasion. In M.P. Zanna, J.M. Olsen and C.P. Herman (eds) *Social Influence: The Ontario Symposium*, Vol. 5. Hillsdale, NJ: Lawrence Erlbaum Associates, Inc.

Cheesman, S. (2006) Promoting concordance: the implications for prescribers. *Nurse Prescribing*, 4(5), 205–208.

Chesterfield, P. (1992) Communicating with dying children. *Nursing Standard*, 6(20), 30–32.

Chisolm, K., Carter, M.C., Ames, E.W. and Morison, S.J. (1995) Attachment security and indiscriminately friendly behaviour in children adopted from Romanian orphanages. *Development & Psychopathology*, 7, 283–294.

Christensen, M. and Hewitt-Taylor, J. (2006) Empowerment in nursing: paternalism or maternalism? *British Journal of Nursing*, 15(1), 695–699.

Churchill, H. (1995) Perceptions of childbirth: are women properly informed? *Nursing Times*, 91(45), 32–34.

Claridge, G. and Davis, C. (2003) *Personality and Psychological Disorders*. London: Arnold.

Claridge, G. and Herrington, R.N. (1960) Sedation threshold, personality and the theory of neurosis. *Journal of Mental Science*, 106, 1568–1583.

Claridge, G. and Herrington, R.N. (1962) Excitation-inhibition and the theory of neurosis: a study of the sedation threshold. In H.J. Eysenck (ed.) *Experiments with Drugs*. New York: Pergamon Press.

Clark, K.E. and Miller, G.A. (eds) (1970) *Psychology: Behavioural and Social Sciences Survey Committee*. Englewood Cliffs, NJ: Prentice Hall.

Clarke, A. and Clarke, A. (2000) *Early Experience and the Life Path*. London: Jessica Kingsley.

Cloninger, C.R. (1987) Neurogenetic adaptive mechanisms in alcoholism. *Science*, 236, 410–416.

Cochrane, R. (1983) *The Social Creation of Mental Illness*. London: Longman.

Coffey, L., Skipper, K. and Jung, F. (1988) Nurses and shift work: effects on job performance and job related stress. *Journal of Advanced Nursing*, 13, 245–254.

Cohen, F. and Lazarus, R.S. (1979) Coping with the stress of illness. In G.C. Stone *et al.* (eds) *Health Psychology: A Handbook*. Washington, DC: Jossey-Bass.

Cohen, J. (1958) *Humanistic Psychology*. London: Allen & Unwin.

Cole, M. (1990) Cultural psychology: a once and future discipline? In J.J. Berman (ed.) *Nebraska Symposium on Motivation: Cross-Cultural Perspectives*. Lincoln, NA: University of Nebraska Press.

Coleman, J.C. (1980) *The Nature of Adolescence*. London: Methuen.

Coleman, J.C. (1995) Adolescence. In P.E. Bryant and A.M. Colman (eds) *Developmental Psychology*. London: Longman.

Coleman, J.C. and Hendry, L.B. (1990) *The Nature of Adolescence* (2nd edition). London: Routledge.

Coleman, J.C. and Roker, D. (1998) Adolescence. *The Psychologist*, 11(12), 593–596.

Coleman, P.G. and O'Hanlon, A. (2004) *Ageing and Development*. London: Arnold.

Collins, J. (1994) What is Pain? In J. Robbins (ed.) *Caring for the Dying Patient and the Family* (2nd edn). London: Chapman & Hall.

Comfort, A. (1977) *A Good Age*. London: Mitchell Beazley.

Compas, B.E., Hinden, B.R. and Gerhardt, C.A. (1995) Adolescent development: pathways and processes of risk and resilience. *Annual Review of Psychology*, 46, 265–293.

Connor, S. (2004) Brain scans prove teenagers are children at heart. *Independent*, 18 May, 12.

Coolican, H. (2004) *Research Methods and Statistics in Psychology* (4th edn). London: Hodder & Stoughton.

Coolican, H., Cassidy, T., Chercher, A., Harrower, J., Penny, G., Sharp, R., Walley, M. and Westbury, T. (1996) *Applied Psychology*. London: Hodder & Stoughton.

Cooper, C. and Faragher, B. (1993) Psychological stress and breast cancer: the interrelationship between stress events, coping strategies and personality. *Psychological Medicine*, 23, 653–662.

Cooper, D. (1995) *NT Guide to Working With People Who Misuse Drugs*. Nursing Times Guides.

Cooper, J., Kelly, K.A. and Weaver, K. (2004) Attitudes, norms and social groups. In M.B. Brewer and M. Hewstone (eds) *Social Cognition*. Oxford: Blackwell Publishing.

Coopersmith, S. (1967) *The Antecedents of Self Esteem*. San Francisco: Freeman.

Costa, P.T. and McCrae, R.R. (1992) *Revised NEO Personality Inventory (NEO-PI-R)*. Odessa, FL: Psychological Assessment Resources.

Cox, T. (1978) *Stress*. London: Macmillan Education.

Craig, G.J. (1992) *Human Development* (6th edn). Englewood Cliffs, NJ: Prentice Hall.

Cramer, D. (1995) Special issue on personal relationships. *The Psychologist*, 8, 58–59.

Crano, W.D. (2000) Milestones in the psychological analysis of social influence. *Group Dynamics*, 4, 68–80.

Crawford, M. and Unger, R.K. (1995) Gender issues in psychology. In A.M. Colman (ed.) *Controversies in Psychology*. London: Longman.

Crouch, D. (2003) Tackling substance abuse. *Nursing Times*, 99(33), 20–23.

Crutchfield, R. (1954) A new technique for measuring individual differences in conformity to group judgement. *Proceedings of the Invitational Conference on Testing Problems*, 69–74.

Crutchfield, R. (1995) Conformity and character. *American Psychologist*, 10, 191–198.

Cumming, E. (1975) Engagement with an old theory. *International Journal of Ageing & Human Development*, 6, 187–191.

Cumming, E. and Henry, W.E (1961) *Growing Old: The Process of Disengagement*. New York: Basic Books.

Curry, C. (1998) Adolescence. In K. Trew and J. Kremer (eds) *Gender and Psychology*. London: Arnold.

Curtiss, A. (1999) The psychology of pain. *Psychology Review*, 5(4), 15–18.

Dacey, J.S. (1982) *Adolescents Today* (2nd edn). Glenview, IL: Scott, Foresman & Co.

Damon, W. and Hart, D. (1988) *Self-Understanding in Childhood and Adolescence*. Cambridge: Cambridge University Press.

Damrosch, S. (1995) Facilitating adherence to preventive and treatment regimes. In D. Wedding (ed.) *Behaviour and Medicine* (2nd edn). St Louis, MO: Mosby-Year Book.

Darbyshire, P. (1986a) 'Can Tiger come, too?' *Nursing Times*, 2 April, 40–42.

Darbyshire, P. (1986b) When the face doesn't fit. *Nursing Times*, 24 September, 28–30.

Darley, J.M. and Huff, C.W. (1990) Heightened damage assessment as a result of the internationality of the damage causing act. *British Journal of Social Psychology*, 29, 181–188.

Dasen, P.R. (1994) Culture and cognitive development from a Piagetian perspective. In W.J. Lonner and R.S. Malpass (eds) *Psychology and Culture*. Boston: Allyn & Bacon.

Dasen, P.R. (1999) Rapid social change and the turmoil of adolescence: a cross-cultural perspective. *World Psychology*, 5.

Davidson, A.R. and Jaccard, J. (1979) Variables that moderate the attitude–behaviour relation: results of a longitudinal survey. *Journal of Personality & Social Psychology*, 37, 1364–1376.

Davidson, L. (1990) A room of their own? *Nursing Times*, *86*(27), 32–33.

Davies, E. and Furnham, A. (1986) Body satisfaction in adolescent girls. *British Journal of Medical Psychology*, *59*, 279–288.

Davison, G.C. and Neale, J.M. (1994) *Abnormal Psychology* (6th edn). New York: Wiley.

Davison, G.C., Neale, J.M. and Kring, A.M. (2004) *Abnormal Psychology* (9th edn). New York: John Wiley & Sons Inc.

Davitz, L.L., Davitz, J.R. and Higuchi, Y. (1977) Cross-cultural inferences of physical pain and psychological distress, 2. *Nursing Times*, 21 April, 556–558.

Dean, A. (2002) Talking to dying patients of their hopes and needs. *Nursing Times*, *98*(43), 34–35.

Deese, J. (1972) *Psychology as Science and Art*. New York: Harcourt Brace Jovanovich.

Deutsch, M. and Gerard, H.B. (1955) A study of normative and informational social influence upon individual judgement. *Journal of Abnormal & Social Psychology*, *51*, 629–636.

Devine, P.G. and Zuwerink, J.R. (1994) Prejudice and guilt: the internal struggle to control prejudice. In W.J. Lonner and R.S. Malpass (eds) *Psychology and Culture*. Boston: Allyn & Bacon.

Devlin, R. (1989) Robertson's revolution. *Nursing Times*, *85*(5), 18.

DeWolff, M.S. and van Ijzendoorn, M.H. (1997) Sensitivity and attachment: a meta-analysis on parental antecedents of infant attachment. *Child Development*, *68*, 571–591.

Dex, S. and Phillipson, C. (1986) Social policy and the older worker. In C. Phillipson and A. Walker (eds) *Ageing and Social Policy: A Critical Assessment*. Aldershot: Gower.

Digman, J.M. (1990) Personality structure: emergence of the five-factor model. *Annual Review of Psychology*, *41*, 417–440.

Dimatteo, M.R., Sherbourne, C., Hays, R., Ordway, L., Kravitz, R., McGlynn, E., Kaplan, S. and Rogers, W.H. (1993) Physicians' characteristics influence patients' adherence to medical treatment: results from the medical outcomes study. *Health Psychology*, *12*, 245–286.

Dimond, B. (2003) *Legal Aspects of Nursing* (3rd edn). Harlow: Pearson Longman, 284.

Dion, K.K. and Dion, K.L. (1995) On the love of beauty and the beauty of love: two psychologists study attraction. In G.G. Brannigan and M.R. Merrens (eds) *The Social Psychologists: Research Adventures*. New York: McGraw-Hill.

Dion, K.K., Berscheid, E. and Walster, E. (1972) What is beautiful is good. *Journal of Personality & Social Psychology*, *24*, 285–290.

Dollard, J., Doob, L.W., Mowrer, O.H. and Sears, R.R. (1939) *Frustration and Aggression*. New Haven, CT: Harvard University Press.

Donaldson, M. (1978) *Children's Minds*. London: Fontana.

Donnelly, C. (1991) Ending the torment. *Nursing Times*, *87*(11), 36–38.

Dovidio, J.F., Brigham, J.C., Johnson, B.T. and Gaertner, S.L. (1996) Stereotyping, prejudice, and discrimination: another look. In C.N. Macrae, C. Stangor and M. Hewstone (eds) *Stereotypes and Stereotyping*. New York: McGraw-Hill.

Dowd, J.J. (1975) Ageing as exchange: a preface to theory. *Journal of Gerontology*, *30*, 584–594.

Downie, C.M. and Basford, P. (eds) (2003) *Mentoring in Practice. A Reader*. London: University of Greenwich.

Duchene, P. (1990) Using biofeedback for childbirth pain. *Nursing Times*, *86*(25), 56.

Duck, S. (1991) *Friends for Life* (2nd edn). Hemel Hempstead: Harvester Wheatsheaf.

Dunn, V. (1988) Life after mastectomy. *Nursing Times* (Community Outlook), August, 34.

Durkin, K. (1995) *Developmental Social Psychology: From Infancy to Old Age*. Oxford: Blackwell.

Dworetzky, J.P. (1981) *Introduction to Child Development*. St Paul, MN: West Publishing Co.

Dyson, J. (1980) Sociopolitical influences on retirement. *Bulletin of the British Psychological Society*, *33*, 128–130.

Eboda, M. (2004) What I said was racist – but I'm not a racist. I am an idiot. *Observer*, 25 April, 3.

Edwards, G. (1986) The alcohol dependence syndrome: a concept as stimulus to enquiry. *British Journal of Addiction*, *81*, 71–84.

Egan, G. (1977) *You and Me*. California: Brooks/Cole.

Eiser, J.R. (1983) From attributions to behaviour. In M. Hewstone (ed.) *Attribution Theory: Social and Functional Extensions*. Oxford: Blackwell.

Eiser, J.R. and van der Pligt, J. (1988) *Attitudes and Decisions*. London: Routledge.

Elkind, D. (1970) Erik Erikson's eight ages of man. *New York Times Magazine*, 5 April.

Engel, G.L. (1977) The need for a new medical model: a challenge for bio-medicine. *Science*, *196*, 129–135.

Engel, G.L. (1980) The clinical application of the biopsychosocial model. *American Journal of Psychiatry*, *137*, 535–544.

Erikson, E.H. (1950) *Childhood and Society*. New York: Norton.

Erikson, E.H. (1963) *Childhood and Society* (2nd edn). New York: Norton.

Evans, D. and Allen, H. (2002) Emotional intelligence: its role in training. *Nursing Times*, *98*(27), 41–42.

Ewins, D. and Bryant, J. (1992) Relative comfort. *Nursing Times*, *88*(52), 61–63.

Eysenck, H.J. (1947) *Dimensions of Personality*. London: RKP.

Eysenck, H.J. (1965) *Fact and Fiction in Psychology*. Harmondsworth: Penguin.

Eysenck, H.J. (1970) *Crime and Personality*. London: Paladin.

Eysenck, H.J. (1980) The biosocial model of man and the unification of psychology. In A.J. Chapman and D.M. Jones (eds) *Models of Man*. Leicester: British Psychological Society.

Eysenck, H.J. (1985) *Decline and Fall of the Freudian Empire*. Harmondsworth: Penguin.

Eysenck, H.J. (1995) Trait theories of personality. In S.E. Hampson and A.M. Colman (eds) *Individual Differences and Personality*. London: Longman.

Eysenck, H.J. and Eysenck, M.W. (1985) *Personality and Individual Differences: A Natural Science Approach*. New York: Plenum.

Eysenck, H.J. and Eysenck, S.B.G. (1975) *Manual of the Eysenck Personality Questionnaire*. London: Hodder & Stoughton.

Eysenck, H.J. and Wilson, G.D. (eds) (1973) *The Experimental Study of Freudian Theories*. London: Methuen.

Fairbairn, R. (1952) *Psychoanalytical Studies of the Personality*. London: Tavistock.

Fancher, R.E. (1979) *Pioneers of Psychology*. New York: Norton.

Fancher, R.E. (1996) *Pioneers of Psychology* (3rd edn). New York: Norton.

Farrelly, R. (1994) The special care needs of adolescents in hospital. *Nursing Times*, *90*(38), 31–33.

Fazio, R.H. (1986) How do attitudes guide behaviour? In R.M. Sorrentino and E.T. Higgins (eds) *Handbook of Motivation and Cognition: Foundations of Social Behaviour.* New York: Guilford.

Fazio, R.H. (1990) Multiple processes by which attitudes guide behaviour: the MODE model as an integrative framework. In M.P. Zanna (ed.) *Advances in Experimental Social Psychology*, Vol. 23. San Diego, CA: Academic Press.

Fazio, R.H. and Zanna, M.P. (1978) Attitudinal qualities relating to the strength of the attitude–behaviour relation. *Journal of Experimental Social Psychology*, *14*, 398–408.

Fazio, R.H., Zanna, M.P. and Cooper, J. (1977) Dissonance and self-perception: an integrative view of each theory's major domain of application. *Journal of Experimental & Social Psychology*, *13*, 464–479.

Fennell, G., Phillipson, C. and Evers, H. (1988) *The Sociology of Old Age.* Milton Keynes: Open University Press.

Fergusson, D.M., Horwood, L.J. and Ridder, E.M. (2006) Abortion in young women and subsequent mental health. *Journal of Child Psychology & Psychiatry*, *47*(1), 16–24.

Fernando, S. (1991) *Mental Health, Race and Culture.* London: Macmillan, in conjunction with MIND.

Festinger, L. (1950) Informal social communication. *Psychological Review*, *57*, 271–282.

Festinger, L. (1954) A theory of social comparison processes. *Human Relations*, *7*, 117–140.

Festinger, L. (1957) *A Theory of Cognitive Dissonance.* New York: Harper & Row.

Festinger, L. and Carlsmith, J.M. (1959) Cognitive consequences of forced compliance. *Journal of Abnormal & Social Psychology*, *58*, 203–210.

Firn, S. and Norman, I.J. (1995) Psychological and emotional impact of an HIV diagnosis. *Nursing Times*, *91*(8), 37–39.

Firth, H., McKeown, P., McIntee, J. and Britton, P. (1987) Burn-out, personality and support in long-stay nursing. *Nursing Times*, *83*(32), 55–57.

Firth, S. (1993) Cross-cultural perspectives on bereavement. In D. Dickenson and M. Johnson (eds) *Death, Dying & Bereavement.* London: Sage, in association with the Open University.

Fishbein, M. (1967) Attitudes and the prediction of behaviour. In M. Fishbein (ed.) *Readings in Attitude Theory and Measurement.* New York: Wiley.

Fishbein, M. and Ajzen, I. (1974) Attitudes towards objects as predictors of single and multiple behavioural criteria. *Psychological Review*, *81*, 59–74.

Fishbein, M. and Ajzen, I. (1975) *Belief, Attitude, Intention and Behaviour: An Introduction to Theory and Research.* Reading, MA: Addison-Wesley.

Fisher, S. and Greenberg, R.P. (1977) *The Scientific Credibility of Freud's Theories.* New York: Basic Books.

Fiske, A.P., Kitayama, S., Markus, H.R. and Nisbett, R.E. (1998) The cultural matrix of social psychology. In D.T. Gilbert, S.T. Fiske and G. Lindzey (ed.) *Handbook of Social Psychology* (4th edn, Vol. 2). New York: McGraw-Hill.

Fiske, S.T. (2004) *Social Beings: A Core Motives Approach to Social Psychology.* New York: John Wiley & Sons, Inc.

Fiske, S.T. and Neuberg, S.L. (1990) A continuum of impression formation, from category-based to individuating processes: influences of information and motivation on attention and interpretation. In L. Berkowitz (ed.) *Advances in Experimental Social Psychology*, Vol. 23. New York: Academic Press.

Fiske, S.T. and Taylor, S.E. (1991) *Social Cognition* (2nd edn). New York: McGraw-Hill.

Flavell, J.H. (1982) Structures, stages and sequences in cognitive development. In W.A. Collins (ed.) *The Concept of Development: The Minnesota Symposia on Child Development*, Vol. 15. Hillsdale, NJ: Erlbaum.

Flavell, J.H. (1986) The development of children's knowledge about the appearance–reality distinction. *American Psychologist*, *41*, 418–425.

Flavell, J.H., Green, F.L. and Flavell, E.R. (1990) Developmental changes in young children's knowledge about the mind. *Cognitive Development*, *5*, 1–27.

Flavell, J.H., Shipstead, S.G. and Croft, K. (1978) What young children think you see when their eyes are closed. Unpublished report, Stanford University.

Fletcher, B.C. (1995) The consequences of stress. In D. Messer and C. Meldrum (eds) *Psychology for Nurses and Health Care Professionals.* Hemel Hempstead: Prentice Hall/Harvester Wheatsheaf.

Folkman, S. and Lazarus, R.S. (1988) *Manual for the Ways of Coping Questionnaire.* Palo Alto, CA: Consulting Psychologists Press.

Foot, H. and Howe, C. (1998) The psycho-educational basis of peer-assisted learning. In K. Topping and S. Ehly (eds) *Peer-Assisted Learning.* Mahwah, NJ: Erlbaum.

Foot, H., Morgan, M.J. and Shute, R.H. (1990) *Children Helping Children.* Chichester: Wiley.

Forshaw, M. (2002) *Essential Health Psychology.* London: Arnold.

Freedman, J.L. (1963) Attitudinal effects of inadequate justification. *Journal of Personality*, *31*, 371–385.

Freedman, J.L. (1965) Long-term behavioural effects of cognitive dissonance. *Journal of Experimental & Social Psychology*, *1*, 145–155.

Freud, A. and Dann, S. (1951) An experiment in group upbringing. *Psychoanalytic Study of the Child*, *6*, 127–168.

Freud, S. (1914) *Remembering, Repeating and Working Through. The Standard Edition of Complete Psychological Works of Sigmund Freud, Volume XII.* London: Hogarth Press.

Freud, S. (1923/1984) *The Ego and the Id.* Pelican Freud Library (11). Harmondsworth: Penguin.

Freud, S. (1926) Inhibitions, symptoms and anxiety. In *Standard Edition of the Complete Psychological Works of Sigmund Freud*, Volume XX. London: Hogarth Press.

Freud, S. (1933) *New Introductory Lectures on Psychoanalysis.* New York: Norton.

Freud, S. (1949) *An Outline of Psychoanalysis.* London: Hogarth Press.

Friedman, M. and Rosenman, R.H. (1974) *Type A Behaviour and Your Heart.* New York: Harper Row.

Frith, M. (2006) Warning: campaigns to promote health are a waste of money. *Independent*, 18 April, 7.

Fromant, S. (1988) Helping each other. *Nursing Times*, *84*(36), 30–32.

Furnham, A. and Heaven, P. (1999) *Personality and Social Behaviour.* London: Arnold.

Fursland, E. (1998) Finding ways to cope. *Nursing Times*, *94*(33), 30–31.

Gahagan, J. (1984) *Social Interaction and its Management.* London: Methuen.

Gallagher, M., Millar, R., Hargie, O. and Ellis, R. (1992) The personal and social worries of adolescents in Northern Ireland: results of a survey. *British Journal of Guidance & Counselling*, *30*(3), 274–290.

Garrett, R. (1996) Skinner's case for radical behaviourism. In W. O'Donohue and R.F. Kitchener (eds) *The Philosophy of Psychology*. London: Sage.

Gaze, H. (1988) Stressed to the limit. *Nursing Times*, *84*(36), 16–17.

Gelder, M., Mayou, R. and Geddes, J. (1999) *Psychiatry* (2nd edn). Oxford: Oxford University Press.

Gelman, R. (1979) Preschool thought. *American Psychologist*, *34*, 900–905.

George, M. (1995) Crisis of silence. *Nursing Standard*, *10*(10), 20–21.

Gerard, H.B., Wilhelmy, R.A. and Connolly, E.S. (1968) Conformity and group size. *Journal of Personality & Social Psychology*, *8*, 79–82.

Gergen, K.J. (1973) Social psychology as history. *Journal of Personality & Social Psychology*, *26*, 309–320.

Gergen, K.J. (1985) The social constructionist movement in modern psychology. *American Psychologist*, *40*, 266–275.

Giedd, J.N., Blumenthal, J., Jeffries, N.O., Castellanos, F.X., Liu, H., Zijdenboss, A., Paus, T., Evans, A.C. and Rapaport, J.L. (1999) Brain development during childhood and adolescence: a longitudinal MRI study. *Nature Neuroscience*, *2*, 861.

Gilbert, D.T. (1995) Attribution and interpersonal perception. In A. Tesser (ed.) *Advanced Social Psychology*. New York: McGraw-Hill.

Gilbert, D.T. (1998) Ordinary personology. In D.T. Gilbert, S.T. Fiske and G. Lindzey (eds) *Handbook of Social Psychology* (4th edn, Vol. 2). New York: McGraw-Hill.

Gilbert, G.M. (1951) Stereotype persistence and change among college students. *Journal of Abnormal & Social Psychology*, *46*, 245–254.

Gilbert, S.J. (1981) Another look at the Milgram obedience studies: the role of the graduated series of shocks. *Personality & Social Psychology Bulletin*, *7*, 690–695.

Gillies, M. (1992) Teenage traumas. *Nursing Times*, *88*(27), 26–29.

Gilligan, C. (1982) *In a Different Voice: Psychological Theory and Women's Development*. Cambridge, MA: Harvard University Press.

Glassman, W.E. (1995) *Approaches to Psychology* (2nd edn). Buckingham: Open University Press.

Glide, S. (1994) Maintaining sensory balance. *Nursing Times*, *27*(90), 33–34.

Goetsch, V.L. and Fuller, M.G. (1995) Stress and stress management. In D. Wedding (ed.) *Behaviour and Medicine* (2nd edn). St Louis, MO: Mosby-Year Book.

Goffman, E. (1971) *The Presentation of Self in Everyday Life*. Harmondsworth: Penguin.

Goldberg, L.R. (1993) The structure of phenotypic personality traits. *American Psychologist*, *48*, 26–34.

Goldberg, S. (2000) *Attachment and Development*. London: Arnold.

Goldfarb, W. (1943) The effects of early institutional care on adult personality. *Journal of Experimental Education*, *12*, 106–129.

Gollwitzer, P.M. (1993) Goal achievement: the role of intentions. In W. Stroebe and M. Hewstone (eds) *European Review of Social Psychology*, Vol. 4. Chichester: John Wiley.

Golombok, S., Cook, R., Bish, A. and Murray, C. (1995) Families created by the new reproductive technologies: quality of parenting and social and emotional development of the children. *Child Development*, *66*, 285–289.

Golombok, S., MacCallum, F. and Goodman, E. (2001) The 'test tube' generation: parent–child relationships and the psychological well-being of *in vitro* fertilisation children at adolescence. *Child Development*, *72*, 599–608.

Golombok, S., Murray, C., Brinsden, P. and Addalla, H. (1999) Social versus biological parenting: family functioning and socioemotional development of children conceived by egg or sperm donation. *Journal of Child Psychology & Psychiatry*, *40*, 519–527.

Gopnik, A. and Astington, J.W. (1988) Children's understanding of representational change and its relation to the understanding of false belief and the appearance–reality distinction. *Child Development*, *59*, 26–37.

Gopnik, A. and Wellman, H.M. (1994) The theory theory. In L.A. Hirschfield and S.A. Gelman (eds) *Mapping the Mind*. Cambridge: Cambridge University Press.

Gosling, J. (1995) Personality. In D. Messer and C. Meldrum (eds) *Psychology for Nurses and Health Care Professionals*. Hemel Hempstead: Prentice Hall/Harvester Wheatsheaf.

Greenwald, A.G. (1980) The totalitarian ego: fabrication and revision of personal history. *American Psychologist*, *35*, 603–613.

Greer, S. (1991) Psychological response to cancer and survival. *Psychological Medicine*, *21*, 43–49.

Greer, S. and Morris, T. (1975) Psychological attributes of women who develop breast cancer: a controlled study. *Journal of Psychosomatic Research*, *19*, 147–153.

Greer, S., Morris, T. and Pettingale, K.W. (1979) Psychological response to breast cancer: effect on outcome. *The Lancet*, *13*, 785–787.

Greer, S., Morris, T., Pettingale, K.W. and Haybittle, J.L. (1990) Psychological responses to breast cancer and fifteen year outcome. *Lancet*, *335*, 49–50.

Griffiths, E. (1989) More than skin deep. *Nursing Times*, *85*(40), 34–36.

Griffiths, M.D. (1995) Technological addictions. *Clinical Psychology Forum*, *76*, 14–19.

Groskop, V. (2004) Minding the parent gap. *Observer*, 25 April, 4.

Gross, R. (2005) *Psychology: The Science of Mind & Behaviour* (5th edn). London: Hodder Arnold.

Gross, R. and Rolls, G. (2006) *Essential Psychology for AS and A2*. London: Hodder Arnold.

Hall, E.T. (1959) *The Silent Language*. New York: Doubleday.

Hall, E.T. (1966) *The Hidden Dimension*. Garden City, NY: Doubleday & Co.

Hall, G.S. (1904) *Adolescence*. New York: Appleton & Co.

Hamilton, L. and Timmons, C.R. (1995) Psychopharmacology. In D. Kimble and A.M. Colman (eds) *Biological Aspects of Behaviour*. London: Longman.

Hamilton, V.L. (1978) Obedience and responsibility: a jury simulation. *Journal of Personality & Social Psychology*, *36*, 126–146.

Hammersley, R. (1999) Substance use, abuse and dependence. In D. Messer and F. Jones (eds) *Psychology and Social Care*. London: Jessica Kingsley Publishers.

Hampson, S. (1995) The construction of personality. In S.E. Hampson & A.M. Colman (eds) *Individual Differences and Personality*. London: Longman.

Harari, H. and McDavid, J.W. (1973) Teachers' expectations and name stereotypes. *Journal of Educational Psychology*, *65*, 222–225.

Harlow, H.F. (1959) Love in infant monkeys. *Scientific American*, *200*, 68–74.

Harlow, H.F. and Zimmerman, R.R. (1959) Affectional responses in the infant monkey. *Science*, *130*, 421–432.

Harré, R. and Secord, P.F. (1972) *The Explanation of Social Behaviour*. Oxford: Blackwell.

Harris, P. and Middleton, W. (1995) Social cognition and health behaviour. In D. Messer and C. Meldrum (eds) *Psychology for Nurses and Health Care Professionals*. Hemel Hempstead: Prentice Hall/Harvester Wheatsheaf.

Hartley, J. and Branthwaite, A. (1997) Earning a crust. *Psychology Review*, 3(3), 24–26.

Hartley, J. and Branthwaite, A. (2000) Prologue: the roles and skills of applied psychologists. In J. Hartley and A. Branthwaite (eds) *The Applied Psychologist* (2nd edn). Buckingham: Open University Press.

Havighurst, R.J. (1964) Stages of vocational development. In H. Borrow (ed.) *Man in a World at Work*. Boston: Houghton Mifflin.

Havighurst, R.J., Neugarten, B.L. and Tobin, S.S. (1968) Disengagement and patterns of ageing. In B.L. Neugarten (ed.) *Middle Age and Ageing*. Chicago, IL: University of Chicago Press.

Hawkins, L.H. and Armstrong-Esther, C.A. (1978) Circadian rhythms and night shift working in nurses. *Nursing Times*, 4 May, 49–52.

Haynes, R.B., Sackett, D.L. and Taylor, D.W. (eds) (1979) *Compliance in Health Care*. Baltimore: Johns Hopkins University Press.

Hayslip, B. and Panek, P.E. (1989) *Adult Development and Ageing*. New York: Harper & Row.

Heather, N. (1976) *Radical Perspectives in Psychology*. London: Methuen.

Hedge, B. (1995) Psychological implications of HIV infection. In D. Messer and C. Meldrum (eds) *Psychology for Nurses and Health Care Professionals*. Hemel Hempstead: Prentice Hall/Harvester Wheatsheaf.

Heenan, A. (1990) Playing patients. *Nursing Times*, 86(46), 46–48.

Hegarty, J. (2000) Psychologists, doctors and cancer patients. In J. Hartley and A. Branthwaite (eds) *The Applied Psychologist* (2nd edn). Buckingham: Open University Press.

Heider, F. (1958) *The Psychology of Interpersonal Relations*. New York: Wiley.

Heine, S.J. and Lehman, D.R. (1997) Culture, dissonance and self-affirmation. *Personality & Social Psychology Bulletin*, 23, 389–400.

Hemingway, H. and Marmot, M. (1999) Psychosocial factors in the aetiology and prognosis of coronary heart disease: systematic review of prospective cohort studies. *British Medical Journal*, 318, 160–167.

Hendry, L.B. (1999) Adolescents and society. In D. Messer and F. Jones (eds) *Psychology and Social Care*. London: Jessica Kingsley.

Hendry, L.B. and Kloep, M. (1999) Adolescence in Europe – an important life phase? In D. Messer and S. Millar (eds) *Exploring Developmental Psychology: From Infancy to Adolescence*. London: Arnold.

Hendry, L.B., Shucksmith, J., Love, J.G. and Glendinning, A. (1993) *Young People's Leisure and Lifestyles*. London: Routledge.

Hennessy, J. and West, M.A. (1999) Intergroup behaviour in organisations: a field test of social identity theory. *Small Group Research*, 30, 361–382.

Hetherington, E.M. and Baltes, P.B. (1988) Child psychology and life-span development. In E.M. Hetherington, R. Lerner and M. Perlmutter (eds) *Child Development in Life-Span Perspective*. Hillsdale, NJ: Erlbaum.

Hewstone, M. (2003) Intergroup contact: panacea for prejudice? *The Psychologist*, 16(7), 352–355.

Hewstone, M. and Fincham, F. (1996) Attribution theory and research: basic issues and applications. In M. Hewstone, W. Stroebe and G.M. Stephenson (eds) *Introduction to Social Psychology* (2nd edn). Oxford: Blackwell.

Hewstone, M., Rubin, M. and Willis, H. (2002) Intergroup bias. *Annual Review of Psychology*, 53, 575–604.

Hill, P. (1993) Recent advances in selected aspects of adolescent development. *Journal of Child Psychology & Psychiatry*, 34(1), 69–99.

Hillan, E. (1991) Caesarean section: psychosocial effects. *Nursing Standard*, 5(50), 30–33.

Hilton, D.J. and Slugoski, B.R. (1986) Knowledge-based causal attribution: the abnormal conditions focus model. *Psychological Review*, 93, 75–88.

Hinsliff, G. and Martin, L. (2006) How the baby shortage threatens our future. *Observer*, 19 February, 8–9.

Hinton, J. (1975) *Dying*. Harmondsworth: Penguin.

Hochschild, A.R. (1983) *The Managed Heart: Commercialisation of Human Feeling*. Berkeley, CA: University of California Press.

Hodges, C. (1998) Easing children's pain. *Nursing Times*, 94 (10), 55–58.

Hodges, J. and Tizard, B. (1989) Social and family relationships of ex-institutional adolescents. *Journal of Child Psychology & Psychiatry*, 30, 77–97.

Hofling, K.C., Brotzman, E., Dalrymple, S., Graves, N. and Pierce, C.M. (1966) An experimental study in the nurse–physician relationship. *Journal of Nervous & Mental Disorders*, 143, 171–180.

Hogg, M.A. and Abrams, D. (1988) *Social Identifications: A Social Psychology of Intergroup Relations and Group Processes*. London: Routledge.

Hogg, M.A. and Abrams, D. (2000) Social psychology. In N.R. Carlson, W. Buskist and G.N. Martin (eds) *Psychology: The Science of Behaviour* (European Adaptation). Harlow: Pearson Education Limited.

Hogg, M.A. and Vaughan, G.M. (1995) *Social Psychology: An Introduction*. Hemel Hempstead: Prentice Hall/Harvester Wheatsheaf.

Hogg, M.A. and Vaughan, G.M. (1998) *Social Psychology: An Introduction* (2nd edn). Hemel Hempstead: Prentice Hall/Harvester Wheatsheaf.

Holahan, C.K. and Sears, R.R. (1995) *The Gifted Group in Later Maturity*. Stanford, CA: Stanford University Press.

Hole, L. (1998) More than skin deep. *Nursing Times*, 94(33), 28–30.

Holland, K. and Hogg, C. (2001) *Cultural Awareness in Nursing and Health Care: An Introductory Text*. London: Arnold.

Holmes, D.S. (1994) *Abnormal Psychology* (2nd edn). New York: HarperCollins.

Holmes, T.H. and Rahe, R.H. (1967) The social readjustment rating scale. *Journal of Psychosomatic Research*, 11, 213–218.

Holyoake, D.-D. (1998) Disentangling caring from love in a nurse–patient relationship. *Nursing Times*, 94(49), 56–58.

Horn, J.L (1982) The ageing of human abilities. In B. Wolman (ed.) *Handbook of Developmental Psychology*. Englewood Cliffs, NJ: Prentice Hall.

Horton, M. (1999) Prejudice and discrimination: group approaches. In D. Messer and F. Jones (eds) *Psychology and Social Care*. London: Jessica Kingsley Publishers.

Hovland, C.I. and Sears, R.R. (1940) Minor studies in aggression, VI: correlation of lynching with economic indices. *Journal of Psychology*, 2, 301–310.

Hovland, C.I. and Janis, I.L. (1959) *Personality and Persuasibility*. New Haven, CT: Yale University Press.

Hovland, C.I., Janis, I.L. and Kelley, H.H (1953) *Communication and Persuasion: Psychological Studies of Opinion Change*. New Haven, CT: Yale University Press.

Howarth, A. (2002) Management of chronic pain. *Nursing Times*, 98(32), 52–53.

Howitt, D. and Owusu-Bempah, J. (1994) *The Racism of Psychology: Time for Change*. Hemel Hempstead: Harvester Wheatsheaf.

Hughes, S.J. (2003) The bio psychosocial aspects of unwanted teenage pregnancy. *Nursing Times*, *99*(12), 32–33.

IASP (International Association for the Study of Pain) (1986) Classification of chronic pain syndrome and definition of pain terms. *Pain*, *3* (Supp.): S1–S226.

Ickes, W.J. and Barnes, R.D. (1977) The role of sex and self-monitoring in unstructured dyadic interactions. *Journal of Personality & Social Psychology*, *35*, 315–330.

Insko, C.A., Drenan, S., Solomon, M.R., Smith, R. and Wade, T.G. (1983) Conformity as a function of the consistency of a positive self-evaluation with being liked and being right. *Journal of Experimental Social Psychology*, *19*, 341–358.

Iyengar, S.S. and Lepper, M.R. (1999) Rethinking the value of choice: a cultural perspective on intrinsic motivation. *Journal of Personality & Social Psychology*, *76*, 349–366.

Jackson, S., Cicogani, E. and Charman, L. (1996) The measurement of conflict in parent–adolescent relationships. In L. Verhofstadt-Deneve, I. Kienhorst and C. Braet (eds) *Conflict and Development in Adolescence*. Leiden: DSWO Press.

Jacobs, M. (1992) *Freud*. London: Sage Publications.

James, T., Harding, I. and Corbett, K. (1994) Biased care? *Nursing Times*, *90*(51), 28–30.

James, W. (1890) *The Principles of Psychology*. New York: Henry Holt & Company.

Jamieson, S. (1996) Altered body image. *Nursing Standard*, *10*(16), 51–53.

Janis, I. and Feshbach, S. (1953) Effects of fear-arousing communication. *Journal of Abnormal & Social Psychology*, *48*, 78–92.

Janis, I. and Terwillinger, R.T. (1962) An experimental study of psychological resistance to fear-arousing communication. *Journal of Abnormal & Social Psychology*, *65*, 403–410.

Janis, I.L, Kaye, D. and Kirschner (1965) Facilitating effects of 'eating-while-reading' on responsiveness to persuasive communications. *Journal of Personality & Social Psychology*, *1*, 181–186.

Janz, N.K. and Becker, M.H. (1984) The health belief model: a decade later. *Health Education Quarterly*, *11*, 1–47.

Jasper, M. (2003) *Beginning Reflective Practice*. Cheltenham: Nelson Thornes.

Jellinek, E.M. (1946) Phases in the drinking history of alcoholics. *Quarterly Journal of Studies on Alcohol*, 7, 1–88.

Jellinek, E.M. (1952) The phases of alcohol addiction. *Quarterly Journal of Studies on Alcohol*, *13*, 673–684.

Jenness, A. (1932) The role of discussion in changing opinion regarding matter of fact. *Journal of Abnormal & Social Psychology*, *27*, 279–296.

Johnson, J.H. and Sarason, I.G. (1978) Life stress, depression and anxiety: internal/external control as a moderator variable. *Journal of Psychosomatic Research*, *22*, 205–208.

Jonas, K., Eagly, A.H. and Stroebe, W. (1995) Attitudes and persuasion. In M. Argyle and A.M. Colman (eds) *Social Psychology*. London: Longman.

Jones, E.E. and Davis, K.E. (1965) From acts to dispositions: the attribution process in person perception. In L. Berkowitz (ed.) *Advances in Experimental Social Psychology*, Vol. 2. New York: Academic Press.

Jones, E.E. and Nisbett, R.E. (1971) *The Actor and the Observer: Divergent Perceptions of the Causes of Behaviour*. Morristown, NJ: General Learning Press.

Jones, F. (1995) Managing stress in health care: issues for staff and patient care. In D. Messer and C. Meldrum (eds) *Psychology for Nurses and Health Care Professionals*. Hemel Hempstead: Prentice Hall/Harvester Wheatsheaf.

Jones, H. (1993) Altered images. *Nursing Times*, *89*(5), 58–60.

Jourard, S.M. (1971) *Self-Disclosure: An Experimental Analysis of the Transparent Self*. New York: Wiley Interscience.

Joynson, R.B. (1980) Models of man: 1879–1979. In A.J. Chapman and D.M. Jones (eds) *Models of Man*. Leicester: British Psychological Society.

Judd, D. (1993) Communicating with dying children. In D. Dickinson and M. Johnson (eds) *Death, Dying & Bereavement*. London: Sage, in association with the Open University.

Jung, C.G. (ed.) (1964) *Man and his Symbols*. London: Aldus-Jupiter Books.

Kagan, J., Kearsley, R.B. and Zelago, P.R. (1978) *Infancy: Its Place in Human Development*. Cambridge, MA: Harvard University Press.

Kalish, R.A. (1982) *Late Adulthood: Perspectives on Human Development* (2nd edn). Monterey, CA: Brooks-Cole.

Karlins, M., Coffman, T.L. and Walters, G. (1969) On the fading of social stereotypes: studies in three generations of college students. *Journal of Personality & Social Psychology*, *13*, 1–16.

Kastenbaum, R. (1979) *Growing Old – Years of Fulfilment*. London: Harper & Row.

Katz, D. (1960) The functional approach to the study of attitudes. *Public Opinion Quarterly*, *24*, 163–204.

Katz, D. and Braly, K. (1933) Racial stereotypes of one hundred college students. *Journal of Abnormal & Social Psychology*, *28*, 280–290.

Kelley, H.H. (1950) The warm–cold variable in first impressions of people. *Journal of Personality*, *18*, 431–439.

Kelley, H.H. (1967) Attribution theory in social psychology. In D. Levine (ed.) *Nebraska Symposium on Motivation*, Vol. 15. Lincoln, NE: Nebraska University Press.

Kelley, H.H. (1972) Causal schemata and the attribution process. In E.E. Jones, D.E. Kanouse, H.H. Kelley, S. Valins and B. Weiner (eds) *Attribution: Perceiving the Causes of Behaviour*. Morristown, NJ: General Learning Press.

Kelley, H.H. (1983) Perceived causal structures. In J.M.F. Jaspars, F.D. Fincham and M. Hewstone (eds) *Attribution Theory and Research: Conceptual, Developmental and Social Dimensions*. London: Academic Press.

Kelly, M. (1994) Mind and body. *Nursing Times*, *90*(42), 48–51.

Kelly, R. (1990) Head and neck surgery. *Nursing Times* (Community Outlook), November, 19–22.

Kenrick, D.T. (1994) Evolutionary social psychology: from sexual selection to social cognition. *Advances in Experimental Social Psychology*, *26*, 75–121.

Khan, S. (2003) New wave of heroin sucks in pre-teens. *Observer*, 6 July, 6.

Kiecolt-Glaser, J.K., Garner, W., Speicher, C.E. Penn, G.M., Holliday, J. and Glaser, R. (1984) Psychosocial modifiers of immunocompetence in medical students. *Psychosomatic Medicine*, *46*, 7–14.

Kitayama, S. and Markus, H.R. (1995) Culture and self: implications for internationalising psychology. In N.R. Goldberger and J.B. Veroff (eds) *The Culture and Psychology Reader*. New York: New York University Press.

Kitzinger, C. and Coyle, A. (1995) Lesbian and gay couples: speaking of difference. *The Psychologist*, *8*, 64–69.

Kitzinger, C., Coyle, A., Wilkinson, S. and Milton, M. (1998) Towards lesbian and gay psychology. *The Psychologist*, *11*(11), 529–533.

Klein, M. (1932) *The Psycho-Analysis of Children*. London: Hogarth.

Kleinman, A. and Kleinman, J. (1985) Somatisation: the interconnections in Chinese society among culture, depressive experiences and the meaning of pain. In A. Kleinman and B. Good (eds) *Culture and Depression: Studies in the Anthropology and Cross-cultural Psychiatry of Affect and Disorder*. Berkeley: University of California Press.

Kleinmuntz, B. (1980) *Essentials of Abnormal Psychology* (2nd edn). London: Harper & Row.

Kline, P. (1984) *Personality and Freudian Theory*. London: Methuen.

Kline, P. (1988) *Psychology Exposed*. London: Routledge.

Kline, P. (1989) Objective tests of Freud's theories. In A.M. Colman and J.G. Beaumont (eds) *Psychology Survey No. 7*. Leicester: British Psychological Society.

Kloep, M. and Hendry, L.B. (1999) Challenges, risks, and coping in adolescence. In D. Messer and S. Millar (eds) *Exploring Developmental Psychology: From Infancy to Adolescence*. London: Arnold.

Kloep, M. and Tarifa, F. (1993) Albanian children in the wind of change. In L.E. Wolven (ed.) *Human Resource Development*. Hogskolan: Ostersund.

Knight, D. (1995) Interacting with patients/clients. In D. Messer and C. Meldrum (eds) *Psychology for Nurses and Health Care Professionals*. Hemel Hempstead: Prentice Hall/Harvester Wheatsheaf.

Koluchova, J. (1972) Severe deprivation in twins: a case study. *Journal of Child Psychology & Psychiatry*, *13*, 107–114.

Koluchova, J. (1991) Severely deprived twins after 22 years' observation. *Studia Psychologica*, *33*, 23–28.

Krebs, D. and Blackman, R. (1988) *Psychology: A First Encounter*. New York: Harcourt Brace Jovanovich.

Kremer, J. (1998) Work. In K. Trew and J. Kremer (eds) *Gender & Psychology*. London: Arnold.

Kroger, J. (1985) Separation-individuation and ego identity status in New Zealand university students. *Journal of Youth & Adolescence*, *14*, 133–147.

Kroll, D. (1990) Equal access to care? *Nursing Times*, *86*(23), 72–73.

Krupat, E. and Garonzik, R. (1994) Subjects' expectations and the search for alternatives to deception in social psychology. *British Journal of Social Psychology*, *33*, 211–222.

Kübler-Ross, E. (1969) *On Death and Dying*. London: Tavistock/Routledge.

Kuhn, H.H. and McPartland, T.S. (1954) An empirical investigation of self attitudes. *American Sociological Review*, *47*, 647–652.

Kuhn, T.S. (1962) *The Structure of Scientific Revolutions*. Chicago: University of Chicago Press.

Kulik, J.A. and Mahler, H.I.M. (1989) Stress and affiliation in a hospital setting: pre-operative room-mate preference. *Personality & Social Psychology Bulletin*, *15*, 183–193.

Kuppens, M., de Wit, J. and Stroebe, W. (1996) Angstaanjagenheid in gezondheids-voorlichting: Een dual process analyse. *Gedrag en Gezondheid*, *24*, 241–248.

Kuykendall, J. (1989) Teenage trauma. *Nursing Times*, *85*(27), 26–28.

Lacey, H. (1998) She's leaving home. *Real Life: Independent on Sunday*, 31 May.

LaPiere, R.T. (1934) Attitudes versus action. *Social Forces*, *13*, 230–237.

Larsen, K.S. (1974) Conformity in the Asch experiment. *Journal of Social Psychology*, *94*, 303–304.

Larsen, K.S., Triplett, J.S., Brant, W.D. and Langenberg, D. (1979) Collaborator status, subject characteristics and conformity in the Asch paradigm. *Journal of Social Psychology*, *108*, 259–263.

Laswell, H.D. (1948) The structure and function of communication in society. In L. Bryson (ed.) *Communication of Ideas*. New York: Harper.

Latané, B. and Wolf, S. (1981) The social impact of majorities and minorities. *Psychological Review*, *88*, 438–453.

Lau, R.R. (1995) Cognitive representations of health and illness. In D. Gochman (ed.) *Handbook of Health Behaviour Research*, Vol. 1. New York: Plenum.

Laurance, J. (2000) Young cocaine users run higher risk of strokes. *Independent*, 13 May, 5.

Lazarus, R.S. and Averill, J. (1978) Emotion and cognition. In C.D. Spielberger (ed.) *Anxiety: Current Trends in Theory and Research*. New York: New York Academy Press.

Lazarus, R.S. (1966) *Psychological Stress and the Coping Process*. New York: McGraw-Hill.

Lazarus, R.S. (1999) *Stress and Emotion: A New Synthesis*. London: Free Association Books.

Lazarus, R.S. and Folkman, S. (1984) *Stress, Appraisal and Coping*. New York: Springer.

Leary, M.R. (2004) The self we know and the self we show: self-esteem, self-presentation and the maintenance of interpersonal relationships. In M.B. Brewer and M. Hewstone (eds) *Emotion and Motivation*. Oxford: Blackwell Publishing.

Leary, M.R. and Kowalski, R.M. (1990) Impression management: a literature review and two-component model. *Psychological Bulletin*, *107*, 34–47.

Leekam, S. (1993) Children's understanding of mind. In M. Bennett (ed.) *The Child as Psychologist: An Introduction to the Development of Social Cognition*. Hemel Hempstead: Harvester Wheatsheaf.

LeFrancois, G.R. (1983) *Psychology*. Belmont, CA: Wadsworth Publishing Co.

Legge, D. (1975) *An Introduction to Psychological Science*. London: Methuen.

Lerner, M.J. (1965) The effect of responsibility and choice on a partner's attractiveness following failure. *Journal of Personality*, *33*, 178–187.

Lerner, M.J. (1980) *The Belief in a Just World: A Fundamental Delusion*. New York: Plenum.

Leslie, J.C. (2002) *Essential Behaviour Analysis*. London: Arnold.

Leventhal, H., Benyamini, Y., Brownlee, S. *et al.* (1997) Illness representations: theoretical foundations. In K.J. Petrie and J.A. Weinman (eds) *Perceptions of Health and Illness*. Amsterdam: Harwood.

Leventhal, H., Meyer, D. and Nerenz, D. (1980) The common sense representation of illness danger. *Medical Psychology*, *2*, 7–30.

Levinson, D.J. (1986) A conception of adult development. *American Psychologist*, *41*, 3–13.

Levinson, D.J., Darrow, D.N., Klein, E.B., Levinson, M.H. and McKee, B. (1978) *The Seasons of a Man's Life*. New York: A.A. Knopf.

Levinson, D.J. and Levinson, J.D. (1997) *The Seasons of a Woman's Life*. New York: Ballantine Books.

Lewis, M. (1990) Social knowledge and social development. *Merrill–Palmer Quarterly*, *36*, 93–116.

Lewis, M. and Brooks-Gunn, J. (1979) *Social Cognition and the Acquisition of Self*. New York: Plenum.

Ley, P. (1981) Professional non-compliance: a neglected problem. *British Journal of Clinical Psychology*, *20*, 151–154.

Ley, P. (1989) Improving patients' understanding, recall, satisfaction and compliance. In A. Broome (ed.) *Health Psychology*. London: Chapman & Hall.

Leyens, J.-P. and Corneille, O. (1999) Asch's social psychology: not as social as you may think. *Personality & Social Psychology Review*, *3*, 345–357.

Likert, R. (1932) A technique for the measurement of attitudes. *Archives of Psychology*, *22*, 140.

Lilienfeld, S.O. (1995) *Seeing Both Sides: Classic Controversies in Abnormal Psychology*. Pacific Grove, CA: Brooks/Cole Publishing Co.

Lippmann, W. (1922) *Public Opinion*. New York: Harcourt.

Lipsedge, M. (1997) Addictions. In L. Rees, M. Lipsedge and C. Ball (eds) *Textbook of Psychiatry*. London: Arnold.

Littlewood, R. and Lipsedge, M. (1989) *Aliens and Alienists: Ethnic Minorities and Psychiatry*. London: Unwin Hyman.

Loehlin, J.C., Willerman, L. and Horn, J.M. (1988) Human behaviour genetics. *Annual Review of Psychology*, *39*, 101–133.

Lorenz, K. (1935) The companion in the bird's world. *Auk*, *54*, 245–273.

Lowe, G. (1995) Alcohol and drug addiction. In A.A. Lazarus and A.M. Colman (eds) *Abnormal Psychology*. London: Longman.

Lowe, L. (1989) Anxiety in a coronary care unit. *Nursing Times*, *85*(45), 61–63.

Luchins, A.S. (1957) Primacy-recency in impression formation. In C. Holland (ed.) *The Order of Presentation in Persuasion*. New Haven, CT: Harvard University Press.

Maccoby, E.E. (1980) *Social Development: Psychological Growth and the Parent–Child Relationship*. New York: Harcourt Brace Jovanovich.

Maddox, G.L. (1964) Disengagement theory: a critical evaluation. *The Gerontologist*, *4*, 80–83.

Maes, S. and van Elderen, T. (1998) Health psychology and stress. In M.W. Eysenck (ed.) *Psychology: An Integrated Approach*. London: Longman.

Maitland, J. and Goodliffe, H. (1989) The Alexander technique. *Nursing Times*, *85*(42), 55–57.

Major, B. (1980) Information acquisition and attribution processes. *Journal of Personality & Social Psychology*, *39*, 1010–1023.

Mann, L. (1969) *Social Psychology*. New York: Wiley.

Manthorpe, J. (1994) Life changes. *Nursing Times*, *90*(18), 66–67.

March, P. (1995) Dying and bereavement. In D. Messer and C. Meldrum (eds) *Psychology for Nurses and Health Care Professionals*. Hemel Hempstead: Prentice Hall/Harvester Wheatsheaf.

March, P. and Doherty, C. (1999) Dying and bereavement. In D. Messer and F. Jones (eds) *Psychology and Social Care*. London: Jessica Kingsley Publishers.

Marcia, J.E. (1998) Peer Gynt's life cycle. In E. Skoe and A. von der Lippe (eds) *Personality Development in Adolescence: A Cross National and Lifespan Perspective*. London: Routledge.

Markus, H. and Nurius, P. (1986) Possible selves. *American Psychologist*, *41*, 954–969.

Marland, G. (1998) Partnership encourages patients to comply with treatment. *Nursing Times*, *94*(27), 58–59.

Marrone, M. (1998) *Attachment and Interaction*. London: Jessica Kingsley Publishers.

Marsland, D. (1987) *Education and Youth*. London: Falmer.

Martin, R. and Hewstone, M. (2001) Conformity and independence in groups: majorities and minorities, In M.A. Hogg and R.S. Tindale (eds) *Blackwell Handbook of Social Psychology: Group Processes*. Malden, MA: Blackwell.

Maslach, C. and Jackson, S.E. (1986) *Maslach Burn-Out Inventory*. San Francisco: Consulting Psychologists Press.

Maslach, C., Stapp, J. and Santee, R.T. (1985) Individuation: conceptual analysis and assessment. *Journal of Personality & Social Psychology*, *49*, 729–738.

Maslach, C. and Jackson, S.E. (1981) The measurement of experienced burnout. *Journal of Occupational Behaviour*, *2*, 99–113.

Maslow, A. (1954) *Motivation and Personality*. New York: Harper & Row.

Maslow, A. (1968) *Towards a Psychology of Being* (2nd edn). New York: Van Nostrand Reinhold.

Mason, P. (1991) Jobs for the boys. *Nursing Times*, *87*(7), 26–28.

Matlin, M.W. and Stang, D.J. (1978) *The Pollyanna Principle*. Cambridge, MA: Schenkman.

Mazhindu, D. (1998) Emotional healing. *Nursing Times*, *94*(6), 26–28.

McCauley, C. and Stitt, C.L. (1978) An individual and quantitative measure of stereotypes. *Journal of Personality & Social Psychology*, *36*, 929–940.

McCrae, R.R. and Costa, P.T. (1989) More reasons to adopt the five-factor model. *American Psychologist*, *44*, 451–452.

McCrone, J. (2000) Rebels with a cause. *New Scientist*, *165*(2222), 22–27.

McCrystal, C. (1997) Now you can live forever, or at least for a century. *Observer*, 15 June, 3.

McDonald, D.D. (1994) Gender and ethnic stereotyping and narcotic analgesic administration. *Research in Nursing and Health*, *17*(1), 45–49.

McEleney, M.(1992) Facing facts. *Nursing Times*, *88*(25), 56–58.

McGlone, F., Park, A. and Roberts, C. (1996) *Relative Values*. Family Policy Centre: BSA.

McGuire, W.J. (1969) The nature of attitudes and attitude change. In G. Lindzey and E. Aronson (eds) *Handbook of Social Psychology*, Vol. 3 (2nd edn). Reading, MA: Addison-Wesley.

McHaffie, H. (1994) Breaking down prejudices. *Nursing Times*, *90*(14), 34–35.

Meadows, S. (1993) *The Child as Thinker: The Acquisition and Development of Cognition in Childhood*. London: Routledge.

Meadows, S. (1995) Cognitive development. In P.E. Bryant and A.M. Colman (eds) *Developmental Psychology*. London: Longman.

Medawar, P.B. (1963) *The Art of the Soluble*. Harmondsworth: Penguin.

Mehrabian, A. (1972) Nonverbal communication. In J. Cole (ed.) *Nebraska Symposium on Motivation*, Vol. 19. Lincoln, NE: University of Nebraska Press.

Meins, E. (2003) Emotional development and early attachment relationships. In A. Slater and G. Bremner (eds) *An Introduction to Developmental Psychology*. Oxford: Blackwell Publishing.

Meltzoff, A. and Moore, M. (1983) Newborn infants imitate adult facial gestures. *Child Development*, *54*, 702–709.

Melzack, R. and Wall, P.D. (1988) *The Challenge of Pain* (2nd edn). Harmondsworth: Penguin.

Melzack, R. and Wall, P.D. (1991) *The Challenge of Pain* (3rd edn). Harmondsworth: Penguin.

Meyer, V. and Chesser, E.S. (1970) *Behaviour Therapy in Clinical Psychiatry*. Harmondsworth: Penguin.

Middleton, W., Moylan, A., Raphael, B., Burnett, P. and Martinek, N. (1993) An international perspective on bereavement-related concepts. *Australian & New Zealand Journal of Psychiatry*, 27, 457–463.

Milgram, S. (1963) Behavioural study of obedience. *Journal of Abnormal & Social Psychology*, 67, 391–398.

Milgram, S. (1965) Liberating effects of group pressure. *Journal of Personality & Social Psychology*, 1, 127–134.

Milgram, S. (1974) *Obedience to Authority*. New York: Harper & Row.

Milgram, S. (1992) *The Individual in a Social World* (2nd edn). New York: McGraw-Hill.

Miller, D.T. and Ross, M. (1975) Self-serving biases in the attribution of causality: fact or fiction? *Psychological Bulletin*, 82, 213–225.

Miller, E. and Morris, R. (1993) *The Psychology of Dementia*. Chichester: Wiley.

Minardi, H.A. and Riley, M. (1988) Providing psychological safety through skilled communication. *Nursing* 27, 990–992.

Moghaddam, F.M., Taylor, D.M. and Wright, S.C. (1993) *Social Psychology in Cross-Cultural Perspective*. New York: W.H. Freeman & Co.

Moos, R.H. and Schaefer, J.A. (1984) The crisis of physical illness: an overview and conceptual approach. In R.H. Moos (ed.) *Coping with Physical Illness: New Perspectives*, 2. New York: Plenum.

Morris, C.G. (1988) *Psychology: An Introduction* (6th edn). London: Prentice Hall.

Morris, M.W. and Peng, K. (1994) Culture and cause: American and Chinese attributions for social and physical events. *Journal of Personality & Social Psychology*, 67, 949–971.

Morrison, R. (1992) Diagnosing spiritual pain in patients. *Nursing Standard*, 6(25), 36–38.

Moscovici, S. (1976) *Social Influence and Social Change*. London: Academic Press.

Moscovici, S. (1980) Towards a theory of conversion behaviour. In L. Berkowitz (ed.) *Advances in Experimental Social Psychology*, 13, 209–239.

Moscovici, S. and Faucheux, C. (1972) Social influence, conforming bias and the study of active minorities. In L. Berkowitz (ed.) *Advances in Experimental Social Psychology*, Vol. 6. New York: Academic Press.

Moscovici, S., Lage, E. and Naffrechoux, M. (1969) Influence of a consistent minority on the responses of a majority in a colour perception test. *Sociometry*, 32, 365–380.

Motluck, A. (1999) Jane behaving badly. *New Scientist*, 164(2214), 28–33.

Much, N. (1995) Cultural psychology. In J.A. Smith, R. Harré and L. Van Langenhove (eds) *Rethinking Psychology*. London: Sage.

Munro, R. (2000) In serious pain or just bellyaching? *Nursing Times*, 96(28), 13.

Murphy, G. (1947) *Personality: A Bio-social Approach to Origins and Structure*. New York: Harper & Row.

Nagayama Hall, G.C. and Barongan, C. (2002) *Multicultural Psychology*. Upper Saddle River, NJ: Prentice Hall.

Nemeth, C., Swedund, M. and Kanki, G. (1974) Patterning of the minority's responses, and their influence on the majority. *European Journal of Social Psychology*, 4, 53–64.

Neugarten, B.L. (1975) The future of the young-old. *The Gerontologist*, 15, 4–9.

Neugarten, B.L. and Neugarten, D.A. (1987) The changing meanings of age. *Psychology Today*, 21, 29–33.

New Scientist (1999) Desperate remedies. *New Scientist*, 164(2214), 34–36.

Nichols, K. (2003) *Psychological Care for Ill and Injured People – A Clinical Guide*. Maidenhead: Open University Press.

Nichols, K. (2005) Why is psychology still failing the average patient? *The Psychologist*, 18(1), 26–27.

Nisbett, R.E. and Ross, L. (1980) *Human Inference: Strategies and Shortcomings of Social Judgement*. Englewood Cliffs, NJ: Prentice Hall.

Nisbett, R.E., Caputo, C., Legant, P. and Maracek, J. (1973) Behaviour as seen by the actor and as seen by the observer. *Journal of Personality & Social Psychology*, 27, 154–165.

Nolan, P., Cushway, D. and Tyler, P. (1995) A measurement tool for assessing stress among mental health nurses. *Nursing Standard*, 9(46), 36–39.

North, N. (1988) Psychosocial aspects of coronary artery bypass surgery. *Nursing Times*, 84(1), 26–29.

Norton, C. (2000) Brains can fight breast cancer. *Independent on Sunday*, 16 April, 12.

Nursing Times (1990) Questionnaire: are you a racist? *Nursing Times*, 86(14), 30–32.

Nye, R.D. (2000) *Three Psychologies: Perspectives from Freud, Skinner and Rogers* (6th edn). Belmont, CA: Wadsworth/Thompson Learning.

Oakes, P.J., Haslam, S.A. and Turner, J.C. (1994) *Stereotyping and Social Reality*. Oxford: Blackwell.

O'Connell, S. (2000) Pain? Don't give it another thought. *Independent Review*, 16 June, 8.

O'Donnell, E. (1996) Stressing the point. *Nursing Standard*, 10(16), 22–23.

O'Donohue, W. and Ferguson, K.E. (2001) *The Psychology of B.F. Skinner*. Thousand Oaks, CA: Sage Publications.

O'Dowd, A. (1998) Handmaidens and battleaxes. *Nursing Times*, 94(36), 12–13.

Offer, D., Ostrov, E., Howard, K.I. and Atkinson, R. (1988) *The Teenage World: Adolescents' Self-Image in Ten Countries*. New York: Plenum Press.

Ogden, J. (2000) *Health Psychology: A Textbook* (2nd edn). Buckingham: Open University Press.

Ogden, J. (2004) *Health Psychology: A Textbook* (3rd edn). Maidenhead: Open University Press/McGraw-Hill Education.

Operario, D. and Fiske, S.T. (2004) Stereotypes: content, structures, processes and context. In M.B. Brewer and M. Hewstone (eds) *Social Cognition*. Oxford: Blackwell Publishing.

Orne, M.T. (1962) On the social psychology of the psychological experiment: with particular reference to demand characteristics and their implications. *American Psychologist*, 17, 776–783.

Orne, M.T. and Holland, C.C. (1968) On the ecological validity of laboratory deceptions. *International Journal of Psychiatry*, 6, 282–293.

Owen, W. (1990) After Hillsborough. *Nursing Times*, 86(25), 16–17.

Palermo, D.S. (1971) Is a scientific revolution taking place in psychology? *Psychological Review*, 76, 241–263.

Parke, R.D. (2002) Fathers and families. In M.H. Bornstein (ed.) *Handbook of Parenting* (2nd edn, Vol. 3). Mahwah, NJ: Erlbaum.

Parkes, C.M. (1972) *Bereavement: Studies of Grief in Adult Life*. Harmondsworth: Penguin.

Parkes, C.M. (1986) *Bereavement: Studies of Grief in Adult Life* (2nd edn). London: Tavistock.

Parkes, C.M. (1993) Bereavement as a psychosocial transition: processes of adaptation to change. In M.S. Stroebe, W. Stroebe and R.O. Hansson (eds) *Handbook of Bereavement: Theory, Research and Intervention*. New York: Cambridge University Press.

Parkes, C.M. (1995) Attachment and bereavement. In T. Lundin (ed.) *Grief and Bereavement: Proceedings from the Fourth International Conference on Grief and Bereavement in Contemporary Society*, Stockholm, 1994. Stockholm: Swedish Association for Mental Health.

Parkes, C.M. and Weiss, R.S. (1983) *Recovery from Bereavement*. New York: Basic Books.

Parkinson, P. (1992) Coping with dying and bereavement. *Nursing Standard*, 6(17), 36–38.

Payne, D. (2000) Shock study triggers call to ban ageist slur. *Nursing Times*, 96(18), 13.

Pediani, R. (1992) Preparing to heal. *Nursing Times*, 88(27), 68–70.

Peek, L. (2000) One in six girls now reaches puberty aged 8. *The Times*, 19 June, 3.

Penny, G. (1996) Health psychology. In H. Coolican, *Applied Psychology*. London: Hodder & Stoughton.

Perrin, S. and Spencer, C. (1981) Independence or conformity in the Asch experiment as a reflection of cultural and situational factors. *British Journal of Social Psychology*, 20, 205–209.

Petersen, A.C. and Crockett, L. (1985) Pubertal timing and grade effects on adjustment. *Journal of Youth & Adolescence*, 14, 191–206.

Petersen, A.C., Sarigiani, P.A. and Kennedy, R.E. (1991) Adolescent depression: why more girls? *Journal of Youth & Adolescence*, 20, 247–271.

Petit-Zeman, S. (2000) Mmm, guilt-free chocolate. *The Times*, 18 July, 10.

Pettigrew, T.F. (1959) Regional differences in antinegro prejudice. *Journal of Abnormal & Social Psychology*, 59, 28–56.

Pettigrew, T.F. (1971) *Racially Separate or Together?* New York: McGraw-Hill.

Pettigrew, T.F. (1998) Intergroup contact theory. In J.T. Spence, J.M. Darley and D.J. Foss (eds) *Annual Review of Psychology*, Vol. 49. Palo Alto, CA: Annual Reviews.

Pettigrew, T.F. and Meertens, R.W. (1995) Subtle and blatant prejudice in western Europe. *European Journal of Social Psychology*, 25, 57–75.

Phillips, J.L. (1969) *The Origins of Intellect: Piaget's Theory*. San Francisco: W.H. Freeman.

Piaget, J. (1952) *The Child's Conception of Number*. London: Routledge & Kegan Paul.

Piaget, J. (1973) *The Child's Conception of the World*. London: Paladin.

Piaget, J. and Inhelder, B. (1956) *The Psychology of the Child*. London: Routledge & Kegan Paul.

Piaget, J. and Szeminska, A. (1952) *The Child's Conception of Number*. New York: Humanities Press.

Pinel, J.P.J. (1993) *Biopsychology* (2nd edn). Boston: Allyn & Bacon.

Plant, S. (1999) *Writing on Drugs*. London: Faber & Faber.

Popper, K. (1959) *The Logic of Scientific Discovery*. London: Hutchinson.

Popper, K. (1972) *Objective Knowledge: An Evolutionary Approach*. Oxford: Oxford University Press.

Potter, J. (1996) Attitudes, social representations and discursive psychology. In M. Wetherell (ed.) *Identities, Groups and Social Issues*. London: Sage, in association with the Open University.

Powell, J. (2000) Drug and alcohol dependence. In L. Champion and M. Power (eds) *Adult Psychological Problems: An Introduction* (2nd edn). Hove: Psychology Press.

Premack, D. and Woodruff, G. (1978) Does the chimpanzee have a theory of mind? *Behavioural & Brain Sciences*, 4, 515–526.

Price, B. (1986) Keeping up appearances. *Nursing Times*, 1 October, 58–61.

Price, B. (1988) What are nurses like? *Nursing Times*, 84(1), 42–43.

Price, B. (1990) *Body Image: Nursing Concepts and Care*. Hemel Hempstead: Prentice Hall.

Price, W.F. and Crapo, R.H. (1999) *Cross-Cultural Perspectives in Introductory Psychology* (3rd edn). Belmont, CA: Wadsworth Publishing Co.

Prochaska, J.A. and DiClemente, D.D. (1984) *The Transtheoretical Approach: Crossing Traditional Boundaries of Therapy*. Homewood, IL: Dow Jones Irwin.

Psychologist, The (2006) Physical therapists providing psychological support. *The Psychologist*, 19(3), 134.

Pullen, M. (1998) Support role. *Nursing Times*, 94(47), 57.

Quinton, D. and Rutter, M. (1988) *Parental Breakdown: The Making and Breaking of Intergenerational Links*. London: Gower.

Rabbitt, P.M.A. (1993) Does it all go together when it goes? *Quarterly Journal of Experimental Psychology*, 46A, 385–434.

Rainey, N. (1998) Old age. In K. Trew and J. Kremer (eds) *Gender & Psychology*. London: Arnold.

Ramachandran, V.S. and Blakeslee, S. (1998) *Phantoms in the Brain*. London: Fourth Estate.

Ramsay, R. and de Groot, W. (1977) A further look at bereavement. Paper presented at EATI conference, Uppsala. Cited in P.E. Hodgkinson (1980) Treating abnormal grief in the bereaved. *Nursing Times*, 17 January, 126–128.

Rank, S.G. and Jacobson, C.K. (1977) Hospital nurses' compliance with medication overdose orders: a failure to replicate. *Journal of Health & Social Behaviour*, 18, 188–193.

Raphael, B. (1984) *The Anatomy of Bereavement*. London: Hutchinson.

Reason, J. (2000) The Freudian slip revisited. *The Psychologist*, 13(12), 610–611.

Rees, M. (1993) He, she or it? *Nursing Times*, 89(10), 48–49.

Reich, B. and Adcock, C. (1976) *Values, Attitudes and Behaviour Change*. London: Methuen.

Resnick, L., Levine, J. and Teasley, S. (eds) (1991) *Perspectives on Socially Shared Cognition*. Washington, DC: American Psychological Association.

Richards, G. (1996) *Putting Psychology in its Place*. London: Routledge.

Richardson, K. (1991) *Understanding Intelligence*. Milton Keynes: Open University Press.

Roberts, Y. (2006) Off your head? *Observer*, 19 February, 21–32.

Robotham, M. (1999) What you think of doctors. *Nursing Times*, 95(2), 24–27.

Roger, D. and Nash, P. (1995) Coping. *Nursing Times*, 91(29), 42–43.

Rogers, C.R. (1951) *Client-Centred Therapy – Its Current Practices, Implications and Theory*. Boston: Houghton Mifflin.

Rogers, C.R. (1959) A theory of therapy, personality and interpersonal relationships as developed in the client-centred framework. In S. Koch (ed.) *Psychology: A Study of Science, Volume III, Formulations of the Person and the Social Context*. New York: McGraw-Hill.

Rogers, J., Meyer, J. and Mortel, K. (1990) After reaching retirement age physical activity sustains cerebral perfusion and cognition. *Journal of the American Geriatric Society*, *38*, 123–128.

Rogers, R.W. (1975) A protection motivation theory of fear appeals and attitude change. *Journal of Psychology*, *91*, 93–114.

Rogers, R.W. (1985) Attitude change and information integration in fear appeals. *Psychological Reports*, *56*, 179–182.

Rogoff, B. (1990) *Apprenticeship in Thinking: Cognitive Development in Social Context*. New York: Oxford University Press.

Rokeach, M. (1960) *The Open and Closed Mind*. New York: Basic Books.

Rose, P. (1993) Out in the open? *Nursing Times*, *89*(30), 50–52.

Rose, P. and Platzer, H. (1993) Confronting prejudice. *Nursing Times*, *89*(31), 52–54.

Rose, S. (1997) *Lifelines: Biology, Freedom, Determinism*. Harmondsworth: Penguin.

Rose, S. (2003) *The Making of Memory: From Molecules to Mind* (revised edn). London: Vintage.

Rose, S.A. and Blank, M. (1974) The potency of context in children's cognition: an illustration through conservation. *Child Development*, *45*, 499–502.

Rosenberg, M.J. and Hovland, C.I. (1960) Cognitive, affective and behavioural components of attitude. In M.J. Rosenberg, C.I. Hovland, W.J. McGuire, R.P. Abelson and J.W. Brehm (eds) *Attitude Organisation and Change: An Analysis of Consistency Among Attitude Components*. New Haven, CT: Yale University Press.

Rosenblatt, P.C. (1993) The social context of private feelings. In M.S. Stroebe, W. Stroebe and R.O. Hansson (eds) *Handbook of Bereavement: Theory, Research and Intervention*. New York: Cambridge University Press.

Rosenthal, R. and Fode, K.L. (1963) The effects of experimenter bias on the performance of the albino rat. *Behavioural Science*, *8*, 183–189.

Rosenthal, R. and Jacobson, L. (1968) *Pygmalion in the Classroom: Teacher Expectation and Pupils' Intellectual Development*. New York: Holt.

Rosenthal, R. and Lawson, R. (1964) A longitudinal study of the effects of experimenter bias on the operant learning of laboratory rats. *Journal of Psychiatric Research*, *2*, 61–72.

Rosnow, I. (1985) Status and role change through the life cycle. In R.H. Binstock and E. Shanas (eds) *Handbook of Ageing and the Social Sciences* (2nd edn). New York: Van Nostrand Reinhold.

Ross, L. (1977) The intuitive psychologist and his shortcomings. In L. Berkowitz (ed.) *Advances in Experimental Social Psychology*, Vol. 10. New York: Academic Press.

Ross, M. and Fletcher, G.J.O. (1985) Attribution and social perception. In G. Lindzey and E. Aronson (eds) *Handbook of Social Psychology* (3rd edn). New York: Random House.

Rotter, J. (1966) Generalised expectancies for internal versus external control of reinforcement. *Psychological Monographs*, *30*(1), 1–26.

Rowe, A. (1999) Spectre at the feast. *Nursing Times*, *95*(2), 28–29.

Rowe, J.W. and Kahn, R.L. (1998) *Successful Ageing*. New York: Plenum.

Royal College of Psychiatrists (1987) *Drug Scenes: A Report on Drugs and Drug Dependence by the Royal College of Psychiatrists*. London: Gaskell.

Rutter, M. (1981) *Maternal Deprivation Reassessed* (2nd edn). Harmondsworth: Penguin.

Rutter, M. (1989) Pathways from childhood to adult life. *Journal of Child & Psychology & Psychiatry*, *30*, 23–25.

Rutter, M. and Rutter, M. (1992) *Developing Minds: Challenge and Continuity across the Life Span*. Harmondsworth: Penguin.

Rutter, M., Graham, P., Chadwick, D.F.D. and Yule, W. (1976) Adolescent turmoil: fact or fiction? *Journal of Child Psychology & Psychiatry*, *17*, 35–56.

Ryan, R.M. and Lynch, J.H. (1989) Emotional autonomy versus detachment: revisiting the vicissitudes of adolescence and young adulthood. *Child Development*, *60*, 340–356.

Salomon, G. (ed.) (1993) *Distributed Cognitions: Psychological and Educational Considerations*. Cambridge: Cambridge University Press.

Samuel, J. and Bryant, P. (1984) Asking only one question in the conservation experiment. *Journal of Child Psychology & Psychiatry*, *25*, 315–318.

Sangiuliano, I. (1978) *In Her Time*. New York: Morrow.

Savage, R. and Armstrong, D. (1990) Effect of a general practitioner's consulting style on patients' satisfaction: a controlled study. *British Medical Journal*, *301*, 968–970.

Sayer, L. (1992) Prejudice pre-empted. *Nursing Times*, *88*(37), 46–48.

Schachter, S. (1964) The interaction of cognitive and physiological determinants of emotional state. In L. Berkowitz (ed.) *Advances in Experimental Social Psychology*, Vol. 1. New York: Academic Press.

Schaffer, H.R. (1971) *The Growth of Sociability*. Harmondsworth: Penguin.

Schaffer, H.R. (1996a) *Social Development*. Oxford: Blackwell.

Schaffer, H.R. (1996b) Is the child father to the man? *Psychology Review*, *2*(3), 2–5.

Schaffer, H.R. (1998) Deprivation and its effects on children. *Psychology Review*, *5*(2), 2–5.

Schaffer, H.R. (2004) *Introducing Child Psychology*. Oxford: Blackwell Publishing.

Schaffer, H.R. and Emerson, P.E. (1964) The development of social attachments in infancy. *Monographs of the Society for Research in Child Development*, *29* (whole No. 3).

Schaie, K.W. and Hertzog, C. (1983) Fourteen-year cohort-sequential analysis of adult intellectual development. *Developmental Psychology*, *19*, 531–543.

Scheer, S.D. and Unger, D.G. (1995) Parents' perceptions of their adolescents – implications for parent–youth conflict and family satisfaction. *Psychological Reports*, *76*(1), 131–136.

Schiffman, R. and Wicklund, R.A. (1992) The minimal group paradigm and its minimal psychology. *Theory & Psychology*, *2*, 29–50.

Schifter, D.E. and Ajzen, I. (1985) Intention, perceived control and weight loss: an application of the theory of planned behaviour. *Journal of Personality & Social Psychology*, *49*, 843–851.

Schlenker, B.R. (1980) *Impression Management*. Monterey, CA: Brooks/Cole.

Schlenker, B.R. (1982) Translating action into attitudes: an identity-analytic approach to the explanation of social conduct. In L. Berkowitz (ed.) *Advances in Experimental Social Psychology*, Vol. 15. New York: Academic Press.

Schliefer, S.J., Keller, S.E., Camerino, M., Thornton, J.C. and Stein, M. (1983) Suppression of lymphocyte stimulation following bereavement. *Journal of the American Medical Association*, *250*, 374–377.

Schlossberg, N.K. (1984) Exploring the adult years. In A.M. Rogers and C.J. Scheirer (eds) *The G. Stanley Hall Lecture Series*, Vol. 4. Washington, DC: American Psychological Association.

Schlossberg, N.K., Troll, L.E. and Leibowitz, Z. (1978) *Perspectives on Counselling Adults: Issues and Skills.* Monterey, CA: Brooks/Cole.

Schott, J. and Henley, A. (1999) *Culture, Religion & Childbearing in a Multi-racial Society.* Oxford: Butterworth Heinemann.

Schuchter, S.R. and Zisook, S. (1993) The course of normal grief. In M.S. Stroebe, W. Stroebe and R.O. Hansson (eds) *Handbook of Bereavement: Theory, Research and Intervention.* New York: Cambridge University Press.

Schwarzer, R. (1992) Self efficacy in the adoption and maintenance of health behaviours: theoretical approaches and a new model. In R. Schwarzer (ed.) *Self Efficacy: Thought Control of Action.* Washington, DC: Hemisphere.

Scodel, A. (1957) Heterosexual somatic preference and fantasy dependence. *Journal of Consulting Psychology, 21,* 371–374.

Segall, M.H., Dasen, P.R., Berry, J.W. and Poortinga, Y.H. (1999) *Human Behaviour in Global Perspective: An Introduction to Cross-Cultural Psychology* (2nd edn). Needham Heights, MA: Allyn & Bacon.

Seligman, M.E.P. (1975) *Helplessness: On Depression, Development and Death.* San Francisco: W.H. Freeman.

Selye, H. (1956) *The Stress of Life.* New York: McGraw-Hill.

Shatz, M. (1994) *A Toddler's Life: Becoming a Person.* New York: Oxford University Press.

Sheahan, P. (1996) Psychological pain and care. *Nursing Times, 92* (17), 63–67.

Sherif, M. (1935) A study of social factors in perception. *Archives of Psychology, 27* (whole No. 187).

Sherif, M. (1966) *Group Conflict and Co-operation: Their Social Psychology.* London: RKP.

Sherr, L. (1989) Death of a baby. In L. Sherr (ed.) *Death, Dying and Bereavement.* Oxford: Blackwell Scientific Publications.

Shweder, R.A. (1990) Cultural psychology: what is it? In J.W. Stigler, R.A. Shweder and G. Herdt (eds) *Cultural Psychology.* Cambridge: Cambridge University Press.

Siegal, M. (2003) Cognitive development. In A. Slater and G. Bremner (eds) *An Introduction to Developmental Psychology.* Oxford: Blackwell Publishing.

Siegel, K., Schrimshaw, E.W. and Dean, L. (1999) Symptom interpretation and medication adherence among late middle-aged and older HIV-affected adults. *Journal of Health Psychology, 4,* 247–257.

Simmons, R.G. and Blyth, D.A. (1987) *Moving into Adolescence: The Impact of Pubertal Change and School Context.* New York: Aldine de Gruyter.

Sinha, D. (1997) Indigenising psychology. In J.W. Berry, Y.H. Poortinga and J. Pandey (eds) *Handbook of Cross-cultural Psychology* (2nd edn, Vol. 1). Boston: Allyn & Bacon.

Skinner, B.F. (1974) *About Behaviourism.* New York: Alfred Knopf.

Skinner, B.F. (1987) Skinner on behaviourism. In R.L. Gregory (ed.) *The Oxford Companion to the Mind.* Oxford: Oxford University Press.

Small, E. (1995) Valuing the unseen emotional labour of nursing. *Nursing Times, 91*(26), 40–41.

Smith, A.D. (1998) Ageing of the brain: is mental decline inevitable? In S. Rose (ed.) *From Brain to Consciousness: Essays on the New Science of the Mind.* Harmondsworth: Penguin.

Smith, J. and Baltes, P.B. (1997) Profiles of psychological functioning in the old and oldest old. *Psychology and Ageing, 12,* 458–472.

Smith, K.R. and Zick, C.D. (1996) Risk of mortality following widowhood: age and sex differences by mode of death. *Social Biology, 43,* 59–71.

Smith, P.B. (1995) Social influence processes. In M. Argyle and A.M. Colman (eds) *Social Psychology.* London: Longman.

Smith, P.B. and Bond, R.A. (1998) *Social Psychology Across Cultures: Analysis and perspectives* (2nd edn). Hemel Hempstead: Prentice Hall Europe.

Smith, S. (1997) A time to die. *Nursing Times, 93*(44), 34–35.

Snell, J. (1995) It's tough at the bottom. *Nursing Times, 91*(43), 55–58.

Snell, J. (1997) Joke over. *Nursing Times, 93*(11), 26–28.

Snyder, M. (1974) Self-monitoring of expressive behaviour. *Journal of Personality & Social Behaviour, 30,* 526–537.

Snyder, M. (1979) Self-monitoring processes. In L. Berkowitz (ed.) *Advances in Experimental Social Psychology,* Vol. 18. New York: Academic Press.

Snyder, M. (1987) *Public Appearance/Private Realities: The Psychology of Self-Monitoring.* New York: W.H. Freeman.

Snyder, M. (1995) Self-monitoring: public appearances versus private realities. In G.G. Brannigan and M.R. Merrens (eds) *The Social Psychologists: Research Adventures.* New York: McGraw-Hill.

Snyder, S. (1977) Opiate receptors and internal opiates. *Scientific American, 236,* 44–56.

Sowell, E.R. *et al.* (1999) In vivo evidence for post-adolescent brain maturation in frontal and striatal regions. *Nature Neuroscience, 2,* 859.

Spencer, C. and Perrin, S. (1998) Innovation and conformity. *Psychology Review, 5*(2), 23–26.

Sperling, H.G. (1946) An experimental study of some psychological factors in judgement, Master's thesis, New School for Social Research.

Spitz, R.A. (1945) Hospitalism: an inquiry into the genesis of psychiatric conditions in early childhood. *Psychoanalytic Study of the Child, 1,* 53–74.

Spitz, R.A. (1946) Hospitalism: a follow-up report on investigation described in Vol. 1, 1945. *Psychoanalytic Study of the Child, 2,* 113–117.

Spitz, R.A. and Wolf, K.M. (1946) Anaclitic depression. *Psychoanalytic Study of the Child, 2,* 313–342.

Stahlberg, D. and Frey, D. (1988) Attitudes 1: structure, measurement and functions. In M. Hewstone, W. Stroebe, J.P. Codol and G.M. Stephenson (eds) *Introduction to Social Psychology.* Oxford: Blackwell.

Stainton Rogers, R., Stenner, P., Gleeson. K. and Stainton Rogers, W. (1995) *Social Psychology: A Critical Agenda.* Cambridge: Polity Press.

Stanley, J. (1998) Mixed messages. *Nursing Times, 94*(49), 58–59.

Starr, B.S. (1995) Approaches to pain control. In D. Messer and C. Meldrum (eds) *Psychology for Nurses and Health Care Professionals.* Hemel Hempstead: Prentice Hall/Harvester Wheatsheaf.

Starr, B.S. and Chandler, C.J. (1995) Common addictive behaviours. In D. Messer and C. Meldrum (eds) *Psychology for Nurses and Health Care Professionals.* Hemel Hempstead: Prentice Hall/Harvester Wheatsheaf.

Stattin, H. and Magnusson, D. (1990) *Pubertal Maturation in Female Development.* Hillsdale, NJ: Erlbaum.

Stephan, W.G. and Stephan, C.W. (1985) Intergroup anxiety. *Journal of Social Issues, 41,* 157–175.

Stevens, R. (1995) Freudian theories of personality. In S.E. Hampson and A.M. Colman (eds) *Individual Differences and Personality.* London: Longman.

Storms, M.D. (1973) Videotape and the attribution process: reversing actors' and observers' points of view. *Journal of Personality & Social Psychology, 27,* 165–175.

Stouffer, S.A., Suchman, E.A., DeVinney, L.C., Starr, S.A. and Williams, R.M. (1949) *The American Soldier: Adjustment During Army Life*, Vol. 1. Princeton, NJ: Princeton University Press.

Stroebe, M.S. and Stroebe, M. (1993) The mortality of bereavement: a review. In M.S. Stroebe, W. Stroebe and R.O. Hansson (eds) *Handbook of Bereavement: Theory, Research and Intervention*. New York: Cambridge University Press.

Stroebe, M.S., Stroebe, W. and Hansson, R.O. (1993) Contemporary themes and controversies in bereavement research. In M.S. Stroebe, W. Stroebe and R.O. Hansson (eds) *Handbook of Bereavement: Theory, Research and Intervention*. New York: Cambridge University Press.

Stroebe, W. (2000) *Social Psychology and Health* (2nd edn). Buckingham: Open University Press.

Stuart-Hamilton, I. (1994) *The Psychology of Ageing: An Introduction* (2nd edn). London: Jessica Kingsley.

Stuart-Hamilton, I. (1997) Adjusting to later life. *Psychology Review*, 4(2), 20–23.

Stuart-Hamilton, I. (2000) Ageing and intelligence. *Psychology Review*, 6(4), 19–21.

Stuart-Hamilton, I. (2003) Intelligence and ageing: is decline inevitable? *Psychology Review*, 9(3), 14–16.

Sumner, W.G. (1906) *Folkways*. Boston: Ginn.

Swensen, C.H. (1983) A respectable old age. *American Psychologist*, 46, 1208–1221.

Sykes, E.A. (1995) Psychopharmacology. In D. Messer and C. Meldrum (eds) *Psychology for Nurses and Health Care Professionals*. Hemel Hempstead: Prentice Hall/Harvester Wheatsheaf.

Tajfel, H. (1969) Social and cultural factors in perception. In G. Lindzey and E. Aronson (eds) *Handbook of Social Psychology*, Vol. 3. Reading, MA: Addison-Wesley.

Tajfel, H. (1972) Experiments in a vacuum. In J. Israel and H. Tajfel (eds) *The Context of Social Psychology: A Critical Assessment*. London: Academic Press.

Tajfel, H. (ed.) (1978) *Differentiation Between Social Groups: Studies in the Social Psychology of Intergroup Relations*. London: Academic Press.

Tajfel, H., Billig, M.G. and Bundy, R.P. (1971) Social categorisation and intergroup behaviour. *European Journal of Social Psychology*, 1, 149–178.

Tajfel, H. and Turner, J.C. (1986) The social identity theory of intergroup behaviour. In S. Worchel and W. Austin (eds) *Psychology of Intergroup Relations*. Monterey, CA: Brooks Cole.

Taylor, G. (1993) Challenges from the margins. In J. Clarke (ed.) *A Crisis in Care*. London: Sage.

Taylor, J., Miller, D., Wattley, L. and Harris, P. (1999) *Nursing Children. Psychology, Research and Practice* (3rd edn). Stanley Thornes (Publishers) Ltd.

Taylor, P. (1994) Beating the taboo. *Nursing Times*, 90(13), 51–53.

Teasdale, K. (1998) *Advocacy in Health Care*. Oxford: Blackwell Science, 1.

Tedeschi, J.T. and Rosenfield, P. (1981) Impression management theory and the forced compliance situation. In J.T. Tedeschi (ed.) *Impression Management Theory and Social Psychological Research*. New York: Academic Press.

Temoshok, L. (1987) Personality, coping style, emotions and cancer: towards an integrative model. *Cancer Surveys*, 6, 545–567 (Supp.).

Thomas, B. (1993) Gender loving care. *Nursing Times*, 89(10), 50–51.

Thomas, R.M. (1985) *Comparing Theories of Child Development* (2nd edn). Belmont, CA: Wadsworth Publishing Company.

Thorne, B. (1992) *Rogers*. London: Sage Publications.

Tizard, B. (1977) *Adoption: A Second Chance*. London: Open Books.

Tizard, B. and Hodges, J. (1978) The effects of early institutional rearing on the development of eight-year-old children. *Journal of Child Psychology & Psychiatry*, 19, 99–118.

Tizard, B. and Phoenix, A. (1993) *Black, White or Mixed Race?* London: Routledge.

Tobin, S.S. (1999) *Preservation of the Self in the Oldest Years: With Implications for Practice*. New York: Springer.

Tobin-Richards, M.H., Boxer, A.M. and Petersen, A.C. (1983) The psychological significance of pubertal change: sex differences in perceptions of self during early adolescence. In J. Brooks-Gunn and A.C. Petersen (eds) *Girls at Puberty: Biological and Psychosocial Perspectives*. New York: Plenum.

Tolman, E.C. (1948) Cognitive maps in rats and man. *Psychological Review*, 55, 189–208.

Toogood, L. (1999) In *Nursing Times*, 95(14), 50–51.

Topping, A. (1990) Sexual activity and the stoma patient. *Nursing Standard*, 4(41), 24–26.

Torrance, C. and Jordan, S. (1995) Bionursing: putting science into practice. *Nursing Standard*, 9(49), 25–27.

Tredre, R. (1996) Untitled article. *Observer Life*, 12 May, 16–19.

Tschudin, V. (2003) *Ethics in Nursing* (3rd edn). Oxford: Butterworth Heinemann.

Turnbull, S.K. (1995) The middle years. In D. Wedding (ed.) *Behaviour and Medicine* (2nd edn). St Louis, MO: Mosby-Year Book.

Turner, J.C. (1991) *Social Influence*. Milton Keynes: Open University Press.

Turner, J.S. and Helms, D.B. (1989) *Contemporary Adulthood* (4th edn). Fort Worth, FL: Holt, Rinehart & Winston.

Turpin, G. and Slade, P. (1998) Clinical and health psychology. In P. Scott and C. Spencer, *Psychology: A Contemporary Introduction*. Oxford: Blackwell.

UKCC (1992) *Code of Professional Conduct*. London: UKCC.

Valentine, E.R. (1992) *Conceptual Issues in Psychology*. London: Routledge.

Van Avermaet, E. (1996) Social influence in small groups. In M. Hewstone, W. Stroebe and G.M. Stephenson (eds) *Introduction to Social Psychology* (2nd edn). Oxford: Blackwell.

Van Ijzendoorn, M.H. and Schuengel, C. (1999) The development of attachment relationships: infancy and beyond. In D. Messer and S. Millar (eds) *Exploring Developmental Psychology: From Infancy to Adolescence*. London: Arnold.

Veitia, M.C. and McGahee, C.L. (1995) Ordinary addictions: tobacco and alcohol. In D. Wedding (ed.) *Behaviour and Medicine* (2nd edn). St Louis, MO: Mosby-Year Book.

Vivian, J. and Brown, R. (1995) Prejudice and intergroup conflict. In M. Argyle and A.M. Colman (eds) *Social Psychology*. London: Longman.

Voss, S. (2002) The winter years: understanding ageing. *Psychology Review*, 8(3), 26–28.

Vygotsky, L.S. (1978) *Mind in Society*. Cambridge, MA: Harvard University Press.

Vygotsky, L.S. (1981) The genesis of higher mental functions. In J.V. Wretch (ed.) *The Concept of Activity in Soviet Psychology*. Armonk, NY: Sharpe.

Vygotsky, L.S. (1987) Thinking and speech. In R.W. Rieber and A.S. Carton (eds) *The Collected Works of L.S. Vygotsky*. New York: Plenum.

Wade, C. and Tavris, C. (1999) *Invitation to Psychology*. New York: Longman.

Walker, J., Payne, S., Smith, P. and Jarrett, N. (2004) *Psychology for Nurses and the Caring Professions* (2nd edn). Maidenhead: Open University Press/McGraw-Hill Education.

Walsh, M. (1995) Why patients get the blame for being ill. *Nursing Standard*, 9(37), 38–40.

Walster, E.M. (1966) The assignment of responsibility for an accident. *Journal of Personality & Social Psychology*, 5, 508–516.

Walters, G.D. (1999) *The Addiction Concept: Working Hypothesis or Self-Fulfilling Prophecy*. Needham Heights, MA: Allyn & Bacon.

Ward, R. (1990) Meeting points. *Nursing Times*, 86(22), 58–60.

Warr, P.B. (1987) Job characteristics and mental health. In P.B. Warr (ed.) *Psychology at Work*. Harmondsworth: Penguin.

Warren, S. and Jahoda, M. (1973) *Attitudes* (2nd edn). Harmondsworth: Penguin.

Waterhouse, R., Macaskill, M. and Bostaz, S. (2000) Young people are drinking to 'get trolleyed' like never before. And trouble is often close behind. *The Sunday Times*, 23 July, 23.

Watson, J.B. (1913) Psychology as the behaviourist views it. *Psychological Review*, 20, 158–177.

Watson, J.B. (1919) *Psychology from the Standpoint of a Behaviourist*. Philadelphia: J.B. Lippincott.

Watson, J.B. and Rayner, R. (1920) Conditioned emotional reactions. *Journal of Experimental Psychology*, 3, 1–14.

Watts, F. (1986) Listening to the client. *Changes*, 4(1), 164–167.

Weiner, B. (1986) *An Attributional Theory of Motivation and Emotion*. New York: Springer-Verlag.

Weiner, B. (1992) *Human Motivation: Metaphors, Theories and Research*. Newbury Park, CA: Sage.

Weinman, J. (1995) Health psychology. In A.M. Colman (ed.) *Controversies in Psychology*. London: Longman.

Weinstein, N. (1983) Reducing unrealistic optimism about illness susceptibility. *Health Psychology*, 2, 11–20.

Weinstein, N. (1984) Why it won't happen to me: perceptions of risk factors and susceptibility. *Health Psychology*, 3, 431–457.

Weisstein, N. (1993) Psychology constructs the female; or, the fantasy life of the male psychologist (with some attention to the fantasies of his friend, the male biologist and the male anthropologist). *Feminism & Psychology*, 3(2), 195–210.

Wellman, H.M. (1990) *The Child's Theory of Mind*. Cambridge, MA: MIT Press.

Wells, G.L. and Harvey, J.H. (1977) Do people use consensus information in making causal attributions? *Journal of Personality & Social Psychology*, 35, 279–293.

Wetherell, M. (1982) Cross-cultural studies of minimal groups: implications for the social identity theory of intergroup relations. In H. Tajfel (ed.) *Social Psychology and Intergroup Relations*. Cambridge: Cambridge University Press.

Wetherell, M. (1996) Group conflict and the social psychology of racism. In M. Wetherell (ed.) *Identities, Groups and Social Issues*. London: Sage, in association with the Open University.

WHO (World Health Organization) (1947) *Constitution of the World Health Organization*. Geneva: WHO.

Whyte, A. (1998) Weight on our minds. *Nursing Times*, 94(14), 29–31.

Wichstrom, L. (1998) Self-concept development during adolescence: do American truths hold for Norwegians? In E. Skoe and A. von der Lippe (eds) *Personality Development in Adolescence: A Cross National and Life Span Perspective*. London: Routledge.

Wiemann, J.M. and Giles, H. (1988) Interpersonal communication. In M. Hewstone, W. Stroebe, J.P. Codol and G.M. Stephenson (eds) *Introduction to Social Psychology*. Oxford: Blackwell.

Willis, J. (1998) Inner strength. *Nursing Times*, 94(40), 36–37.

Willis, R.H. (1963) Two dimensions of conformity–nonconformity. *Sociometry*, 26, 499–513.

Wilson, G.D. (1976) Personality. In H.J. Eysenck and G.D. Wilson (eds) *A Textbook of Human Psychology*. Lancaster: MTP.

Wilson, G.T., O'Leary, K.D., Nathan, P.E. and Clark, L.A. (1996) *Abnormal Psychology: Integrating Perspectives*. Needham Heights, MA: Allyn & Bacon.

Wood, C. (1988) Type-casting: is disease linked with personality? *Nursing Times*, 84(48), 27–29.

Wood, D. and Wood, H. (1996) Vygotsky, tutoring and learning. *Oxford Review of Education*, 22, 5–16.

Wood, D.J., Bruner, J.S. and Ross, G. (1976) The role of tutoring in problem-solving. *Journal of Child Psychology & Psychiatry*, 17, 89–100.

Wood, W. (2000) Attitude change: persuasion and social influence. In S.T. Fiske, D.L. Schanchter and C. Zahn-Waxler (eds) *Annual Review of Psychology*, Vol. 51. Palo Alto, CA: Annual Reviews.

Wood, W., Lundgren, S., Ouellette, J.A., Busceme, S. and Blackstone, T. (1994) Minority influence: a meta-analytic review of social influence processes. *Psychological Bulletin*, 115, 323–345.

Worden, J.W. (1991) Grief counselling and grief therapy: a handbook for the mental health practitioner. In M.F. Alexander, J.N. Fawcett and P.J. Runciman (eds) (2006) *Nursing Practice Hospital and Home* (3rd edn). London: Churchill Livingstone.

Zanna, M.P. and Cooper, J. (1974) Dissonance and the pill: an attribution approach to studying the arousal propensities of dissonance. *Journal of Personality & Social Psychology*, 29, 703–709.

Zborowski, M. (1952) Cultural components in response to pain. *Journal of Social Issues*, 8, 16–30.

Zebrowitz, L.A. (1990) *Social Perception*. Milton Keynes: Open University Press.

Zeldow, P.B. (1995) Psychodynamic formulations of human behaviour. In D. Wedding (ed.) *Behaviour and Medicine* (2nd edn). St Louis, MO: Mosby-Year Book.

Zimbardo, P.G. (1992) *Psychology and Life* (13th edn). New York: HarperCollins.

Zimbardo, P.G. and Leippe, M. (1991) *The Psychology of Attitude Change and Social Influence*. New York: McGraw-Hill.

Zimbardo, P.G., Banks, W.C., Craig, H. and Jaffe, D. (1973) A Pirandellian prison: the mind is a formidable jailor. *New York Times Magazine*, 8 April, 38–60.

INDEX

Note: page numbers in **bold** refer to diagrams and information contained within tables.